Recent Advances in Environmental and Occupational Medicine

Recent Advances in Environmental and Occupational Medicine

Edited by Charlotte Lance

hayle
medical

New York

Hayle Medical,
750 Third Avenue, 9th Floor,
New York, NY 10017, USA

Visit us on the World Wide Web at:
www.haylemedical.com

ISBN: 978-1-63241-747-3

Cataloging-in-Publication Data

Recent advances in environmental and occupational medicine / edited by Charlotte Lance.
    p. cm.
Includes bibliographical references and index.
ISBN 978-1-63241-747-3
1. Medicine, Industrial. 2. Environmentally induced diseases--Treatment.
3. Occupational diseases. 4. Environmental health. I. Lance, Charlotte.
RC963 .R43 2019
613.62--dc23

Table of Contents

Permissions

List of Contributors

Index

Preface

Environmental medicine is the study of the interactions between the environment and human health. The role of the environment in causing diseases also comes under the scope of this field. It may be considered a sub-field of environmental health. Some of the current issues in focus under the branch of environmental medicine include mercury poisoning, lead poisoning, food poisoning, indoor air quality, water-borne diseases and effects of ozone depletion. The field of medicine concerned with the prevention and treatment of illnesses and injuries in the workplace, along with the maintenance and increase in the productivity and social adjustment is called occupational medicine. The various advancements in environmental and occupational medicine are glanced at in this book and their applications as well as ramifications are looked at in detail. The various studies that are constantly contributing towards advancing technologies and evolution of these fields are examined in detail. In this book, using case studies and examples, constant effort has been made to make the understanding of the difficult concepts of these disciplines as easy and informative as possible, for the readers.

The information contained in this book is the result of intensive hard work done by researchers in this field. All due efforts have been made to make this book serve as a complete guiding source for students and researchers. The topics in this book have been comprehensively explained to help readers understand the growing trends in the field.

I would like to thank the entire group of writers who made sincere efforts in this book and my family who supported me in my efforts of working on this book. I take this opportunity to thank all those who have been a guiding force throughout my life.

Editor

Consequences of tuberculosis among asylum seekers for health care workers in Germany

Roland Diel[1*], Robert Loddenkemper[2] and Albert Nienhaus[3,4]

Abstract

Background: Immigrants have been contributing to the incidence of tuberculosis (TB) in Germany for many years. The current wave of migration of asylum seekers to Germany may increase that figure. Healthcare workers (HCW) who look after refugees not only in hospitals and medical practices but also in aid projects may be exposed to cases of TB.

Methods: The incremental TB cases arising from imported TB as well as from TB cases that developed later in refugees were calculated in a Markov model over a period of 5 years. Infectious and non-infectious susceptible TB and multidrug-resistant TB (MDR-TB) cases were determined separately. In addition, the total amount of latent TB in contact persons and the risk of infection by HCW were estimated. Due to uncertainty of future refugee flows to Europe, different scenarios were considered in univariate and multivariate sensitivity analysis.

Results: Assuming a decrease in immigration by half each year to the bottom line of 2014, and in light of the current number of 800,000 asylum seekers, we calculated an additional 10,090 TB cases by the end of the fifth year (5976 cases of infectious pulmonary TB and 143 cases of pulmonary MDR-TB). In case of an unchanging influx of asylum seekers over the 5-year period, 19,031 TB cases would arise, 377 of which infectious MDR-TB. Eighty -seven ensuing TB cases would develop in HCW in the same period, 3 of which MDR-TB cases.

Conclusions: Although the total number of TB cases in HCW expected to ensue from the current influx of asylum seekers is rather small, the 3 MDR-TB cases we calculated have to be taken seriously. We consider it essential to increase awareness of protective measures such as respiratory masks and, in the event of documented exposure, of supply-oriented occupational health screening.

Keywords: Health care workers, Asylum seekers, Tuberculosis, MDR-TB

Background

Immigrants have been contributing toward the incidence of tuberculosis (TB) in Germany for many years. TB incidence is now more than thirteen times higher among residents who are foreign nationals than among persons born here [1], and in 2014 more than half (62.4 %) of all TB patients were foreign born. Not only is there a comparatively high frequency among first-generation immigrants, but a cross-sectional study conducted in 2012 in Berlin found TB incidence in the second generation to be at least twice as high as that found in Germans born of native parents. (10.4 versus 4.6 TB cases per 100,000 residents) [2]. At present, more than 1000 people arrive in Germany every day (a total of 54,877 refugees only in October 2015 (http://www.bamf.de/DE/Infothek/Aktuelles/aktuelles-node.html)), most of them from Syria, Afghanistan, Iraq, Eritrea and different Balkan states; no end to the influx is foreseen. The prevalence of active TB and consequently latent TB infection (LTBI) is known to be quite high in most of these countries, markedly different from the low rates found in Germany.

Many of these asylum seekers arrive after a dangerous journey on which they have suffered hunger, exposure, overcrowded accommodation and intolerable sanitary

* Correspondence: roland.diel@epi.uni-kiel.de
[1]Institute for Epidemiology, University Medical Hospital Schleswig-Holstein, Airway Research Center North (ARCN), Niemannsweg 11, 24015 Kiel, Germany
Full list of author information is available at the end of the article

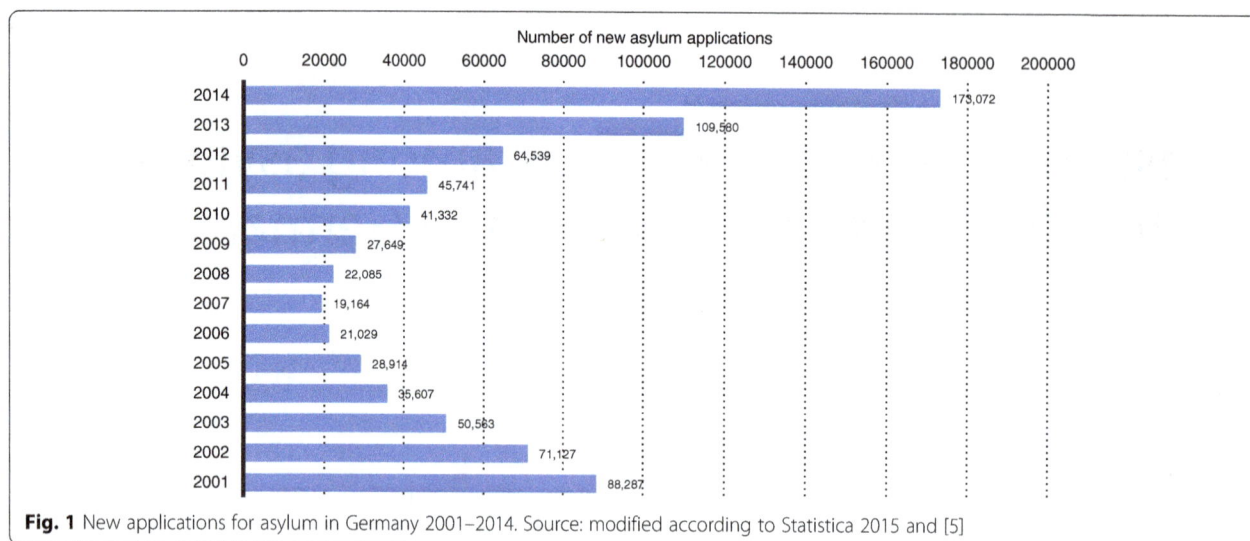

Fig. 1 New applications for asylum in Germany 2001–2014. Source: modified according to Statistica 2015 and [5]

conditions, all of which place LTBI cases at elevated risk for progression to active, transmissible TB disease. Refugees are cared for in Germany by healthcare workers not only as TB patients in hospitals and medical practices but also from aid agencies. Transmission of TB from immigrants to persons born in Germany is statistically rare [3], but with the expected arrival of TB disease with refugees the incidence of TB infections leading to illness can be expected to rise among healthcare workers (HCW), who are often the first point of contact with immigrants and most exposed. It is therefore of special interest to accident insurers to understand how an increase in TB infections via immigrants may have impact on the number of TB cases among HCW in the future. This study models the possible development over the next 5 years and discusses the associated consequences.

Methods

a) Statutory examination of asylum seekers at the place of residence

Under Section 36 (4) of the German Infectious Diseases Law (Infektions-schutzgesetz, IfSG), persons who are to be admitted to shared accommodation sites for refugees or asylum seekers[1] must produce a medical certificate stating that there are no signs of potentially infectious pulmonary TB. In the case of individuals aged 15 or older, with the exception of pregnant women, the certificate must be based on a chest X-ray [4].

Neither the number of chest X-ray examinations done in the months since the flood of refugees began nor the number and country of birth of persons whose X-rays

Table 1 Input variables for the dynamic disease model

Category of variable	Name of variable	Basic value	Reference
Number of refugees arriving per year	T_refugees	Decreasing number from 1st to 4th year, then plateau	Federal Ministry of the Interior estimate of 19 August 2015 (http://www.bamf.de/DE/Infothek/Aktuelles/aktuelles-node.html)
Probability of deportation per year	pExit	0.0628	Calculated from data in [13] and (https://www.tagesschau.de/inland/abschiebungen-103.html)
Probability of TB ascertained on entry screening	pSick_Entry	0.0025	Diel et al. [3]
Probability of infectious pulmonary TB	pInfect_TB	0.6121	RKI 2015 [8]
Probability of later development of TB in refugees (up to 5 years after entry)	T_active	Decreasing probability from 1st to 5th year	Calculated from data in Diel et al. [3]
Probability of MDR-TB in cases of infectious pulmonary TB	pInfect_MDR_TB	0.0324	Calculated from RKI data 2015 [9]
Probability of MDR-TB in cases of non-infectious TB	pMDR_TB	0.010	RKI 2015 [9]

show signs of TB are known, as it is not mandatory for German health authorities, reception centres performing the X-rays or contractual practices to record these data. Although Section 11 Paragraph 8 of the IfSG stipulates that the relevant state authorities must be notified of the citizenship and nationality of any person with the disease, the wording "admission to shared accommodation" does not distinguish between refugee accommodation, hostels for homeless persons, or care homes, and there is no separate "asylum seekers" category.

b) The risk of TB occurrence among asylum seekers over time

173,072 applications for asylum were lodged in Germany in 2014 [5] (see Fig. 1).

In the same year, 409 persons were recorded as having been diagnosed with TB upon admission to shared accommodation for asylum seekers [6]. Taking this figure as the denominator, there were 236 TB cases per 100,000 new applications, a ratio of 0.236 %.

This ratio seems to have changed hardly in recent years. The study by Diel et al. [3], until now the only one to have examined the results of screening in accordance with Section 36 (4) of the IfSG – carried out on asylum seekers in Hamburg over a long period (from 1997 to 2003) – found a ratio of 0.25 %. In the absence of other valid surveys and for the sake of simplicity, for

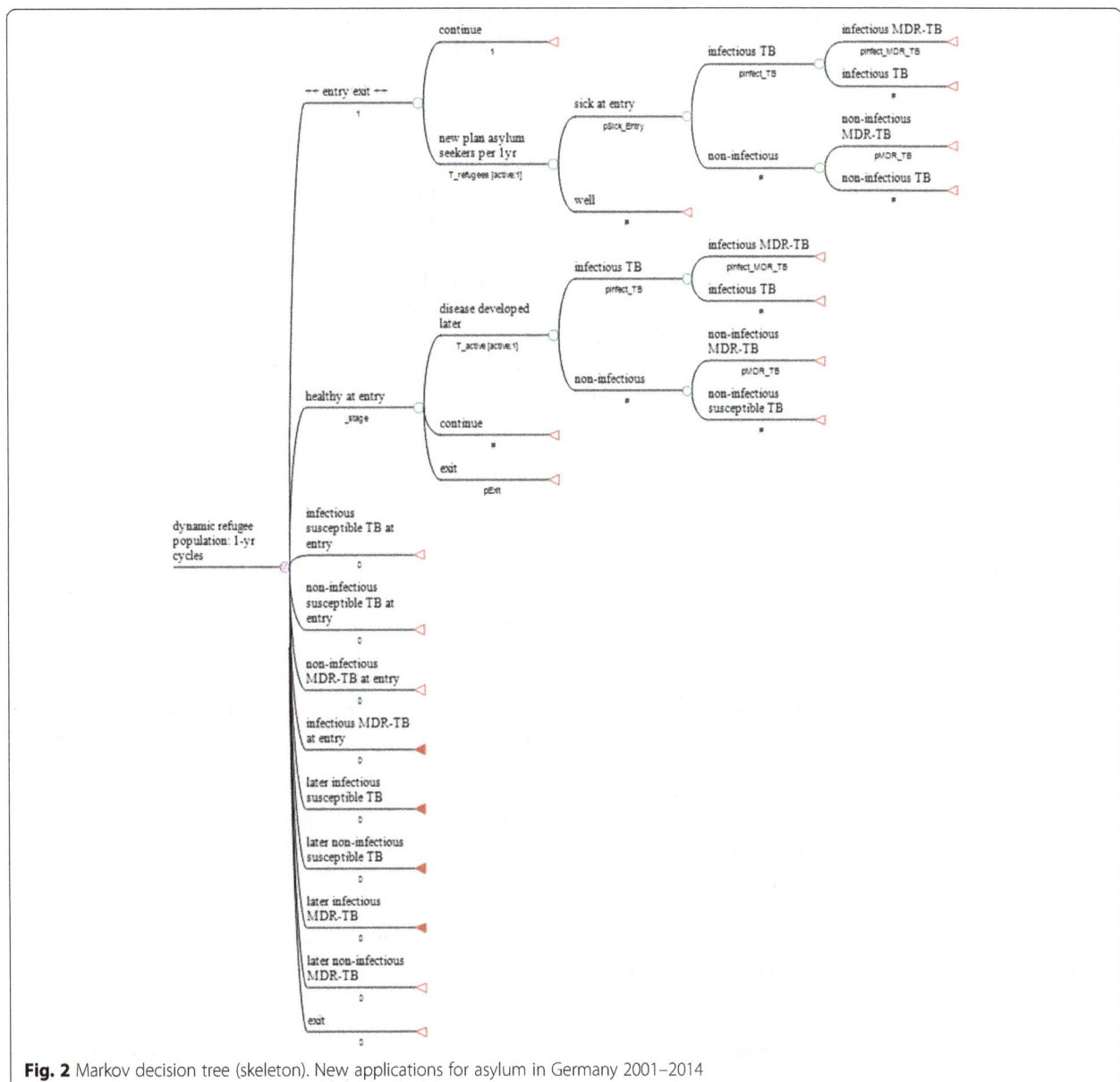

Fig. 2 Markov decision tree (skeleton). New applications for asylum in Germany 2001–2014

our modelling we took this figure (probability of TB ascertained on entry screening [pSick_Entry], see Table 1) as the annual probability in the base year analysis. Arithmetically, with an assumed number of 800,000 refugees per year throughout Germany, this results in 2000 cases of TB diagnosed on at- entry screening.

A recent meta-analysis [7], summarizing the findings of 22 studies that reported cases of active pulmonary tuberculosis among 2,620,739 screened refugees, asylum seekers and regular immigrants, even reported a yield for pulmonary TB of 3.5 cases (95 % CI 2.9.-4.1) per 1000 persons screened.

Diel et al. [3] also found that asylum seekers who stayed in the country ran a considerable risk of suffering TB disease in the four subsequent years (1.64 %% in the first year, 1.56 %% in the second, 0.99 %% and 0.57 %% in the third and fourth, and 0.41 %% in the fifth year). These probabilities of contracting TB within 5 years [T_active] were used for modelling.

c) Infectious tuberculosis

In 2013, 76.9 % of all notified TB cases in Germany (3298/4287) were pulmonary tuberculosis [8], of which 79.6 % (2624/3298), that is, 61.21 % of the total, were open (confirmed by culture) (probability of infectious pulmonary TB [pInfect_TB]). Of these, 45 % showed positive in sputum smears (1181/2624) and 55 % (1443/2624) negative. Open pulmonary tuberculosis accounted for 85 of the 102 notified multi-drug-resistant TB (MDR-TB) cases, that is, 83.3 %. Of these, 63.5 % (54/85) showed positive in sputum smears [9]. One can therefore assume that 3.2 % of all cases of open pulmonary TB are open pulmonary MDR-TB (probability of MDR-TB in cases of infectious pulmonary TB [pInfect_MDR_TB]). As a consequence there will be secondary cases among contact persons.

d) Non-infectious tuberculosis

The number of cases of non-infectious tuberculosis, regardless of organ manifestation, was calculated from the difference between the total number of cases and the number of open pulmonary tuberculosis infections (1-pInfect_TB). Seventeen out of 1663 cases of non-open tuberculosis in 2013, that is, 1 %, were cases of MDR-TB (probability of MDR-TB in cases of non-infectious TB [pMDR_TB]) [8].

e) Contact persons and probability of progression to tuberculosis

The average number of contact persons that a patient with open pulmonary TB will infect cannot be precisely predicted, as the literature shows it to be a highly situation-dependent phenomenon. If one assumes that on average a sputum-smear-positive index case infects five contact persons [10] and a sputum-smear-negative case one [11], the weighted mean value amounts to three infected contact persons per case of open pulmonary TB taking into account the above-mentioned distribution of sputum-smear positive and sputum-smear negative pulmonary TB that was also found in previous years [12].

f) Deportations of asylum seekers who have entered the country

When considering how the influx of asylum seekers may effect TB incidence in the coming years, one needs to take into account the proportion of new applicants who are deported. Officially, in 2014, of the 128,911 asylum applications on which a ruling was given, 68.6 % were rejected (88,348 in all) [13], but, in fact, only 10,884 individuals were deported. Applying this historic percentage of applicants deported to the number of new applications, the percentage of those leaving the pool of persons who may develop tuberculosis after 1 year is just 6.28 % (10,884 out of the 173,072 applications for asylum in 2014).

According to media reports (https://www.tagesschau.de/inland/abschiebungen-103.html), 8178 rejected asylum seekers were deported in the first half of 2015. Given the marked year-on-year increase in the number of refugees, it is not anticipated that the percentage will be higher in 2015.

Model structure

We used TreeAge software (Version 2015) to develop a dynamic Markov decision tree, in which the duration of each cycle is 1 year (Fig. 2). To do this we had to make several assumptions on the following key parameters:

In the base model, the decision tree assumes that, in 2015, 800,000 asylum seekers arriving in Germany will be X-rayed in accordance with Section 36 (4) of the IfSG, and that 6.28 % of the asylum seekers arriving between 2015 and 2019 will be deported; the latter can therefore not develop TB in Germany in the years ahead. Indeed, currently up to 1,500,000 refugees are expected to arrive in Germany in 2015. As many, though, may fail to register and can therefore not be screened, our estimate of 800,000 refugees is deliberatively conservative. It will further be assumed that all asylum seekers who develop the disease will remain in Germany

In the absence of reliable trending data on immigration of non-EU citizens into Germany, we made a further conservative estimate and assumed a year-on-year halving of

Table 2 Results and sensitivity analyses

a) Base case

Year	Healthy at entry	Infectious TB at entry	Non-infectious TB at entry	Non-infectious MDR-TB at entry	Infectious MDR-TB at entry	Later infectious TB	Later non-infectious TB	Later infectious MDR-TB	Later non-infectious MDR-TB	Exit
1	798,000.00	1184.54	768.04	7.76	39.66	775.11	251.60	12.99	2.54	0.00
2	1,145,576.88	1776.80	1152.06	11.64	59.50	1833.55	595.37	30.75	6.01	50,177.20
3	1,271,347.55	2072.94	1344.07	13.58	69.41	2575.24	836.41	43.19	8.45	122,250.73
4	1,362,893.97	2329.20	1510.23	15.25	77.99	3038.57	987.03	50.97	9.97	202,286.12
5	1,449,161.25	2585.46	1676.39	16.93	86.57	3390.47	1101.44	56.88	11.13	288,111.21

10,090 cases (5976 infectious drug-susceptible TB cases, 143 infectious MDR-TB cases)

b) 800,000 asylum seekers every year

Year	Healthy at entry	Infectious TB at entry	Non-infectious TB at entry	Non-infectious MDR-TB at entry	Infectious MDR-TB at entry	Later infectious TB	Later non-infectious TB	Later infectious MDR-TB	Later non-infectious MDR-TB	Exit
1	798,000.00	1184.54	768.04	7.76	39.66	775.11	502.58	25.95	5.08	0.00
2	154,4576,88	2369.07	1536.08	15.52	79.33	2202.21	1427.89	73.74	14.42	5,0114.40
3	2,243,167.91	3553.61	2304.13	2327	118.99	3510.83	2276.39	117.56	22.99	147,113.83
4	2,898,087.45	4738.14	3072.17	31.03	158.66	4496.07	2915.21	150.55	29.45	287,984.77
5	3,512,424.05	5922.68	3840.21	38.79	198.32	5348.99	3468.24	179.11	35.03	469,984.66

19,031 cases (11,272 infectious drug-susceptible TB cases, 377 infectious MDR-TB cases)

c) Halved TB prevalence at chest X-ray screening and 800,000 asylum seekers every year

Year	Healthy at entry	Infectious TB at entry	Non-infectious TB at entry	Non-infectious MDR-TB at entry	Infectious MDR-TB at entry	Later infectious TB	Later non-infectious TB	Later infectious MDR-TB	Later non-infectious MDR-TB	Exit
1	799,000.00	592.27	384.02	3.88	19.83	776.08	502.58	25.95	5.08	0.00
2	1,546,512.44	1184.54	768.04	7.76	39.66	2204.97	1427.89	73.74	14.42	50,114.40
3	2,245,978.90	1776.80	1152.06	11.64	59.50	3515.23	2276.39	117.56	22.99	147,113.83
4	2,901,719.14	2369.07	1536.08	15.52	79.33	4,501,71	2915.21	150.55	29.45	287,984.77
5	3,516,825.59	2961.34	1920.11	19.40	99.16	5355.70	3468.24	179.11	35.03	469,984.66

14,043 cases (8317 infectious drug-susceptible TB cases, 278 infectious MDR-TB cases)

d) Halved TB prevalence at chest X-ray screening, halved probabilities of developing TB in the following 5 years and 800,000 asylum seekers every year

Year	Healthy at entry	Infectious TB at entry	Non-infectious TB at entry	Non-infectious MDR-TB at entry	Infectious MDR-TB at entry	Later infectious TB	Later non-infectious TB	Later infectious MDR-TB	Later non-infectious MDR-TB	Exit
1	7,990,00.00	592.27	384.02	3.88	19.83	388.04	503.21	25.99	5.08	0.00
2	1,547,167.62	1184.54	768.04	7.76	39.66	1102.79	1429.68	73.83	14.44	50,177.20
3	2,247,798.70	1776.80	1152.06	11.64	59.50	1758.45	2279.24	117.71	23.02	147,298.18
4	2,904,529.90	2369.07	1536.08	15.52	79.33	2252.17	2918.87	150.74	29.48	288,345.66
5	3,520,291.83	2961.34	1920.11	19.40	99.16	2679.58	3472.58	179.34	35.08	470,573.62

9524 cases (5641 infectious drug-susceptible TB cases, 279 infectious MDR-TB)

e) Halved TB prevalence at chest X-ray screening and halved probabilities of developing TB in the following 5 years

Year	Healthy at entry	Infectious TB at entry	Non-infectious TB at entry	Non-infectious MDR-TB at entry	Infectious MDR-TB at entry	Later infectious TB	Later non-infectious TB	Later infectious MDR-TB	Later non-infectious MDR-TB	Exit
1	7,990,00.00	592.27	384.02	3.88	19.83	388.04	251.60	12.99	2.54	0.00
2	1,147,667.62	888.40	576.03	5.82	29.75	918.23	595.37	30.75	60.10	50,177.20

Table 2 Results and sensitivity analyses *(Continued)*

3	1,274,448.91	1036.47	672.04	6.79	34.71	1289.98	836.41	43.19	8.45	122,250.73
4	1,366,641.51	1164.60	755.12	7.63	39.00	1522.28	987.03	50.97	9.97	202,286.12
5	1,453,279.86	1292.73	838.19	8.47	43.29	1698.73	1101.44	56.88	11.13	288,111.21

5051 cases (2991 infectious drug-susceptible TB cases, 100 infectious MDR-TB cases)

numbers for 2016 and 2017, i.e. that there will be 400,000 refugees in 2016 and 200,000 in 2017, and that in 2018 and 2019 the figure will remain at the 2014 level (173,072 asylum applications). Given the current increase in the number of refugees from Afghanistan, a high-incidence country, and that more than 4 million Syrians have had to flee to neighbouring countries whilst around 7.6 million Syrians have been displaced within Syria (http://www.unhcr.de/home/artikel/b0843b46d8393e8e4bf87511f f1c7b1c/zahl-der-syrien-fluechtlinge-uebersteigt-4-millionen.html), we assumed for the sensitivity analysis a worst-case scenario of an unchanging influx of registered 800,000 refugees in each of the 5 years.

According to our base probability described above, asylum seekers present with TB at the rate of 2.5 per 1000 persons initially X-rayed. Those refugees who do not have the disease and are not deported in subsequent years may go on to develop TB in line with the probability for each year as stated in the Table (T_active). The number of TB cases found on X-ray examination of new immigrants and those falling sick later are added up over 5 years. Table 1 provides an overview on all input variables finally programmed.

Due to uncertainty over a) the number of asylum seekers per year, b) the probability of discovering TB by at-entry screening, and c) the probabilities of contracting the disease in the next few years, we conducted several univariate and multivariate sensitivity analyses for these parameters, both singly and in combination. In one analysis, the probability of "pSick_Entry" was halved, as were all probabilities in the Table for "T_active". As a worst-case scenario, the number of 800,000 immigrants per year was not reduced in the sensitivity analysis, but held constant for all 5 years. In the multivariate sensitivity analyses we either simultaneously halved the probabilities for "pSick_entry" and "T_active" and also halved the yearly numbers of immigrants or left the number of immigrants constant at 800,000 per year.

Results

The results of our calculations are in Table 2. There are three different scenarios taken into consideration: The base analysis (scenario 1) shows 10,090 cases of tuberculosis by the end of the fifth year, of which 5976 are cases of infectious drug-susceptible pulmonary TB and 143 are cases of infectious pulmonary MDR-TB. If one assumes an unchanging influx of asylum seekers over the 5-year period, there are 19,031 TB cases, of which 11,272 have infectious drug-susceptible pulmonary TB and 377 have infectious pulmonary MDR-TB (worst-case scenario). The most favourable scenario, which assumes that TB cases found on chest X-ray screening are halved and that the probability of developing the disease over time is also halved, results in 5051 TB cases among immigrants, with 2991 cases of infectious drug-susceptible pulmonary TB and 100 cases of pulmonary MDR-TB (best-case scenario).

In line with the results of the base analysis, this would mean an average number of 6119×3 infected contact persons (18,529). Unfortunately there are no officially reported data, but with a conservative estimate, assuming that only one in ten contact persons is a HCW, arrives at 1853 infected healthcare workers. With a risk of 5 % of developing the disease in the first 2 years after a fresh infection [12], one can expect 84 consequential cases of drug-susceptible active TB and 3 cases of MDR-TB by the end of the fifth year. In our best-case scenario still 42 cases of drug-susceptible TB and 1 case of MDR-TB would occcur, whereas the worst-case scenario results in 156 and 5 drug-susceptible TB and MDR-TB cases, respectively.

Discussion

Asylum seekers can be assumed to have a higher risk of TB, for several reasons:

1. They are often from countries with a high prevalence of TB [14].
2. A high proportion is of age groups that are particularly affected in the country of origin (in particular young adults aged between 25 and 34) [15].
3. The acute psychosocial and/or physical strains of fleeing their home country are among the factors known to promote reactivation of a previously acquired LTBI [7].
4. They may have been exposed to TB during the various stages of a journey that has often taken months or years.

Eight of the nine main countries of origin of immigrants worldwide are countries with a high TB incidence > 20 per 100.000 population (Fig. 3).

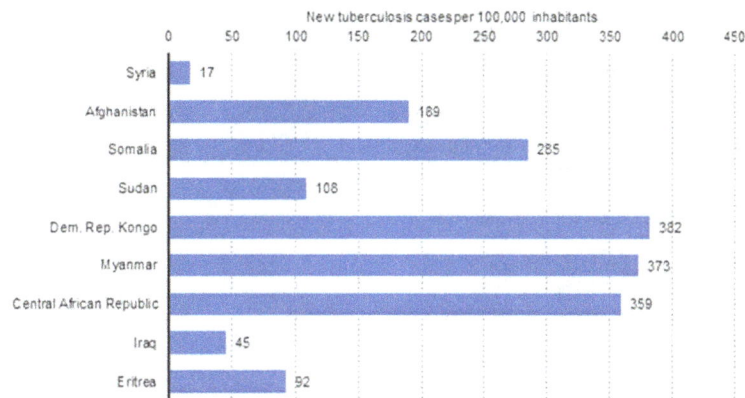

Fig. 3 TB incidence in asylum seekers' nine main countries of origin. Source: modified according to [19] and [20]

For many years, there was a declining trend in new cases of TB notified to the German Robert Koch Institute (RKI), but this decline had ceased even before the current rise in refugee numbers [16]: In 2014, 4448 cases were notified and the incidence significantly increased with 5.6/100,000 [1], as against 4210 cases of TB and an incidence of 5.2/100,000 in 2012 [8].

In 2013, the Institute for Statutory Accident Insurance and Prevention in the Health and Welfare Services (BGW) alone received notification of 160 cases of active TB in HCW. That is 3.7 % of the 4318 cases reported to the RKI. A further 383 notifications were related to detected latent infections. However, one can assume that the actual number of TB cases to be currently expected among healthcare workers in Germany is higher because the TB cases notified to other accident insurers have not been taken into account.

Without any doubt, the risk of progression to TB is highest in the first year following the arrival of an immigrant in Germany and decreases as time goes on [3]. Nonetheless, the risk after several years of residency should certainly not be ignored and is therefore included in our calculation: Marx et al. [2] observed a significantly high number of TB cases among Berlin migrants in the first 9 years after immigration. While 28.4 % of cases occurred in the first year, the median period of latency between immigration and notification of TB was 8 years.

An earlier Danish study [17] on Somali asylum seekers found that the initially high rate of TB (3.0 % of all Somali immigrants) declined only gradually and that after 7 years 9.5 % of Somalis had suffered TB disease in their new country.

Conclusions

Although the number of consequential TB cases in HCW to be expected in our base analysis is rather small, having been calculated at 87 cases in the next 5 years,

one still has to expect 3 complicated MDR-TB cases requiring protracted treatment. It is therefore essential to increase awareness of protective measures such as respiratory masks and, in the event of documented exposure, of supply-oriented occupational health screening [18].

Endnote

[1]The term "asylum seekers" covers asylum applicants, refugees who are unaccompanied minors, other refugees and tolerated persons.

Competing interests

R.D. was supported by Riemser Pharma GmbH for building the Markov model. Riemser had no role in study design, data calculation, decision to publish and preparation of the manuscript. R.L. and A.N. declare no conflict of interest.

Authors' contributions

RD planned and managed the work and produced the first draft of the manuscript. AN and RL reviewed and revised the manuscript, including essential amendments. RD finalized the paper. All authors read and approved the final submitted version.

Author details

[1]Institute for Epidemiology, University Medical Hospital Schleswig-Holstein, Airway Research Center North (ARCN), Niemannsweg 11, 24015 Kiel, Germany. [2]German Central Committee against Tuberculosis, Berlin, Germany. [3]Institute for Health Services Research in Dermatology and Nursing, University Medical Center, Hamburg-Eppendorf, Germany. [4]Institution for Statutory Accident Insurance and Prevention in the Health and Welfare Services (BGW), Hamburg, Germany.

References

1. Koch-Institut R. Bericht zur Epidemiologie der Tuberkulose in Deutschland für 2014. Berlin: Robert Koch-Institut; 2016.
2. Marx FM, Fiebig L, Hauer B, Brodhun B, Glaser-Paschke G, Magdorf K, et al. Higher rate of tuberculosis in second generation migrants compared to native residents in a metropolitan setting in Western Europe. PLoS One. 2015;10(6), e0119693.
3. Diel R, Rüsch-Gerdes S, Niemann S. Molecular epidemiology of tuberculosis among immigrants in Hamburg, Germany. J Clin Microbiol. 2004;42: 2952–60.

4.   Gesetz zur Verhütung und Bekämpfung von Infektionskrankheiten beim
     Menschen (Infektionsschutzgesetz - IfSG) vom 20. Juli 2000 (BGBl. I S. 1045),
     zuletzt geändert Art. 70 V v. 31.8.2015 I 1474.
5.   Bundesamt für Migration und Flüchtlinge. Aktuelle Zahlen zu Asyl. Ausgabe:
     August 2015, p 9.
6.   Robert Koch-Institut. Epidemiologisches Bulletin 43/2015, 26 October 2015
7.   Arshad S, Gajari K, Paget SNJ, Baussano I. Active screening at entry for
     tuberculosis among new immigrants: a systematic review and meta-analysis.
     Eur Respir J. 2010;35:1336–45.
8.   Koch-Institut R. Bericht zur Epidemiologie der Tuberkulose in Deutschland
     für 2013. Berlin: Robert Koch-Institut; 2015.
9.   Robert Koch-Institut, Bonita Brodhun. Special calculation, 15 April 2015
10. Salpeter EE, Salpeter SR. Mathematical model for the epidemiology of
     tuberculosis, with estimates of the reproductive number and infection-delay
     function. Am J Epidemiol. 1998;142:398–406.
11. Behr MA, Warren SA, Salamon H, et al. Transmission of *Mycobacterium
     tuberculosis* from patients smear-negative for acid-fast bacilli. Lancet. 1999;
     353:444–9.
12. Diel R, Nienhaus A, Loddenkemper R. Cost-effectiveness of interferon-
     gamma release assay screening for latent tuberculosis infection treatment
     in Germany. Chest. 2007;131:1424–34.
13. Deutscher Bundestag Drucksache 18/4025, 18. Wahlperiode 16.02.2015.
     Antwort der Bundesregierung auf die Kleine Anfrage der Abgeordneten Ulla
     Jelpke, Jan Korte, Sevim Dağdelen, weiterer Abgeordneter und der Fraktion
     DIE LINKE. – Drucksache 18/3896 – Abschiebungen im Jahr 2014.
14. Erkens C, Slump E, Kamphorst M, et al. Coverage and yield of entry and
     follow-up screening for tuberculosis among new immigrants. Eur Respir J.
     2008;32:153–61.
15. Tomás BA, Pell C, Cavanillas AB, et al. Tuberculosis in migrant populations. A
     systematic review of the qualitative literature. PLOS one. 2013;8(12):e82440.
16. Fiebig L, Hauer B, Brodhun B, Altmann D, Haas W. Tuberculosis in Germany:
     a declining trend coming to an end? Eur Resp J. 2016;47:667–670.
17. Lillebaek T, Andersen AB, Dirksen A, Smith E, Skovgaard LT, Kok-Jensen A.
     Persistent high incidence of tuberculosis in immigrants in a low-incidence
     country. Emerg Infect Dis. 2002;8:679–84.
18. Verordnung zur arbeitsmedizinischen Vorsorge (ArvMedVV) vom 18.
     Dezember 2008 (BGBl. I S. 2768), letzte Änderung durch Artikel 1 der
     Verordnung vom 23. Oktober 2013 (BGBl. I, S. 3882).
19. UNHCR. Global Trends 2014, pp 49–53. unhcr.org/556725e69.html
20. WHO. Global tuberculosis report. Geneva: World Health Organization; 2014.

2

Work-related floors as injury hazards – a nationwide pilot project analyzing floors in theatres and education establishments in Germany

Eileen M. Wanke[1]*, Mike Schmidt[2], Doris Klingelhöfer[1], Jeremy Leslie-Spinks[3], Daniela Ohlendorf[1] and David A. Groneberg[1]

Abstract

Background: An adequate dance floor is said to prevent injuries. On the basis of scientific research, numerous recommendations regarding an adequate dance floor have been developed. Up to the present, however, studies have still been lacking into how far these recommendations have already been implemented in theatres with regular dance productions and/or in-house dance ensembles. The aim of this study is to analyze a nationwide survey on dance floors of theatres and education establishments in Germany.

Methods: A questionnaire-based survey on existence and type of floors in the various dance-related working areas was carried out at theatres and education establishments institutions ($n = 86$ institutions ($n = 76$ theatres, $n = 10$ education establishments). References as to region, size of dance ensembles and dance styles performed were created.

Results: Of all education establishments, 75.3% were equipped with a sprung sub-floor in the ballet studios. In contrast, sprung sub-floors were only found in 29.7% of the working areas, the stage AND ballet studios in theatres. The percentage of theatres providing sprung sub-floors in all rooms used by dancers is even lower. Considering all dance-related work areas, larger ensembles (>30 dancers) were offered better conditions regarding floors than smaller ensembles ($p > 0.001$). No significant tendencies were found regarding regions or dance styles.

Conclusion: Recommendations concerning an appropriate dance floor have only partly been realized. Besides secured finances for reinstallation, further education of responsible officials and artists is essential. However, accrediting dance as own genre in theatres is the indispensable prerequisite.

Keywords: Work related risks, Dance, Floor, Theatres, Injury prevention

Background

A dance floor is a very important element of the working environment in dance. If the floor is in accordance with the existing standards it can contribute to minimize or even better avoid traumatic injuries as well as chronic work- and floor-related health problems of the musculo-skeletal system [1–8]. In cases where the floor is defective (e.g. folds in the performance surface) [9] or even inappropriate (e.g. absent/lacking sprung sub-floor), it may be a health hazard and precipitate incapacity for work [10]. While performance surfaces can be significant in the case of traumatic injuries or occupational accidents, respectively, the properties of a sub-floor play an important role in the occurrence of chronic misuse and overload injury [8, 11].

Although a detailed description of the components of an adequate dance floor is not part of this article, it should be mentioned that in principle a dance floor should include a performance surface (preferably one that meets the requirements of the various dance styles performed), a sprung sub-floor and an underlying

* Correspondence: wanke@med.uni-frankfurt.de
[1]Institute of Occupational Medicine, Social Medicine and Environmental Medicine, Goethe-University, Theodor-Stern-Kai 7, 60590 Frankfurt am Main, Germany
Full list of author information is available at the end of the article

sub-floor onto which the sprung sub-floor as well as the performance surface are fitted. This concept is based on several national and international recommendations and standards [12], fine tuning, however, should be done in co-operation with all the parties (e.g. technical staff, theatre management) involved (including dancers) [8].

The same is valid for the performance surface which is to be chosen specifically for the dance styles to be performed [8, 10, 12]. Currently, there is a vast variety of offers available (e.g. point elastic, area elastic, combi-elastic, cushioned or not cushioned Vinyl surface). Depending on various requirements, these offers should be carefully tested in order to be sure of installing the optimal dance floor[11].

For reasons of occupational health and safety numerous authors of relevant studies as well as statutory accident insurers recommend an especially purpose-constructed sprung sub-floor meeting all requirements determined by dance style, age and organization for the work-related activities of professional dancers [9, 12, 13]. Furthermore, an – ideally identical - sprung sub-floor should be fitted in all working areas used by dancers [10], because it is an additional challenge for the body to individually adjust to different types of floors. Even if the existing floors are basically appropriate it would take time to adjust to another floor and in reality there is no time [6]. The same applies to different floor types in one working area such as a basket system with varying area deflection[6].

Objective of the present study

On the one hand, the number of studies dealing with the effects of different types of floors on the musculoskeletal system of dancers has considerably increased. On the other hand, published data on the status quo scenario at theatres with regular dance production are still lacking.

Similar to a pilot study, this is the first analysis of dance floors at theatres in Germany. The primary focus was on the sub-floor costing far more and requiring more handling than the performance surface. It was the aim to find out whether, to what extent and by what means (types of floors) the existing recommendations on injury prevention, mis- or overload concerning floors in dance have already been realized [8, 11, 13, 14]. A relative assessment based on region, size of dance ensemble and dance style was created.

Methods

In the theatre season 2016/17 (August–June/July) a survey was conducted in all theatres in Germany.

Inclusion criteria were as follows:

1. Theatres with own dance company
2. Theatres with scheduled dance performances

3. (University-) Educational establishments with a dance department

A total of $n = 86$ institutions (theatre and education establishments) with that criteria were identified and chosen for the survey. Direct contact persons were either the responsible technical staff or the management of each institution. In order to achieve the highest possible response rate and, thus, attain reliable results, this study was beforehand announced at a nationwide meeting with theatre managements attending.

The survey comprised the following floor key aspects:

- Aspect 1: Construction type of sub floor in the training area(s) (ballet studio(s),
- Aspect 2: Construction type of sub floor on stage,
- Aspect 3: Existence of a mobile floor for touring purposes
- Aspect 4: Total number of dancers in the dance genre/ size of dance ensemble
- Aspect 5: Region/federal province
- Aspect 6: Dance style (classical/neo-classical and/or contemporary/modern)

A pre-test was carried out in a total of $n = 6$ theatres of various sizes without dance genre.

The aspects were limited to keep the utilization of the participants in this pilot project as low as possible. Digital and printed versions of the questionnaire were available.

Data Analysis

Results were calculated using the PASW Statistics software package, version 21.0 and Excel 2010. Predominantly, the evaluation was carried out in the form of frequency analyses. Chi-Square Tests were used at crucial points to evaluate the differences between the groups. The significance level was set at $\alpha = 0.05$.

The theatres were categorized according the size of their dance company for the analysis. Dance ensembles with up to 30 dancers were categorized as 'small to medium', ensembles with more than 30 dancers as 'big'.

With regard to dance styles a simplified categorization with either classical/neo classical and contemporary focus was chosen.

Questions concerning raked stages were intentionally neglected even when here and there a possible relation between raked floor and incidence of injuries was stated [14–18]. The types of floors were categorized in ‚dance floors', sports floors' and ‚other floors' (not dance appropriate).

Working areas comprised ballet studios as locations for daily dance classes and rehearsals, resp., as well as the stage as location for dance performances and preceding stage rehearsals.

The various types of floors were categorized into dance specific sprung sub-floors and other sprung floors (basket, sports floor etc.) [11, 12]. One point worthy of note is that - among others - a (batten) basket construction is also customary for special dance floors. Therefore, in replying to this question, subjects could assign a basket-construction to dance specific floors. In cases, where that was not done it was presumed that the basket floor used in their establishment was not a dance specific one.

Results

There were regular dance performances and/or an employed dance company as in-house genre at a total of $n = 76$ theatres and other locations during the theatre season 2016/17 in Germany. In addition to that, there were a total of $n = 10$ education establishments for professional dance. The response rate of the survey was 90% ($n = 9$) from the education establishments and 86.7% ($n = 65$) from the theatres. Not to be discounted was the lack of answers of up to 16.7% depending on the question. Due to the fact that there were no stages at the education establishments and only few guest performances just the ballet studios were analyzed.

Theatres equipped with sprung sub-floors suitable for dancers

Ballet studio only

On the whole, 75.3% of all institutions (theatres and education establishments) were equipped with a sprung sub-floor, 9.4% did not dispose of one, with 15.3% not furnishing any particulars. With the theatres the results were similar: 73.3% were fitted with a dance appropriate floor, 10.7% did not dispose of one, and 16% did not furnish any particulars.

9 in 10 of the education establishments were equipped with a sprung sub-floor with $n = 1$ not furnishing particulars.

Stage only

The situation 'on stage' was completely different: a mere 30.3% of all stages were equipped with a sprung sub-floor with 57.9 not being equipped with one and 11.8% not furnishing particulars. Educational establishments remained neglected as they were not equipped with a separate stage.

Ballet studio AND stage

Less than one in three theatres (29.7) was equipped with a floor suitable for dance in all areas used by dancers in training, rehearsals and performances, with 54.1% not

being equipped with one and 16.2% not furnishing particulars.

Ballet studio, stage AND touring

As even fewer theatres were equipped with a mobile dance floor for touring, the percentage of the institutions equipped with a floor suitable for dance in all working areas decreased to 23.3% compared to 60.5% of the institutions not disposing of a mobile dance floor with 16.3% not furnishing particulars (Fig. 1).

Type of floors in ballet studios and on stages

Of all institutions equipped with a sprung sub-floor, 33.9% of all ballet studios were equipped with a dance specific sprung sub-floor whereas 66.1% were equipped with another sprung sub-floor (e.g. sports, basket, alternate construction). On the contrary, the stages of the majority of theatres were equipped with a dance (sprung) floor (66.1%) compared to 33.9% equipped with an alternate constructed sprung sub-floor.

Significance of ensemble size in relation to dance appropriate floors

Big ensembles (> 30 dancers) usually in larger regional capitals or metropolises, respectively, have an advantage over smaller ensembles (< 30 dancers). All theatres (100%) with an own dance genre in regional capitals or metropolises were equipped with a dance appropriate floor in the ballet studio compared to a mere 85% of the smaller ensembles (< 30 dancers)($p = 0.150$).

Of all big ensembles, 58% offered a sprung sub-floor both in the ballet studio and on stage in contrast to only 30% of the smaller ensembles ($p = 0.073$). The differences relating to size of the ensemble and existence of dance appropriate floors in ballet studio, on stage and while touring ($p = 0.002$) (> 30 dancers: 50%, < 30 dancers: 11%) is significant. Comparing big and small ensembles with regard to stage there is a tendency (> 30 dancers: 58%, < 30 dancers: 31%, $p = 0.073$) (Fig.2).

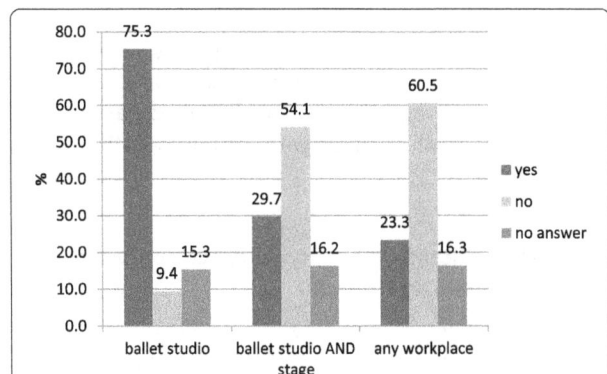

Fig. 1 Sprung floors in German theatres with dance productions ($n = 76$)

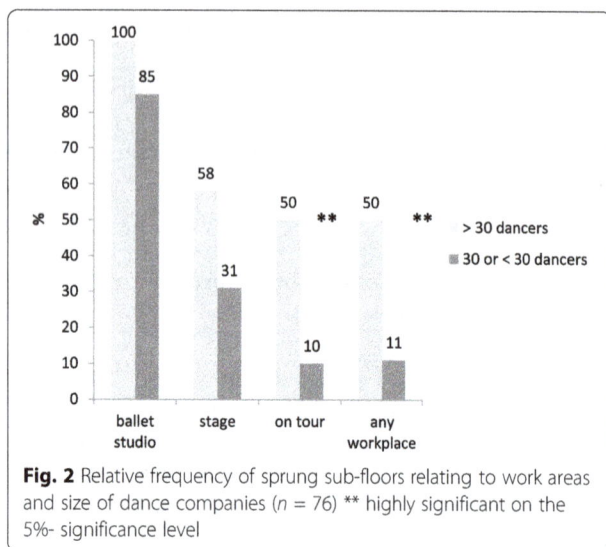

Fig. 2 Relative frequency of sprung sub-floors relating to work areas and size of dance companies (*n* = 76) ** highly significant on the 5%- significance level

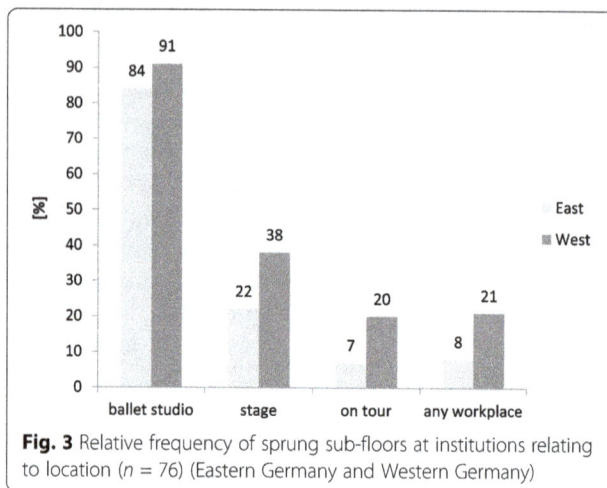

Fig. 3 Relative frequency of sprung sub-floors at institutions relating to location (*n* = 76) (Eastern Germany and Western Germany)

Significance of dance style in relation to dance appropriate floors

Of all contemporary company, 89% and 85% of the classical and neo-classical ensembles were equipped with a dance appropriate floor in the ballet studio (*p* = 0.610). Generally speaking, as a tendency more classical and neo-classical ensembles (44%) than contemporary ensembles (33%) were furnished with appropriate floorings on stage (*p* = 0.390). In the ballet studio and on stage, an appropriate dance floor is provided for 36% of the contemporary companies and 42% of the classical and neo-classical companies (*p* = 0.619). Nevertheless, the percentage of appropriate flooring in all working areas was with 27% (classical or neo-classical companies) compared to 14% (contemporary companies almost twice as high, however, as described above, still very low (*p* = 0.249). Hence, ensembles with classical and neo-classical focus were generally speaking – not significantly – better equipped than dance ensembles with contemporary focus.

Regional significance in relation to dance appropriate floors (East-West Germany)

There were not significantly more sprung sub-floors in theatres of West Germany compared to East Germany (the former German Democratic Republic), even when the percentage of theatres with sprung sub-floors was slightly higher (Fig.3).

Regional significance in relation to dance appropriate floors (East-West-North-South)

Ballet studio only

With an average of 22.7% not furnishing any particulars and strong regional deviations (East: 12%, West: 27%, North: 27.8%, South: 24%), a comparable percentage of

theatres was equipped with sprung sub-floors in ballet studios (Fig.4).

Ballet studio and stage

17.6% of all institutions did not furnish any particulars. Significant regional deviations were found with respect to provision of a sprung sub-floor on stage (Fig.4)

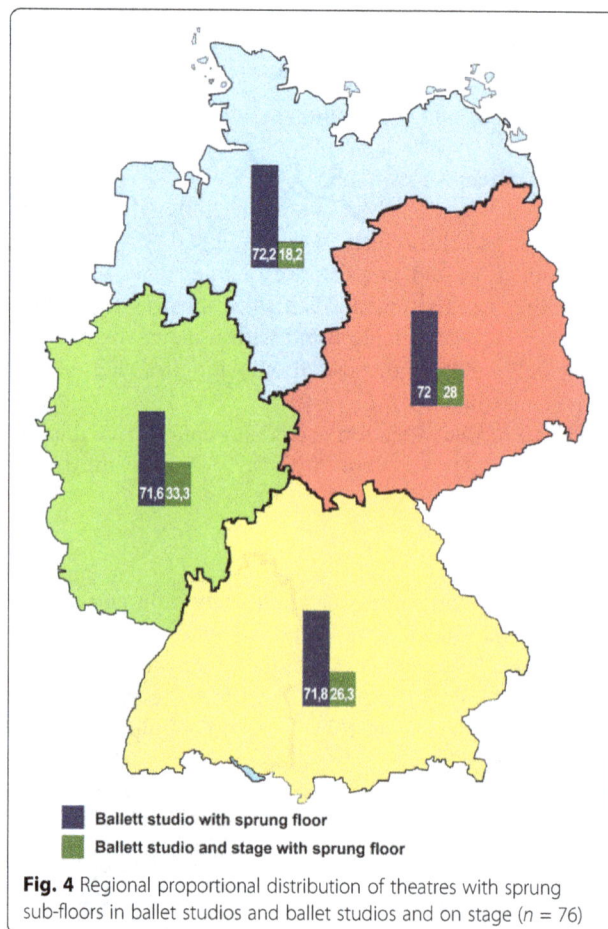

Fig. 4 Regional proportional distribution of theatres with sprung sub-floors in ballet studios and ballet studios and on stage (*n* = 76)

Discussion

The occupational activities of a dancer are accompanied by maximum loads to the musculoskeletal system. Those are repetitive movements, forced postures, slightly limited movements of joints, spine as well as static stop- and support activities or carrying loads (in this case, the dance partner). Over the past 20 years the loads have significantly increased [18]. There is hardly any technical support. As the loads directly affect the dancers' body a healthy body is essential for the profession. Even minor deficits in the musculoskeletal system can hardly be compensated. A healthy working environment is therefore all the more important in terms of primary preventive measures.

Dance or sports floors are not simply a work tool in dance or other types of sports but also an important contribution towards injury prevention [19, 20]. From a quality point of view, even standardized (after DIN or EN) sports floors are not all equally appropriate for the dance compared to special dance floors due to the existing requirements to a floor and the characteristics of dance (e.g. lack of cushioned footwear) and the anthropometry of female dancers (< 70 kg/11 stones).

The objective of this pilot project was to analyze the present equipment of dance appropriate floors at German theatres by a nationwide survey.

While on the one hand a high percentage of training areas (ballet studios) are equipped with appropriate floors there is on the other hand a great need for this type of flooring on stages and for touring purposes. Fewer than one in four theatres offering regular dance performances are equipped with a dance appropriate floor in all areas and for touring purposes; this results in very variable conditions within the theatre as a work place. Furthermore, the results show that due to the inappropriate floors found in smaller theatres, working conditions are worse for dance ensembles than in bigger theatres (>30 dancers). Concerning dance style and region within Germany just tendencies without any significant value were found.

As a whole, the results show that recommendations in terms of dance floors have only roughly been realized in the ballet studio but not – as recommended - in all other working areas for dancers. Of all theatres surveyed, 75% are not equipped with floors in accordance with the existing recommendations despite their regular dance productions or even own dance companies. The reasons seem to be versatile.

A good sub floor is expensive and long lasting. The first aspect may be the reason why it is the bigger theatres (with big ensembles) in mostly bigger cities and municipalities which have initiated installation of appropriate dance floors. Bigger theatres simply dispose of more financial resources than smaller ones.

The second aspect makes clear that long-lasting floors are much older in relation to the relatively recent research findings and have not yet been replaced because it was not necessary.

The extent to which a lack of information on possible physical effects on working dancers constitutes the reason why so few theatres dispose of dance appropriate floors is yet to be determined. However, the significance of a sprung sub- floor for other theatre genres (drama/opera) is definitely underestimated. As for portable sprung sub-floors, it cannot be excluded that particularly the technical management would like to avoid shifting the physical load from dancers to stagehands in cases where a mobile sprung sub-floor consisting partly of heavy panels for dance productions was installed.

Inappropriate floors may be significantly responsible for chronic misuse and overuse complaints sustained by dancers. It is conceivable that these chronic complaints appear years later far beyond any contractual connection. Regarding the causal chain between floor and chronic diseases no research findings have been presented to date. A primary preventive approach towards a dance appropriate floor in all working areas is therefore all the more important.

Hitherto, there seem to have been many – by and large inadequately– explanatory approaches as to why the recommendations relating to appropriate dance floors have been realized in ballet studios but not on stage and or for touring purposes. Further research seems to be inevitable here.

Conclusion

Recommendations concerning an appropriate dance floor have only partly been realized. Besides secured finances for reinstallation, further education of responsible officials and artists is essential. However, accrediting dance as own genre in theatres is the indispensable prerequisite.

Acknowledgements
Not applicable.

Funding
Neither direct or indirect financial support nor any donations of equipment, services, supplies, specimens, use of testing facilities, etc. have been granted for this investigation.

Authors' contributions
EMW drafted the manuscript and has made substantial intellectual contributions to the interpretation of data. MS has made substantial contributions to statistical evaluation. DK has been involved in creating figures and Tables. DO has been involved in revising the manuscript critically for important intellectual content. JLS has been involved in English proof reading. DAG has made substantial contributions to conception and design of this study and has given final approval of the version to be published. All authors read and approved the final manuscript.

Competing interests

The authors declare that they have no competing interests.

Author details

[1]Institute of Occupational Medicine, Social Medicine and Environmental Medicine, Goethe-University, Theodor-Stern-Kai 7, 60590 Frankfurt am Main, Germany. [2]Department of Sports and Exercise Medicine, Institute of Human Movement Science University of Hamburg, Mollerstraße 10, 20148 Hamburg, Germany. [3]School of Performing Arts, University of Wolverhampton, Gorway Rd, Walsall, West Midlands WS1 3BD, England.

References

1. Hackney J, Brummel S, Newman M, Scott S, Reinagel M, Smith J. Effect of reduced stiffness dance flooring on lower extremity joint angular trajectories during a ballet jump. J Dance Med Sci. 2015 Sep;19(3):110–7.
2. Hackney J, Brummel S, Becker D, Selbo A, Koons S, Stewart M. Effect of sprung (suspended) floor on lower extremity stiffness during a force-returning ballet jump. Med Probl Perform Art. 2011 Dec;26(4):195–9.
3. Hopper LS, Alderson JA, Elliott BC, Ackland TR. Dance floor force reduction influences ankle loads in dancers during drop landings. J Sci Med Sport. 2015 Jul;18(4):480–5.
4. Hackney J, Brummel S, Becker D, Chenoweth A, Koons S, Stewart M. Follow-up study to "The effect of sprung (suspended) floors on leg stiffness during grand jeté landings in ballet". J Dance Med Sci. 2011 Sep;15(3):134–5.
5. Hackney J, Brummel S, Jungblut K, Edge C. The effect of sprung (suspended) floors on leg stiffness during grand jeté landings in ballet. J Dance Med Sci. 2011 Sep;15(3):128–33.
6. Hopper LS, Wheeler TJ, Webster JM, Allen N, Roberts JR, Fleming PR. Dancer perceptions of the force reduction of dance floors used by a professional touring ballet company. J Dance Med Sci. 2014;18(3):121–30.
7. Hopper LS, Alderson JA, Elliott BC, Ackland TR, Fleming PR. Dancer perceptions of quantified dance surface mechanical properties Proceedings of the Institution of Mechanical Engineers. Part P: Journal of Sports Engineering and Technology. 2011;225(2):65–73.
8. Wanke EM: Rahmenempfehlungen zur Prävention von Verletzungen im professionellen Bühnentanz. 2. überarbeitete und ergänzte Auflage. [Basic recommendations on injury prevention in professional dance. 2nd revised and enlarged version] Unfallkasse Berlin und Deutsche gesetzliche Unfallversicherung (Hrsg.), 2013.
9. Wanke EM, Mill H, Wanke A, Davenport J, Koch F, Groneberg DA. Dance floors as injury risk: Analysis and evaluation of acute injuries caused by dance floors in professional dance with regard to preventative aspects. Med Probl Perform Art. 2012;27(3):137–42.
10. Seals JG. A study of dance surfaces (1983). Clin Sports Med. 1983;2(3):557–61.
11. Morrin N. Dance Floors. Dance UK Information sheet Nr. 2013;6
12. https://www.sportengland.org/media/4553/floors-for-indoor-sports.pdf. Accessed 23 Jan 2017.
13. Looseleaf V. The silent partner. Dance magazine, New York. 2006;80(1):88–93.
14. Pappas E, Hagins M. The effects of "raked" stages on standing posture in dancers. J Dance Med Sci. 2008;12(2):54–8.
15. Pappas E, Orishimo KF, Kremenic I, Liederbach M, Hagins M (2012).The effects of floor incline on lower extremity biomechanics during unilateral landing from a jump in dancers. J Appl Biomech 2012 May;28(2):192-199.
16. Hagins M, Pappas E, Kremenic I, Orishimo KF, Rundle A. The effect of an inclined landing surface on biomechanical variables during a jumping task. Clin Biomech. (Bristol, Avon). 2007;22(9):1030–6.
17. Pappas E, Kremenic I, Liederbach M, Orishimo KF, Hagins M. Time to stability differences between male and female dancers after landing from a jump on flat and inclined floors. Clin J Sport Med. 2011;21(4):325–9.
18. Wanke EM, Arendt M, Mill H, Groneberg DA. Occupational accidents in professional dance with focus on gender differences. J Occup Med Toxicol. 2013 Dec 17;8(1):35.
19. Orchard JW, Powell JW. Risk of knee and ankle sprains under various weather conditions in American football. Med Sci Sports Sci. 2003 Jul;35(7):1118–23.
20. Naunheim R, McGurren M, Standeven J, Fucetola R, Lauryssen C, Deibert E. Does the use of artificial turf contribute to head injuries? J Trauma. 2002 Oct;53(4):691–4.

3

Textile industry and occupational cancer

Zorawar Singh[1*] and Pooja Chadha[2]

Abstract

Background and summary: Thousands of workers are engaged in textile industry worldwide. Textile industry involves the use of different kinds of dyes which are known to possess carcinogenic properties. Solvents used in these industries are also associated with different health related hazards including cancer. In previous studies on textile and iron industries, the authors have reported genotoxicity among them and observed occurrence of cancer deaths among textile industry workers. Thus, an attempt has been made to compile the studies on the prevalence of different types of cancers among textile industry workers.

Literature search: A wide literature search has been done for compiling the present paper. Papers on cancer occurrence among textile industry workers have been taken from 1976 to 2015. A variety of textile dyes and solvents, many of them being carcinogenic, are being used worldwide in the textile industry. The textile industry workers are therefore, in continuous exposure to these dyes, solvents, fibre dusts and various other toxic chemicals. The present study evaluates the potential of different chemicals and physical factors to be carcinogenic agents among occupationally exposed workers by going through various available reports and researches. Papers were collected using different databases and a number of studies report the association of textile industry and different types of cancer including lung, bladder, colorectal and breast cancer. After going through the available reports, it can be concluded that workers under varied job categories in textile industries are at a higher risk of developing cancer as various chemicals used in the textile industry are toxic and can act as potential health risk in inducing cancer among them. Assessing the cancer risk at different job levels in textile industries may be found useful in assessing the overall risk to the workers and formulating the future cancer preventive strategies.

Keywords: Textile industries, Cancer, Occupational cancer, Mutagenic, Mortality

Abbreviations: BTC, Biliary Tract Cancer; HR, Hazard Ratio; IRR, Incident Rate Ratios; MFs, Magnetic Fields; OR, Odds Ratio; PRR, Proportional Registration Ratios; SIR, Standardized Incidence Ratios; SMRs, Standardized Mortality Ratios

Background

Textile is one of the leading industries in the world. The textile industry workers are exposed to a number of chemicals including dyes, solvents, optical brighteners, finishing agents and numerous types of natural and synthetic fibre dusts which affect their health. Various dyes and solvents used by the textile industry have been found to have mutagenic and carcinogenic properties. Workers engaged in finishing processes are frequently exposed to crease-resistance agents. These agents may release formaldehyde which is known for its toxicity. Workers are also exposed to flame retardants including organophosphorus and organobromine compounds. The textile industries use different kinds of dyes including the most commonly used azo dyes which are aromatic hydrocarbon derivatives of benzene, toluene, naphthalene, phenol and aniline. The solvents used by the workers in different sections result in a major carcinogenic effect by direct contact with the subjects. A number of studies have been put forward emphasizing the occurrence of different types of cancers among textile industry workers [1–34]. Keeping in view the importance of the issue, a brief review of the same is presented herewith.

Bladder cancer

Different studies have pointed out the occurrence of bladder cancer among textile industry workers [35–37]. Gonzales et al. [35] presented results from a case-control study carried out in the county of Mataro, Spain.

* Correspondence: zorawarsinghs@rediffmail.com
[1]Department of Zoology, Khalsa College, G.T. Road, Amritsar, Punjab 143001, India
Full list of author information is available at the end of the article

The study was based on 57 cases that were hospitalized for or died from bladder cancer between 1978 and 1981. An increased risk for past employment in the textile industry (Odds ratio, OR = 2.2; $p = 0.038$) was found among a group of common occupational sectors. Further analyses in the study indicated that the risk for subjects who worked in dyeing or printing sectors and who were exposed to azo-dyes was particularly elevated (OR = 4.41; 95 % confidence limits; 1.15–16.84). Similarly, Zheng et al. [36] conducted a study on 1,219 incident bladder cancer cases based on gender which were diagnosed during the period 1980 to 1984. The bladder cancer cases were compared with 1982 census data on employment. Standardized incidence ratios (SIR) for bladder cancer were estimated for occupation and industry classifications and significant excess risks were observed for dyers, textile bleachers, and finishers (male: SIR = 169); metal refining and processing workers (male: SIR = 139; female: SIR = 197); apparel industry workers and workers engaged in other textile products manufacturing (female: SIR = 204). Serra et al. [37] also investigated the risk of bladder cancer in Spanish textile workers and analyzed the data from a multicenter hospital-based case-control study in Spain. The data included 1219 bladder cancer cases and 1271 controls. Out of those cases, 126 cases and 122 controls reported a history of previous employment in the textile industry. Increased risks were observed for weavers and workers engaged in winding, warping and sizing. Higher risk was also found for workers who were exposed to synthetic materials. Table 1 shows the incidence of different types of cancers among textile industry workers.

Lung cancer

A number of studies report the association of textile industry and lung cancer. The association between endotoxin exposure and lung cancer risk was found in a cohort of female textile workers [23]. Bacterial endotoxin which is a contaminant of raw cotton fibre and cotton dust, has been proposed as a protective agent against cancer. The action of endotoxin may be through the innate and acquired immune systems. Long-term and high-level exposure to endotoxin, compared with no exposure was found to be associated with a reduced risk of lung cancer in this cohort. Similarly, Checkoway et al. [38] investigated the associations of various exposures like wool, synthetic fibre dusts, formaldehyde, silica, dyes and metals with lung cancer in the textile industry. But in this study, no associations were observed for lung cancer with wool, silk, synthetic fibre dust or with other agents. Agalliu et al. [39] investigated the associations between contiguous windows of endotoxin exposure and risk of lung cancer, and reported that endotoxin is consistently associated with a reduced risk of lung cancer. Data from 602 cases of female textile workers was

evaluated in Shanghai, China and an inverse risk trend of lung cancer with increasing levels of endotoxin exposure was found. In a study of Italian textile workers ($N = 1966$), on the basis of 68 deaths from mesothelioma, the standardized mortality ratio (SMR) was found to be 6627 for workers employed only under the age of 30 years. SMR was found to be 8019 for workers those were employed both under the age of 30 years and at the age of 30–39 years. SMR was 5891 for those employed both under the age of 30 years and at the age of 40 years or more. The results of the study also indicated that stopping the exposure of the workers does not modify the subsequent mesotheliomas risk [40].

Elliott et al. [41] conducted a study in North and South Carolina on two US cohorts of asbestos textile workers exposed to chrysotile. The study found an increasing risk of lung cancer mortality with cumulative fibre exposure. Similarly, Wang et al. [42] determined the mortality associated with exposure to chrysotile asbestos from a textile factory in China. The study was done from 1972 to 2008 and a total 577 workers were followed. Follow-up rate for the study was 98.5 % over 37 years. The follow-up of the workers generated a data of 17,508 persons including 259 deaths (from all causes), 2 mesotheliomas and 53 lung cancers. The highest cancer mortality was observed in the high exposure group, with 1.5-fold age-adjusted mortality from all cancers and 2-fold from lung cancer when compared to the low exposure group. Both smokers and non-smokers at the high exposure level had a high death risk from lung cancer. A clear exposure-response trend was seen in smokers which confirmed an increased mortality from lung cancer and all cancers in asbestos workers and the cancer mortality was found to be associated with exposure levels. Deng et al. [43] described mortality in workers exposed to chrysotile asbestos and determined exposure-response relationships between asbestos exposure and mortality from lung cancer. A cohort of 586 workers in an asbestos textile factory was followed. Individual cumulative asbestos exposure was estimated as the product of fibre concentrations and duration of employment in each job and expressed as fibre-years/ml (e.g., 30 fibre-years/ml is an exposure equivalent to 30 years of exposure at 1 fibre/ml concentration or 15 years at 2 fibres/ml; and so on). It was found that out of the 226 deaths, 51 deaths were from lung cancer and 37 from asbestosis. A significant exposure-response relationship between asbestosis and lung cancer ($p < 0.001$) was observed. Applebaum et al. [44] also examined the relationship between endotoxin and lung cancer in a study of Chinese female textile workers. Enrollment of the workers was done between 1989 and 1991 and the workers were followed till 1998. In the study, 3038 sub-cohort members and 602 incident lung cancer cases

Table 1 Studies based on occurrence of different types of cancers among textile industry workers

Sr. No.	Study	Subjects	Type of cancer studied	Output of the study
1	Serra et al., 2008 [37]	Textile industry workers	Bladder cancer	Increased cancer risks were observed for weavers and for workers in winding, warping and sizing. Job more than 10 years appeared to be associated with an increased risk for weavers.
2	Li et al., 2015 [33]	Female textile workers	Breast cancer	No positive association between night shift work and breast cancer.
3	Li et al., 2013 [48]	Female textile workers	Breast cancer	No association was observed between cumulative exposure to MFs and overall risk of breast cancer.
4	Ray et al., 2007 [25]	Female textile workers	Breast cancer	Endotoxin or other components of cotton dust exposures may be associated with reduced risks for breast cancer
5	Fang et al., 2013 [46]	Textile workers	Cancer mortality	Mortality risk from gastrointestinal cancers and all cancers combined, with the exclusion of lung cancer, were increased in cotton workers as compared to silk workers.
6	Wang et al., 2012 [42]	Asbestos textile workers	Cancer mortality	Highest cancer mortality was observed in the high exposure group, with 1.5-fold age-adjusted mortality from all cancers and 2-fold from lung cancer compared to the low exposure group.
7	Kuzmickiene and Stukonis, 2010 [49]	Female flax textile workers	Oral cavity and pharynx cancer	Risk of oral cavity and pharynx cancer was significantly increased in spinning-weaving unit workers with <10 years of employment (SIR 5.71, 95 % CI 1.56 to 14.60).
8	Gunay and Beser, 2011 [50]	Turkish textile workers	Early breast cancer	91.6 % of the women working in a textile factory in Turkey had no education about breast cancer.
9	Kwon et al., 2015 [32]	Female textile workers	Lung cancer	No increased risk of lung cancer among rotating shift workers.
10	Checkoway et al., 2015 [51]	Female textile workers	Lung cancer	Reply to [34]: Exposure–response association may change over time owing to complex, yet poorly understood, underlying mechanisms. Endotoxin is a highly variable exposure, and as we noted in the paper, some exposure misclassification was inevitable.
11	Rylander and Jacobs, 2015 [34]	Female textile workers	Lung cancer	In comment to [30]: The result should be "no relation between endotoxin exposure and lung cancer risk could be detected"
12	Checkoway et al., 2014 [30]	Female textile workers	Lung cancer	The study did not support a protective effect of endotoxin, but is suggestive of possible lung cancer promotion with increasing time since first exposure.
13	Wang et al., 2014 [31]	Textile and mining workers	Lung cancer	A clear exposure-response relationship between lung cancer mortality and exposure levels.
14	Applebaum et al., 2013 [44]	Female textile workers	Lung cancer	A reduced cancer risk in workers exposed to endotoxin, hired >35 years before enrolment [IRR = 0.74, 95 % CI (0.51 to 1.07)] as compared to hired </=35 years.
15	Gallagher et al., 2013 [52]	Female textile workers	Lung cancer	Cancer risk was higher in women with a surgical menopause (HR = 1.64, 95 % CI 0.96–2.79) than in those with a natural menopause (HR = 1.35, 95 % CI 0.84–2.18) demonstrating biological role of hormones in lung carcinogenesis.
16	Agalliu et al., 2011 [39]	Female textile workers	Lung cancer	Endotoxin exposure that occurred 20 years or more before risk confers the strongest protection against lung cancer, indicating a possible early anti-carcinogenic effect.

Table 1 Studies based on occurrence of different types of cancers among textile industry workers *(Continued)*

17	Checkoway et al., 2011 [38]	Female textile workers	Lung Cancer	No associations were observed for lung cancer with wool, silk or synthetic fibre dusts. Increased risks were noted for >/= 10 year exposures to silica (adjusted HR 3.5, 95 % CI 1.0 to 13) and >/= 10 year exposures to formaldehyde (adjusted HR 2.1, 95 % CI 0.4 to 11).
18	Astrakianakis et al., 2010 [53]	Female textile workers	Lung Cancer	A dose-related inverse lung cancer risk was associated with cumulative endotoxin exposure but a possible anti-carcinogenic effect at early stages of lung cancer pathogenesis was not evident.
19	Lenters et al., 2010 [29]	Agriculture industry and cotton textile workers	Lung Cancer	Occupational exposure to endotoxin in cotton textile production and agriculture is protective against lung cancer
20	Loomis et al., 2009 [28]	Asbestos textile workers	Lung Cancer	Mortality from all causes, all cancers and lung cancer was significant higher than expected, with SMRs of 1.47 for all causes, 1.41 for all cancer and 1.96 (95 % CI 1.73 to 2.20) for lung cancer.
21	Kuzmickiene and Stukonis, 2007 [24]	Textile workers	Lung Cancer	Exposure to cotton textile dust at workplaces for male is associated with adverse lung cancer risk effects but lung cancer risk decreased with level of exposure to textile dust.
22	Loomis et al., 2012 [54]	Asbestos textile workers	Lung Cancer	Lung cancer is associated most strongly with exposure to long thin asbestos fibres. Fibres 5–10 μm long and <0.25 μm in diameter were associated most strongly with lung cancer mortality.
23	Elliott et al., 2012 [41]	Asbestos textile workers	Lung Cancer	Increased rates of lung cancer were significantly found to be associated with overall cumulative fibre exposure.
24	Wernli et al., 2008a [27]	Textile workers	Endometrial cancer	An increased risk of endometrial cancer was detected among women who had worked for > or =10 years in silk production (HR = 3.8, 95 % CI 1.2–11.8).
25	Wernli et al., 2008b [55]	Textile workers	Ovarian cancer	An increasing risk of ovarian cancer associated with cumulative exposure to silica dust (for <10 years exposure, HR = 6.8 [CI = 0.6–76]; for > or =10 years, 5.6 [1.3–23.6]).

SIR standardized incidence ratios, *MFs* magnetic fields, *HR* hazard ratio, *IRR* incident rate ratios, *SMRs* standardized mortality ratios

were analyzed. Among the workers, who were never exposed to endotoxin, a comparison was made between lung cancer rates in workers hired more than 35 years before enrolment and workers hired less than or 35 years before enrolment. In the former group, a reduced risk (Incidence rate ratio, IRR = 0.74, 95 % CI) was found. An increased risk of lung cancer among workers hired for more than 50 years ago was also reported.

Dement and Brown [12] investigated the causes of deaths among textile workers and found 185 excess deaths (SMR = 1.44) out of a mortality of 1200 South Carolina textile workers. These excess deaths included 41 lung cancers (SMR = 2.25), 43 non-malignant respiratory diseases (SMR = 2.25) and 71 cardiovascular diseases (SMR = 1.37). In whole of the study, only two mesotheliomas cases were observed. Simpson et al. [45] examined the relation between women's health and their occupation. The study analyzed the data of

381,915 women cancer cases which were registered in England from 1971 to 1990, over the period of 20-year. For exploring the value of the data, five sites (lung, pleura, bladder, breast and stomach) under two occupations including agriculture and textile were selected. The association between stomach cancer and "dusty" occupations were found to as PRR (Proportional registration ratios) = 198, 95 % (CI = 126–298) for textile finishers. Similarly, Mastrangelo et al. [14] analyzed textile industry workers to evaluate the cancer risk within the textile industry in relation to the textile fibre being used or the specific type of job held in the industry. The decrease in the cases of upper respiratory tract cancer paralleled with a corresponding increase in the cases of lung cancer. Conclusively, the importance of preventive measures to reduce the lung cancer burden in the textile workers was emphasized.

Other cancer types

Apart from occurrence of bladder and lung cancer cases in textile industry workers, various other cancer types are also reported in different studies. Camp et al. [15] assessed the development of a cancer study among Shanghai textile workers. The results of the study indicated that women employed in wool, cotton, mixed-fiber and machine-maintenance sectors have a significantly increased risk for breast cancer. De Roos et al. [17] investigated the probable risks of rectum and colon cancers in relation to different types of exposures in textile industry. The investigation revealed that certain long term exposures in textile industry may pose an increased risk of colorectal cancers. Hazard ratio for exposures especially to textile dyes and their intermediates with colon cancer was found to be HR = 3.9; 95 % CI: 1.4–10.6 (> or =20 years exposure versus never). In the same way, Chang et al. [19] investigated the associations between biliary tract cancer (BTC) and occupational exposures to various chemicals and textile dusts in a cohort of 267,400 women textile workers. For employment in maintenance jobs, an increased risk of BTC was found (HR = 2.92, 95 % CI: 1.48, 5.73) with a significant trend by duration of exposure. It was also suggested that long-term exposures to different metals and employment in maintenance sector in the textile industry may have played a role in elevating the BTC risks among textile industry workers. Fang et al. [46] investigated the cancer mortality in relation to cotton dust and endotoxin exposure in a cohort from Shanghai textile workers by assessing 444 cotton textile workers. A reference group of 467 persons who were unexposed silk workers was also recruited. Both the groups were followed for 30 years. Hazard ratios for all cancers (with and without lung cancer) and gastrointestinal cancer were estimated in Cox regression models. In comparison to silk workers, cotton workers were found to have increased risks of mortality from gastrointestinal cancers and all cancers combined [gastrointestinal cancer HR = 4.1 (1.8–9.7); all cancers HR = 2.7 (95 % CI 1.4–5.2)]. A previous study by the present author also demonstrated genotoxic risk among textile industry workers [47].

Conclusion

Textile industry workers are exposed to a number of chemicals which are known to have carcinogenic properties. Reviewing the data of 54 research papers on textile industry workers revealed the occurrence of different types of cancers among them. Exposure to different sets of chemicals and physical factors in textile industry may induce occupational cancer as a long term effect among textile industry workers. Formulation and use of alternate non-toxic textile chemicals for different processes should be encouraged. Conclusively, proper protection equipments and other precautionary measures should be used by the workers while dealing with toxic chemicals in these industries.

Acknowledgements
Not applicable.

Funding
There is no funding source for the present study.

Authors' contribution
SZ conceived the study. CP participated in the design of the study. Both the authors drafted the manuscript. Both authors read and approved the final manuscript.

Competing interest
The authors declare that they have no competing interest.

Financial support and sponsorship
None.

Author details
[1]Department of Zoology, Khalsa College, G.T. Road, Amritsar, Punjab 143001, India. [2]Department of Zoology, Guru Nanak Dev University, Amritsar, Punjab, India.

References
1. Moss E. Oral and pharyngeal cancer in textile workers. Ann N Y Acad Sci. 1976;271:301–7.
2. Buiatti E, Baccetti S, Cecchi F, Tomassini A, Dolara P. Evidence of increased lung cancer rate among textile workers. Med Lav. 1979;70:21–3.
3. Heyden S, Pratt P. Exposure to cotton dust and respiratory disease. Textile workers, 'brown lung', and lung cancer. JAMA. 1980;244:1797–8.
4. Dement JM, Harris Jr RL, Symons MJ, Shy C. Estimates of dose-response for respiratory cancer among chrysotile asbestos textile workers. Ann Occup Hyg. 1982;26:869–87.
5. Delzell E, Grufferman S. Cancer and other causes of death among female textile workers, 1976–78. J Natl Cancer Inst. 1983;71:735–40.
6. Levin LI, Gao YT, Blot WJ, Zheng W, Fraumeni Jr JF. Decreased risk of lung cancer in the cotton textile industry of Shanghai. Cancer Res. 1987;47:5777–81.
7. O'Brien TR, Decoufle P. Cancer mortality among northern Georgia carpet and textile workers. Am J Ind Med. 1988;14:15–24.
8. Pearce N. Multistage modelling of lung cancer mortality in asbestos textile workers. Int J Epidemiol. 1988;17:747–52.
9. Sebastien P, McDonald JC, McDonald AD, Case B, Harley R. Respiratory cancer in chrysotile textile and mining industries: exposure inferences from lung analysis. Br J Ind Med. 1989;46:180–7.
10. Frumin E, Velez H, Bingham E, Gillen M, Brathwaite M, LaBarck R. Occupational bladder cancer in textile dyeing and printing workers: six cases and their significance for screening programs. J Occup Med. 1990;32:887–90.
11. Zappa M, Paci E, Seniori CA, Kriebel D. Lung cancer among textile workers in the Prato area of Italy. Scand J Work Environ Health. 1993;19:16–20.
12. Dement JM, Brown DP. Lung cancer mortality among asbestos textile workers: a review and update. Ann Occup Hyg. 1994;38:525–32. 412.
13. Serra C, Bonfill X, Sunyer J, Urrutia G, Turuguet D, Bastus R, Roque M, 't Mannetje A, Kogevinas M. Bladder cancer in the textile industry. Scand J Work Environ Health. 2000;26:476–81.
14. Mastrangelo G, Fedeli U, Fadda E, Milan G, Lange JH. Epidemiologic evidence of cancer risk in textile industry workers: a review and update. Toxicol Ind Health. 2002;18:171–81.

15. Camp JE, Seixas NS, Wernli K, Fitzgibbons D, Astrakianakis G, Thomas DB, Gao DL, Checkoway H. Development of a cancer research study in the Shanghai textile industry. Int J Occup Environ Health. 2003;9:347–56.

16. Lange JH, Mastrangelo G, Fedeli U, Rylander R, Christiani DC. A benefit of reducing lung cancer incidence in women occupationally exposed to cotton textile dust. Am J Ind Med. 2004;45:388–9.

17. De Roos AJ, Ray RM, Gao DL, Wernli KJ, Fitzgibbons ED, Ziding F, Astrakianakis G, Thomas DB, Checkoway H. Colorectal cancer incidence among female textile workers in Shanghai, China: a case-cohort analysis of occupational exposures. Cancer Causes Control. 2005;16:1177–88.

18. Pira E, Pelucchi C, Buffoni L, Palmas A, Turbiglio M, Negri E, Piolatto PG, La VC. Cancer mortality in a cohort of asbestos textile workers. Br J Cancer. 2005;92:580–6.

19. Chang CK, Astrakianakis G, Thomas DB, Seixas NS, Camp JE, Ray RM, Gao DL, Wernli KJ, Li W, Fitzgibbons ED, Vaughan TL, Checkoway H. Risks of biliary tract cancer and occupational exposures among Shanghai women textile workers: a case-cohort study. Am J Ind Med. 2006;49:690–8.

20. Fang SC, Eisen EA, Dai H, Zhang H, Hang J, Wang X, Christiani DC. Cancer mortality among textile workers in Shanghai, China: a preliminary study. J Occup Environ Med. 2006;48:955–8.

21. Li W, Ray RM, Gao DL, Fitzgibbons ED, Seixas NS, Camp JE, Wernli KJ, Astrakianakis G, Feng Z, Thomas DB, Checkoway H. Occupational risk factors for pancreatic cancer among female textile workers in Shanghai, China. Occup Environ Med. 2006;63:788–93.

22. Tse LA, Yu IT. Re: 'Occupational exposures and risks of liver cancer among Shanghai female textile workers–a case-cohort study'. Int J Epidemiol. 2006;35:1359.

23. Astrakianakis G, Seixas NS, Ray R, Camp JE, Gao DL, Feng Z, Li W, Wernli KJ, Fitzgibbons ED, Thomas DB, Checkoway H. Lung cancer risk among female textile workers exposed to endotoxin. J Natl Cancer Inst. 2007;99:357–64.

24. Kuzmickiene I, Stukonis M. Lung cancer risk among textile workers in Lithuania. J Occup Med Toxicol. 2007;2:14.

25. Ray RM, Gao DL, Li W, Wernli KJ, Astrakianakis G, Seixas NS, Camp JE, Fitzgibbons ED, Feng Z, Thomas DB, Checkoway H. Occupational exposures and breast cancer among women textile workers in Shanghai. Epidemiology. 2007;18:383–92.

26. Reul NK, Li W, Gallagher LG, Ray RM, Romano ME, Gao D, Thomas DB, Vedal S, Checkoway H. Risk ofPancreatic Cancer in Female Textile Workers in Shanghai, China, Exposed to Metals, Solvents, Chemicals, and Endotoxin: Follow-Up to a Nested Case-Cohort Study. J Occup Environ Med. 2016;58: 195-99.

27. Wernli KJ, Ray RM, Gao DL, Fitzgibbons ED, Camp JE, Astrakianakis G, Seixas N, Li W, De Roos AJ, Feng Z, Thomas DB, Checkoway H. Occupational risk factors for endometrial cancer among textile workers in Shanghai, China. Am J Ind Med. 2008;51:673–9.

28. Loomis D, Dement JM, Wolf SH, Richardson DB. Lung cancer mortality and fibre exposures among North Carolina asbestos textile workers. Occup Environ Med. 2009;66:535–42.

29. Lenters V, Basinas I, Beane-Freeman L, Boffetta P, Checkoway H, Coggon D, Portengen L, Sim M, Wouters IM, Heederik D, Vermeulen R. Endotoxin exposure and lung cancer risk: a systematic review and meta-analysis of the published literature on agriculture and cotton textile workers. Cancer Causes Control. 2010;21:523–55.

30. Checkoway H, Lundin JI, Costello S, Ray R, Li W, Eisen EA, Astrakianakis G, Seixas N, Applebaum K, Gao DL, Thomas DB. Possible pro-carcinogenic association of endotoxin on lung cancer among Shanghai women textile workers. Br J Cancer. 2014;111:603–7.

31. Wang X, Lin S, Yano E, Yu IT, Courtice M, Lan Y, Christiani DC. Exposure-specific lung cancer risks in Chinese chrysotile textile workers and mining workers. Lung Cancer. 2014;85:119–24.

32. Kwon P, Lundin J, Li W, Ray R, Littell C, Gao D, Thomas DB, Checkoway H. Night shift work and lung cancer risk among female textile workers in Shanghai, China. J Occup Environ Hyg. 2015;12:334–41.

33. Li W, Ray RM, Thomas DB, Davis S, Yost M, Breslow N, Gao DL, Fitzgibbons ED, Camp JE, Wong E, Wernli KJ, Checkoway H. Shift work and breast cancer among women textile workers in Shanghai, China. Cancer Causes Control. 2015;26:143–50.

34. Rylander R, Jacobs R. Comment on 'Possible pro-carcinogenic association of endotoxin on lung cancer among Shanghai women textile workers'. Br J Cancer. 2015;112:1840.

35. Gonzales CA, Riboli E, Lopez-Abente G. Bladder cancer among workers in the textile industry: results of a Spanish case–control study. Am J Ind Med. 1988;14:673–80.

36. Zheng W, McLaughlin JK, Gao YT, Silverman DT, Gao RN, Blot WJ. Bladder cancer and occupation in Shanghai, 1980–1984. Am J Ind Med. 1992;21:877–85.

37. Serra C, Kogevinas M, Silverman DT, Turuguet D, Tardon A, Garcia-Closas R, Carrato A, Castano-Vinyals G, Fernandez F, Stewart P, Benavides FG, Gonzalez S, Serra A, Rothman N, Malats N, Dosemeci M. Work in the textile industry in Spain and bladder cancer. Occup Environ Med. 2008;65:552–9.

38. Checkoway H, Ray RM, Lundin JI, Astrakianakis G, Seixas NS, Camp JE, Wernli KJ, Fitzgibbons ED, Li W, Feng Z, Gao DL, Thomas DB. Lung cancer and occupational exposures other than cotton dust and endotoxin among women textile workers in Shanghai, China. Occup Environ Med. 2011;68:425–9.

39. Agalliu I, Costello S, Applebaum KM, Ray RM, Astrakianakis G, Gao DL, Thomas DB, Checkoway H, Eisen EA. Risk of lung cancer in relation to contiguous windows of endotoxin exposure among female textile workers in Shanghai. Cancer Causes Control. 2011;22:1397–404.

40. La VC, Boffetta P. Role of stopping exposure and recent exposure to asbestos in the risk of mesothelioma. Eur J Cancer Prev. 2012;21:227–30.

41. Elliott L, Loomis D, Dement J, Hein MJ, Richardson D, Stayner L. Lung cancer mortality in North Carolina and South Carolina chrysotile asbestos textile workers. Occup Environ Med. 2012;69:385–90.

42. Wang XR, Yu IT, Qiu H, Wang MZ, Lan YJ, Tse LY, Yano E, Christiani DC. Cancer mortality among Chinese chrysotile asbestos textile workers. Lung Cancer. 2012;75:151–5.

43. Deng Q, Wang X, Wang M, Lan Y. Exposure-response relationship between chrysotile exposure and mortality from lung cancer and asbestosis. Occup Environ Med. 2012;69:81–6.

44. Applebaum KM, Ray RM, Astrakianakis G, Gao DL, Thomas DB, Christiani DC, LaValley MP, Li W, Checkoway H, Eisen EA. Evidence of a paradoxical relationship between endotoxin and lung cancer after accounting for left truncation in a study of Chinese female textile workers. Occup Environ Med. 2013;70:709–15.

45. Simpson J, Roman E, Law G, Pannett B. Women's occupation and cancer: preliminary analysis of cancer registrations in England and Wales, 1971–1990. Am J Ind Med. 1999;36:172–85.

46. Fang SC, Mehta AJ, Hang JQ, Eisen EA, Dai HL, Zhang HX, Su L, Christiani DC. Cotton dust, endotoxin and cancer mortality among the Shanghai textile workers cohort: a 30-year analysis. Occup Environ Med. 2013;70:722–9.

47. Singh Z, Chadha P. Human health hazard posed by textile dyes: a genotoxic perspective. J Hum Health. 2015;1:42–5.

48. Li W, Ray RM, Thomas DB, Yost M, Davis S, Breslow N, Gao DL, Fitzgibbons ED, Camp JE, Wong E, Wernli KJ, Checkoway H. Occupational exposure to magnetic fields and breast cancer among women textile workers in Shanghai, China. Am J Epidemiol. 2013;178:1038–45.

49. Kuzmickiene I, Stukonis M. Cancer incidence among women flax textile manufacturing workers in Lithuania. Occup Environ Med. 2010;67:500–2.

50. Gunay E, Beser A. Sociodemographic characteristics of women who engage in early breast cancer diagnostic behaviors: the case of Turkish women working in a textile factory. AAOHN J. 2011;59:421–8.

51. Checkoway H, Lundin JI, Costello S, Ray RM, Li W, Eisen EA, Astrakianakis G, Applebaum K, Gao DL, Thomas DB. Reply to comment on: 'Possible pro-carcinogenic association of endotoxin on lung cancer among shanghai women textile workers'. Br J Cancer. 2015;112:1840-1.

52. Gallagher LG, Rosenblatt KA, Ray RM, Li W, Gao DL, Applebaum KM, Checkoway H, Thomas DB. Reproductive factors and risk of lung cancer in female textile workers in Shanghai, China. Cancer Causes Control. 2013;24:1305–14.

53. Astrakianakis G, Seixas NS, Ray R, Camp JE, Gao DL, Feng Z, Li W, Wernli KJ, Fitzgibbons ED, Thomas DB, Checkoway H. Re: lung cancer risk among female textile workers exposed to endotoxin. J Natl Cancer Inst. 2010;102:913–4.

54. Loomis D, Dement JM, Elliott L, Richardson D, Kuempel ED, Stayner L. Increased lung cancer mortality among chrysotile asbestos textile workers is more strongly associated with exposure to long thin fibres. Occup Environ Med. 2012;69:564–8.

55. Wernli KJ, Ray RM, Gao DL, Fitzgibbons ED, Camp JE, Astrakianakis G, Seixas N, Wong EY, Li W, De Roos AJ, Feng Z, Thomas DB, Checkoway H. Occupational exposures and ovarian cancer in textile workers. Epidemiology. 2008;19:244–50.

4

Use of moulded hearing protectors by child care workers

Peter Koch[1*], Johanna Stranzinger[2], Jan Felix Kersten[1] and Albert Nienhaus[1,2]

Abstract

Background: Employees of a multi-site institution for children and adolescents started to wear moulded hearing protectors (MHPs) during working hours, as they were suffering from a high level of noise exposure. It was agreed with the institutional physician and the German Institution for Statutory Accident Insurance and Prevention in the Health and Welfare Services (BGW) that this presented an opportunity to perform a scientific study to investigate potential beneficial effects on risk of burnout and subjective noise exposure at work when child care workers wear MHPs.

Methods: This was an intervention study which compared the initial values with those after a follow-up of 12 months. All teaching child care workers employed by the multi-site institution were offered the opportunity to take part. Forty-five (45) employees in 16 institutions participated. The subjects were provided with personally adapted MHPs and documented the periods of wear in a diary. At the start and end of the intervention, the subjects had to answer a questionnaire related to subjective noise exposure and burnout risk. In parallel, employees were surveyed who had not taken part in the intervention.

Results: Thirty-three (33) subjects took part in the follow-up after 12 months (follow-up rate 73 %). The median period of wear of MHPs was 34.6 h. During the period of observation, the mean subjective noise exposure increased by 2.7 %, and mean burnout risk by 2.5 scale points (baseline: 55.2, follow-up 57.7). Neither difference was statistically significant. 67 % of the participants reported that they were still capable of fulfilling their teaching duties when wearing the MHPs. In the reference group without the intervention, the increase in burnout risk was 3.9 points, which was even less favourable (baseline: 50.6, follow-up: 54.5).

Conclusions: Within the working environment of the child care workers, wearing MHPs did not reduce subjective noise exposure or burnout risk; the satisfaction of the study subjects with wearing MHPs decreased over time. There were however signs that the level of stress increased over time and that this might have been alleviated in the intervention group by wearing MHPs.

Keywords: Moulded hearing protectors, Child care worker, Burnout, Personal hearing protector, Noise exposure

Background

Child care workers in day care centres or other institutions for children and adolescents are continuously exposed to noise from children throughout the working day. Objective measurements have found that the peak sound pressure in these institutions is greater than 85 dB(A) [1–5], which confirms the employees' subjective impression [1, 6, 7]. This noise is mostly caused by the children's voices and their playing [4]. This may be exacerbated by poor conditions, for example, if the ratio of children to child care workers is high, or if the structure of the building is unsuitable. Studies have shown that staff report fewer health problems when they work in institutions with closed rooms than in those with large half open or open rooms [8]. In this setting, symptoms associated with noise include headache, exhaustion, burnout, stress, voice problems, hearing difficulties and tinnitus [4, 7–12]. In environments with continuous background noise, small children are even at risk of disturbances in speech development [13]. A study with preschool children has shown that children who are exposed to a higher level of noise are more likely to have problems in learning to read [14].

* Correspondence: p.koch@uke.de
[1]Centre of Excellence for Epidemiology and Health Services Research for Healthcare Professionals (CVcare), University Medical Centre Hamburg-Eppendorf, Martinistraße 52, Hamburg 20246, Germany
Full list of author information is available at the end of the article

The most usual interventions to reduce noise in child day care centres are technical or organisational. These include, for example, increased noise insulation, the selection of special toys and furniture, using noise warning lights, noise education for children or designating withdrawal rooms for the staff. However, studies on these interventions show that they have little efficacy on subjective noise exposure suffered by employees [11, 15].

In the industrial working environment, the efforts to reduce hearing damage are not only technical or organisational, but may be individualised. In Germany, a personal hearing protector is required if noise exposure exceeds 80 dB(A); this is based on EU Directive 2003/10/EU [16] and was incorporated in the Noise and Vibration Occupational Safety Health Ordinance [17]. In workplaces with technical noise, many employees wear a capsule hearing protector, e.g. soldiers, farmers and industrial workers [18–22]; moulded hearing protectors (MHPs) are often worn by professional musicians. In comparison to capsule hearing protectors, MHPs with adjustable otoplasty filter systems have the advantage that speech is still comprehensible with the hearing protector. For example, in occupational medicine, they are selectively used for teachers and child care workers with hyperacusis. We are unaware of any scientific studies on the use of MHPs in child care workers.

In this context, the following questions were examined in our study:

1a. Does the use of MHPs reduce subjective noise exposure among child care workers?
1b. Does the use of MHPs reduce risk of burnout among child care workers?
2. Do child care workers find the use of MHPs to be comfortable and feasible?
3. What are the acoustics (reverberation time) of critical rooms that were identified by an experienced acoustician and are there associations between acoustic properties of the rooms and subjective noise exposure and risk of burnout respectively?

Methods

As part of stress monitoring for child care workers in a multi-site institution for children and adolescents [7], parallel groups of subjects were recruited for an interventional study on reduction in risk of burnout and subjective noise exposure by MHPs. The participation in the study was offered all 400 child care workers in 26 different facilities (Fig. 1). The multi-site institution bears the responsibility for caring for children in three different types of institutions: 1) day care centres for children aged up to 6 years, 2) school partnerships for school children and 3) facilities to support children and adolescents, e.g. sheltered housing groups. A total of 45

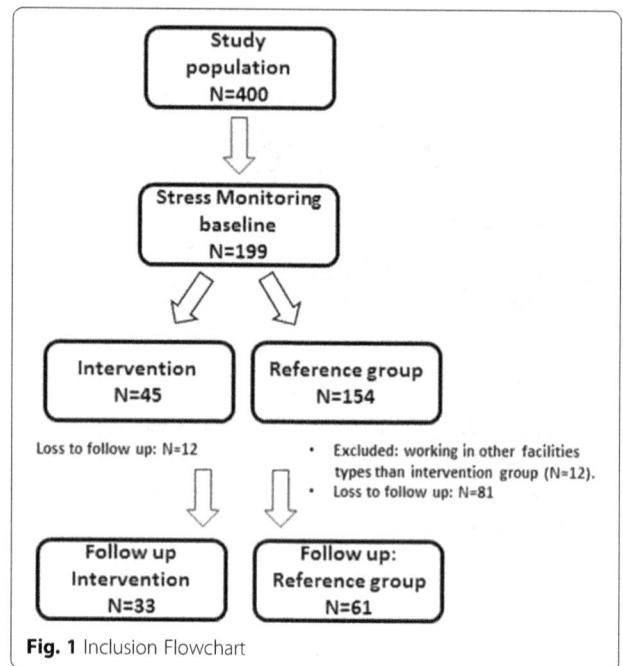

Fig. 1 Inclusion Flowchart

subjects were recruited for the intervention study and also participated in stress monitoring at the same time. The efficacy and practicability of the MHPs were assessed by comparing the initial measurements with those after one year of observation. Post hoc, to examine the results from another perspective, a comparator group was made up of subjects who only took part in stress monitoring. This comparison was carried out so that it would be possible to assess whether the stress potential in the institutions had remained constant or changed over time. As this is not a classical control group, it will be referred to below as the "reference group". 12 subjects working in facilities to support children and adolescents have been excluded from the reference group as in the intervention group no one was working in this type of institution. Overall the reference group comprised 61 subjects. There were no statistically significant differences in demographic characteristics between the intervention and reference group. The inclusion criteria for participation in the intervention were as follows: a) participation in stress monitoring, b) employment in teaching, c) intended employment for at least another year, d) minimum age of 18 years. In order to avoid windfall effects, each subject had to contribute 20 Euros towards their personal hearing protector. The subjects came from 16 different institutions; 11 of these were kindergartens and 5 were school partnerships, in which children from fulltime schools were looked after during teaching breaks.

The pseudoanonymous questionnaire was agreed with the multi-site institution's data protector officer. All study documents including the study protocol were reviewed and approved by the Ethics Committee of the Hamburg

Medical Association (Reference Number: PV4792). Each subject provided a signed declaration of consent.

Intervention

After taking the imprints of the outer ear, the audiologist presented the 45 subjects with a workshop on dealing with MHPs and on the issue of noise. A central recommendation of the workshop was to use the MHPs punctually in situations with high noise exposure (e.g. during lunch). The intervention started in October 2014 (T0) and the subjects were then sent their individually prepared MHPs (Variphone "MEP-2G" Hearing Protector) by post and completed the form on stress monitoring. At the same time, they were given a diary, in which they had to document the times they used the personal hearing protector each day. After five months (T1), the subjects had the opportunity of visiting the audiologist again, in order to modify the fit and the filter strength of their MHPs. At this time, the user satisfaction was recorded with a short questionnaire. After a total of 12 months (T2) follow-up, questionnaires were distributed again on stress monitoring and user satisfaction.

Questionnaire

The questionnaire on stress monitoring collected data on the following factors that could potentially influence the effect of the intervention: three standardized questionnaires components (effort reward imbalance [23], physical stress [24], work-related stress and resources from the Short Questionnaire on Work Analysis (KFZA) [25]). The effort reward imbalance (ERI) questionnaire consists of three dimensions, *effort, reward* and *Overcommitment.* The ERI questionnaire assesses the psychosocial situation of the worker. In studies internal consistencies were satisfactory and varied between 0.70 and 0.91 (Cronbach's alpha) [26, 27]. The KFZA questionnaire comprises different work-related strains and resources. The following scales have been chosen for our questionnaire: *control, variety, entirety, cooperation, qualitative workload, quantitative workload, work disruption and information.* For qualitative workload and work disruption internal consistencies were 0.40 and 0.44 (Cronbachs alpha). For all other scales Cronbachs alpha was between 0.51 and 0.71 [25]. For the questionnaire on physical stress, no study on reliability was available. *Subjective noise exposure* was determined from a cumulative score (range 13–65 points) out of 13 self-developed rating items. Questions such as "There are rooms where I hear particularly poorly" or "This level of noise bothers me" were answered on a 5-point scale, ranging from *strongly agree* to *strongly disagree.* Regarding everyday working life situations for child care workers nine self-developed questions have been added to the questionnaire. To assess situations that might

include a stress potential, questions such as "Breaks and possibilities for recovery are missing" or "There are conflicts with parents" were answered on a 4-point scale ranging from *strongly agree* to *strongly disagree.*

Two outcome variables were examined: burnout risk and subjective noise exposure; the latter may be a factor that influences burnout risk. Burnout risk was assessed on the basis of the subscale *personal burnout* of the Copenhagen Burnout Inventory [28]. In the German version of the Copenhagen Psychosocial Questionnaire (COPSOQ) questionnaire the subscale *personal burnout* shows a Cronbach's alpha of 0.91 [29]. The self-developed questionnaire on user satisfaction collected information on wearing comfort, acoustic perception and the reasonableness of wearing MHPs at work. The answers were rated on the basis of a 5-point rating scale and were then dichotomised due to presentational reasons (yes = absolutely or predominantly true; no = partially correct, predominantly incorrect, absolutely incorrect).

Acoustic measurements

In order to have not only subjective but also objective data on room acoustics, reverberation times were measured in the various institutions during the observation period. The measurements were in the frequency range of 125–4000 Hz and were carried out in rooms with different functions - playrooms, group rooms, classrooms, movement rooms, flights of stairs and restaurants for children. The results were compared with the target values in DIN Norm 18041 on acoustic properties in rooms of small or intermediate size [30]. On the basis of the reverberation times and building properties, an expert in room acoustics performed a final evaluation of the selected rooms. Between 1 and 4 rooms were evaluated for each institution, except one institution of school partnership without any measurement.

Power estimation

During the run-up, it was assumed that about 50 child care workers would be interested in taking part in the study.

On the basis of this number of evaluable cases, it was postulated that the outcome parameter of mean subjective noise exposure would exhibit the necessary normal distribution. With an assumed difference in the means of 2 points before and after the intervention, with a standard deviation of 5 points and an alpha of 5 %, the power of 80 % was calculated.

Statistical analysis

The difference in the means for the comparison before and after the intervention was calculated with the *t* test for dependent samples, for not normally distributed and dependent data the Wilcoxon signed-rank test was used. Group comparisons were based on the *t* test for independent samples. Analysis of variance (ANOVA) and multivariate linear regression were used to test potential factors for the differences in the means of the outcome variables - subjective noise exposure and burnout risk (T2-T0), all analyses were performed on the individual level. The following factors were measured at T0 and were considered as factors potentially influencing the outcome variable *subjective noise exposure*: *work-related resources, everyday situations at work, effort reward imbalance, overcommitment, physical stress, weekly working hours, type of institution, physical exercise,* and time of *wearing MHPs*. To characterize the cohort demographic variables like age, gender and BMI were assessed too. For the analysis of the outcome variable *burnout risk*, the additional variable *subjective noise exposure* was investigated as a covariate. Independent variables with a level of significance of $p > 0.2$ in the bivariate analysis were excluded from the analyses. In addition, a drop-out analysis with all variables was performed by logistic regression. If there were statistically significant predictors, these were included as covariates in the linear model. Level of significance was set to two-tailed $p < 0.05$. Statistical analysis was performed with the program SPSS Version 22.

Results

After the follow-up period of 12 months, questionnaires had been received from 33 subjects (follow-up rate: 73 %). Table 1 describes the demographic characteristics of the cohort at time T0. Most subjects were women (91 %). The largest age group consisted of subjects between 40 and 50 years old (38 %). 40 % had a BMI of over 25 and 56 % were regularly engaged in sporting activities. At that point in time, 40 % were working fulltime; most worked in child day care centres.

Figure 2 shows the cumulative wearing time in hours; there were no entries for 6 persons in the diaries. The median of the cumulative wearing time was 34.6 h (range: 0–326). The median cumulative number of days on which the MHPs were worn was 25 days (range 0–174 days).

There were no statistically significant differences between the intervention and reference group with respect to the demographic and all other independent variables e.g. effort reward imbalance. Among the outcome variables, only the difference of the baseline values in subjective noise exposure was statistically significant ($p = 0.004$). Table 2 shows the changes in the outcome variables for the two groups. In the intervention group, mean subjective noise exposure increased from 44.5 to 45.7 points over time (reference group: from 38.1 to 39.7). The difference in subjective noise exposure was greater in the reference group than in the intervention group ($\Delta = 1.6$ vs. 1.2). The difference in the development of subjective noise exposure between the two groups was not statistically significant. In

Table 1 Demographic characteristics of the subjects

Variable	N	Percentage
Gender		
Women	41	91.1 %
Men	4	8.9 %
Age in years		
18 to <30	9	20 %
30 to <40	12	26.7 %
40 to <50	17	37.8 %
50+	7	15.6 %
Nationality		
German	43	95.6 %
Other	2	4.4 %
BMI		
< 25	25	55.6 %
≥ 25	18	40 %
Missing	2	4.4 %
Physical exercise		
Regularly	25	55.6 %
None	20	44.4 %
Weekly working hours		
Fulltime	18	40 %
Part time	27	60 %
Institution		
Child day care centre	36	80 %
School partnership	9	20 %
Support for children and adolescents	0	0 %
Total	45	100 %

the intervention group, the burnout risk increased from 55.2 to 57.7 ($\Delta = 2.5$) points. The increase in the reference group was greater - from 50.6 to 54.5 points ($\Delta = 3.9$). None of the differences between the groups was statistically significant.

Table 3 shows the means of the outcome variables subjective noise exposure and burnout risk for the institutions with or without a recommendation for improvements in room acoustics. For subjective noise exposure at time T0, there was a small difference between the two groups (45.8 vs. 42.2, $\Delta = 3.6$). The difference was slightly greater on follow-up (47.7 vs. 42.8, $\Delta = 4.9$). After 12 months, the difference (Δ T2-T0) for participants from institutions with recommendation was greater than for the other group ($\Delta = 1.9$ vs. 0.7) but statistically not significant. The differences in burnout risk were greater: at time point T0 (59.2 vs. 48.3), the difference was 10.9 and, at time point T2 (60.8 vs. 52.1), the difference was 8.7 points on the burnout scale. At time point T2 the differences in burnout risk (Δ T2-T0) for

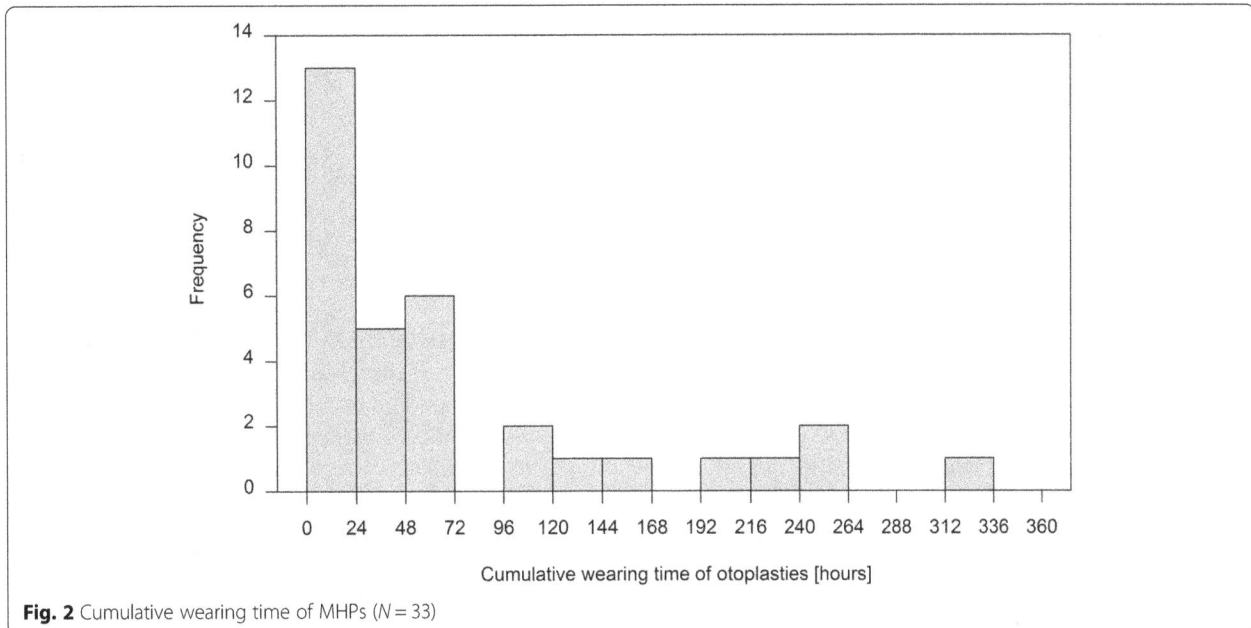

Fig. 2 Cumulative wearing time of MHPs (N = 33)

workers from institutions without a recommendation was more than double high than for the comparison group (Δ = 3.8 vs. 1.6) However, none of these differences was statistically significant.

Multivariate analysis demonstrated that the feature *Breaks and possibilities for recovery are missing* had a significant effect on subjective noise exposure (B = 5.7, $p = 0.013$) (Table 4). According to this, the effect on subjective noise exposure for this subgroup became even less favourable over time. All other potential factors exhibited no significant effects and were therefore excluded from the model. No statistically significant effects on burnout were identified.

Figure 3 shows the information on the satisfaction of the study subjects with wearing MHPs at just over the half of the observation period (T1) and at the end of the period (T2). Satisfaction tended to decrease over time. For example, the fraction of those who found it unpleasant to wear hearing protection in the presence of parents rose from 18 to 35 %. The fraction of those who thought

it was reasonable to wear MHPs sank from 69 to 47 %. The fraction of those who experienced relaxation after work remained constant over time (48 %). The fraction of subjects who missed information slightly improved over time - from 27 to 23 %. Almost three quarter of study subjects (72 %) thought that they could fulfil their teaching duties at time point T1. At time point T2 this value decreased to 67 %. None of these changes over time in the dichotomous variables was statistically significant.

Table 5 describes the distribution of study subjects over the 16 different institutions at T0 and T2. The number of subjects at T0 was between one and seven employees per institution. At time point T2, there was no longer any subject from two of the institutions. The number per institution varied between 1 and 5 persons.

Reverberation times were measured between one and a maximum of four rooms in the different institutions (Table 5). No improvements in the room acoustics were evaluated in 6 institutions, as indicated by the reverberation time measurements and other room characteristics.

Table 2 Description of the outcome variables in the intervention and reference groups

	Intervention group (N = 33)*			Reference group (N = 61)*		
	T0	T2	p	T0	T2	p
Subjective Noise Exposure	44.5 (8.8)	45.7 (7.9)	0.30	38.1 (10.3)	39.7 (10.5)	0.08
Δ Subjective Noise Exposure T2-T0	1.2 (7.4)		NA	1.6 (6.8)		0.80
Burnout Risk Scale	55.2 (19.4)	57.7 (17.7)	0.40	50.6 (19.7)	54.5 (22.1)	0.05
Δ Burnout Risk Scale T2-T0	2.5 (18.3)		NA	3.9 (15.3)		0.70
Burnout Risk Scale ≥ 50	66.7 %	72.7 %	0.62	54.1 %	62.3 %	0.22

*given values are means (standard deviations), rates and p-values

Table 3 Outcome variables for subjects in institutions with or without a recommendation for improvement in room acoustics

| | Acoustic improvements recommended? Yes ($N = 20$), No ($N = 12$) | | | | | |
| | Subjective Noise Exposure* | | | Burnout Risk Scale* | | |
	Yes	No	p	Yes	No	p
T0	45.8 (9.3)	42.2 (8.2)	0.26	59.2 (19.9)	48.3 (19.8)	0.13
T2	47.7 (7.2)	42.8 (8.8)	0.12	60.8 (19.6)	52.1 (14.1)	0.15
Δ T2-T0	1.9 (8.2)	0.7 (7.6)	0.67	1.6 (20.7)	3.8 (15.4)	0.75

*given values are means (standard deviations) and p-values

For the other institutions, improvements in room acoustics were recommended for at least one room. In one institution, no measurement could be performed for organisational reasons. The target values for reverberation times depend on the functions and sizes of the rooms; these values were exceeded in 29/39 measurements (74 %).

Discussion

When child care workers used MHPs in the present setting, their subjective noise exposure and risk of burnout was not reduced over the period of observation.

It was also observed that most of the subjects did not consider it to be very reasonable to wear MHPs and that this reduced their ability to fulfil their teaching duties over time.

As regards the room acoustics, improvements in room acoustics were recommended for more than half of the institutions on the basis of the measured reverberation times and the structural properties of the rooms.

Limitations

This study is a scientific investigation of the effect of MHPs. On the other hand, it is also a preventive measure in occupational medicine, which is intended to be available to all employees. In contrast to a classical RCT, this study was performed without a control group or randomisation and without monitoring of other conditions. As a post-hoc analysis the reference group was included to show to what extent the study was performed under changing overall conditions. As the burnout risk was even greater in the reference group, it is clear that there were uncontrolled factors that influenced these outcome variables in both groups. As the threshold for inclusion was low, it can also be assumed that the group was relatively heterogeneous. At the start of the study, the subjects were not subjected to audiometric controls with respect to, for example, hardness of hearing, tinnitus or ear noises, so

that the status of their hearing is unknown. Thus, it remains possible that their hearing was heterogeneous. This has the advantage that an occupational preventive measure should be open to as many employees as possible.

A failure of unknown reason in the implementation of the intervention conclusively led to little cumulative wearing time. Consequently it was statistically unlikely to detect any potential dose–response relationship between the wearing time and outcome variables. Qualitative interviews, that could have shed light upon the reasons for the failed implementation of the intervention, were not performed in this pilot study. Because of the size of the sample and the follow-up rate of 73 %, it was hardly possible to demonstrate statistically significant effects; the expected power of 0.80 was not reached in this study, apart from the unforeseen development of the outcome variables. This also applied to the drop-out analysis. This did not allow any conclusion as to whether there was no selection bias, or whether the low number of participants prevented the demonstration of statistically significant variables. Moreover, the non-responders survey (3 of 12 questionnaires returned) did not permit any reliable conclusion about the reasons for non-participation either.

Measurements of sound pressure would have provided an objective estimate of noise exposure, and there are already reference values from German kindergartens. These measurements - including audiometry - had originally been planned for the start of the study. However, they were postponed for organisational reasons and would finally have had to be carried out a long time after the end of the observational period. We therefore eventually decided to dispense with these measurements.

Intervention

The entry of the wearing times in the diary is intended to be a sort of quality assurance for the intervention. For 6 persons (18 %), there were no entries in the diaries for

Table 4 Results of multivariate linear regression ($N = 32$), adjusted for subjective noise exposure at time point T0

| Dependent variable: Difference in subjective noise exposure T2-T0 | | | |
Factor	Effect	95 % CI	P
Breaks and possibilities for recovery are missing (1 = yes, 0 no)	5.7	1.29–10.13	0.013
	$R^2 = 0.42$		

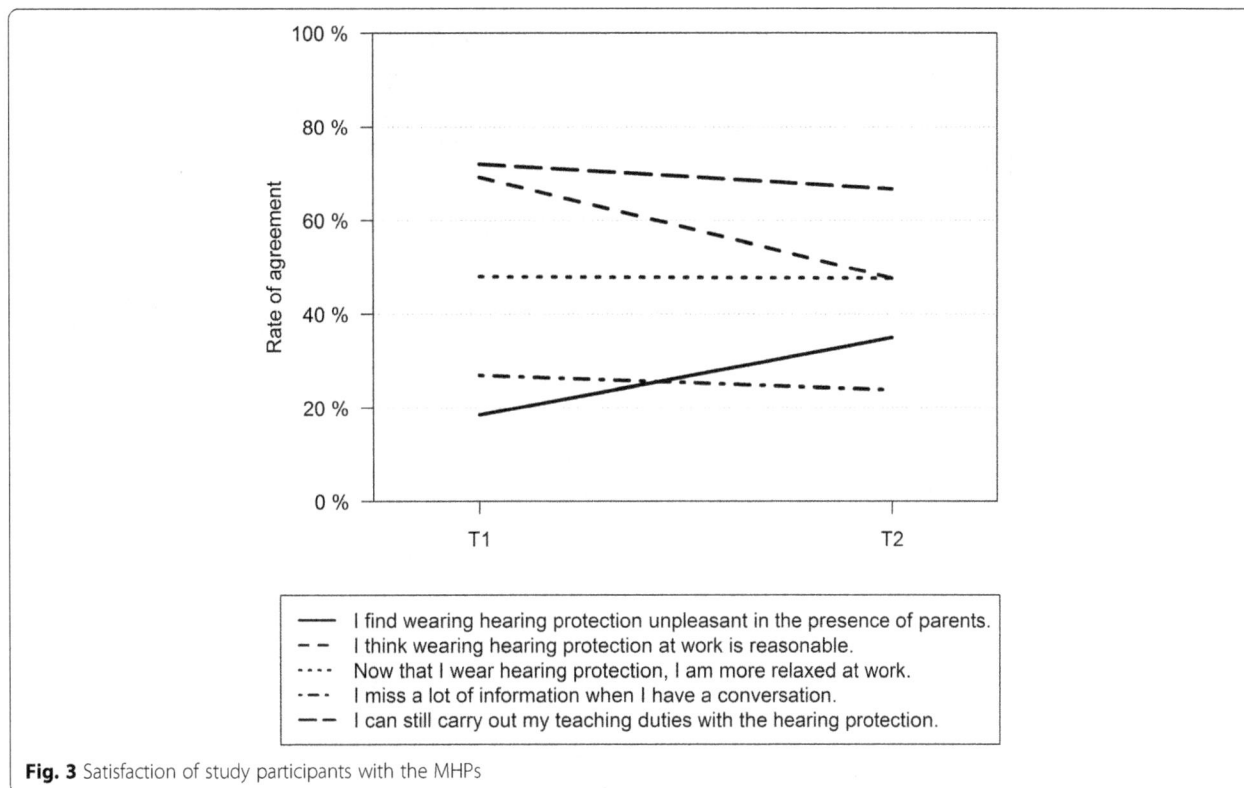

Fig. 3 Satisfaction of study participants with the MHPs

The chart legend:
- — I find wearing hearing protection unpleasant in the presence of parents.
- – – I think wearing hearing protection at work is reasonable.
- · · · · Now that I wear hearing protection, I am more relaxed at work.
- · – · I miss a lot of information when I have a conversation.
- – – I can still carry out my teaching duties with the hearing protection.

Table 5 Overview of room acoustic measurements

Institutions		Participants		Mean reverberation time in seconds (T0): (actual) (target)	Room acoustic improvements recommended by the room acoustics expert
		T0 (N)	T2 (N)		
Child day care centres	C_1	2	2	**0.48** (0.50)	No
	C_2	3	1	**0.46** (0.40), **0.47** (0.40), **0.73** (0.50)	Yes
	C_3	3	3	**0.60** (0.50), **0.45** (0.40), **0.60** (0.40)	No
	C_4	1	0	**0.48** (0.50), **0.60** (0.45), **0.50** (0.40)	No
	C_5	3	2	**0.38** (0.45)	No
	C_6	3	2	**0.48** (0.40), **0.56** (0.50)	Yes
	C_7	3	3	**0.35** (0.40), **0.44** (0.50)	Yes
	C_8	5	4	**0.64** (0.55), **0.49** (0.40), **0.37** (0.40), **0.58** (0.50)	Yes
	C_9	7	5	**0.70** (0.55), **0.54** (0.50), **0.61** (0.50)	Yes
	C_{10}	2	1	**0.53** (0.40), **0.45** (0.40), **0.89** (0.50)	Yes
	C_{11}	4	4	**0.42** (0.50)	No
School partnerships	S_1	1	1	**0.57** (0.55), **0.66** (0.55)	No
	S_2	3	2	**0.47** (0.50), **0.60** (0.50), **0.69** (0.50), **0.73** (0.80)	Yes
	S_3	2	0	**0.85** (0.65), **0.88** (0.65), **0.50** (0.50)	Yes
	S_4	2	2	**0.64** (0.60), **0.82** (0.60), **0.57** (0.50), **0.97** (0.70)	Yes
	S_5	1	1	No measurements	No information

Bold: actual, not bold: target

the wearing times, i.e. it was not known whether these persons had actually worn the MHPs. In accordance with the *intention to treat* principle, these persons were included in the analysis. With the median cumulative wearing time of 34.6 h over 12 months and full employment (224 working days in 2015), this corresponds to a mean daily wearing time of maximally 9 min for half of the participants. As there are no other studies on this type of intervention, there are no reference values and it is difficult to assess whether this is an effective period of time with respect to noise exposure. In the initial workshop, it was emphasised that the participants should wear MHPs at times of peak noise. If time dependent measurements of sound pressure had been performed in the different institutions over the shifts, it might have been possible to relate these to the wearing times. On the other hand, if you consider the statements on satisfaction with MHPs (teaching duties, reasonableness, relaxation effect etc.), it seems more likely that in a substantial number of cases the MHPs were not worn much, because they were disturbing at work.

Comparison with the reference group makes it clear that, at baseline, the intervention group exhibited higher values for both noise exposure and burnout. Especially the difference in subjective noise exposure indicates self-selection of the intervention group. In both groups, burnout risk increased over time. The mean burnout risk and the prevalence in the intervention group (T2: 57.7 and 72.7 %, respectively) appear to be comparatively high. The 2013 COPSOQ database gives a mean reference value of 48 for German child care workers (data in Supporting Information); Buch and Frieling give a burnout prevalence of 30 % [1]. The increase in the burnout risk was smaller in the intervention group, which might indicate that the intervention had a favourable alleviating effect. No factors which might have influenced the intervention effect could be identified in the multivariate analyses. In contrast, it was observed that changes in noise exposure over time were less favourable for subjects who stated in the questionnaire that breaks and possibilities for recovery were missing; thus, the increase in the mean noise exposure values was 5.7 points greater for these persons.

The room acoustic evaluation, including measurements of reverberation time, showed that improvements were possible in 9 of 15 institutions. In some cases, the reverberation times were too high, but in other cases the room acoustics could be improved even though the reverberation times were moderate. Possible problems include wrongly mounted shock absorber elements, missing impact sound insulation, metal doors or too many window surfaces. These assessments make it clear that room acoustics may be suboptimal even when the reverberation times are moderate in accordance with the DIN standard. It was striking - albeit not statistically significant - that employees from institutions where the room acoustics could be improved exhibited higher values of the outcome variables - particularly burnout risk - at both time points. Specific improvements, particularly in these institutions, would therefore benefit the group of employees under the greatest stress. Studies have shown that improvements in room acoustics in schools can reduce reverberation times and, in some cases, also subjective noise exposure [8, 11, 15]. The use of special toy containers can also bring a major reduction in the level of sound pressure [31]. Aside from structural changes, noise exposure can also be reduced at the organisational level. This includes the use of recovery rooms, noise warning lights, light regulation, teaching that increases sensitivity to noise and speech training for child care workers. However, Sjödin et al. have shown that organisational measures are less effective than room acoustic measures, as they require more work [11].

In summary, this study was based on an idea that was initiated by stressed employees and which was implemented as a behavioural preventive measure with scientific support. Due to this frame several characteristics like lack of randomization and control, use of post-hoc reference group, missing compliance in the intervention group and underpowered conditions limit the validity in this study. Further studies should be also designed in a mixed method approach with additional qualitative research. Overall the results suggest that, in this specific setting, wearing MHPs is not an appropriate occupational measure and therefore could not be effectively implemented. In this context it seems that prevention by technical engineering might be more important than the use of personal protective equipment. Qualitative interviews would have been able to identify the reasons for the lack of compliance here more precisely. In contrast to employees in industry, child care workers are exposed to informative noise that has to be heard and which accordingly includes a high level of potential stress. Perhaps the employees' feelings of responsibility to the children prevented them from wearing the MHPs regularly.

The structural causes of the noise exposure and possibly also burnout risk in this group are presumably inadequate numbers of employees, excessively large groups and, especially, too few trained child care workers [7]. These issues have long been discussed by politicians with expertise in employment and could only be modified at another level. In general, the motivation for this study was typical of the overall conditions for child care workers in Germany, with unfavourable ratios of children to child care workers and lack of expert staff.

Conclusion

The use of MHPs by child care workers in child day care centres is not an appropriate measure to prevent noise exposure if it is widely employed. For groups of employees with specific problems such as hyperacusis after acute hearing loss further studies are needed. Within the institutions, a careful analysis should be performed of the room acoustics, followed by modification as necessary. In addition, organisational measures e.g. noise education for children should be implemented that have a favourable effect on the initiation and development of noise and its effects on health.

Acknowledgements
We thank Dr. Matthias Nübling for assistance with unpublished data of the Copenhagen Psychosocial Questionnaire (COPSOQ) database.

Funding
The study was funded by the German Institution for Statutory Accident Insurance and Prevention in the Health and Welfare Services (BGW).

Authors' contributions
PK, performed the survey, carried out the statistical analyses and wrote the manuscript. JS read the draft critically and gave substantial comments for the improvement of the first draft. JFK supported the statistical analysis and supported the writing process. AN revised the manuscript critically for important intellectual content and gave final approval for the version to be published. All authors read and approved the final manuscript.

Competing interests
The authors declare that they have no competing interests.

Author details
[1]Centre of Excellence for Epidemiology and Health Services Research for Healthcare Professionals (CVcare), University Medical Centre Hamburg-Eppendorf, Martinistraße 52, Hamburg 20246, Germany. [2]Health Protection Division (FBG), Institution for Statutory Accident Insurance and Prevention in the Health and Welfare Services (BGW), Pappelallee 33, Hamburg 22089, Germany.

References
1. Buch M, Frieling E. Belastungs- und Beanspruchungsoptimierung in Kindertagesstätten. Kassel: Eigenverlag Universität Kassel, Institut für Arbeitswissenschaft; 2001.
2. Eysel-Gosepath K, Pape HG, Erren T, Thinschmidt M, Lehmacher W, Piekarski C. Sound levels in nursery schools. HNO. 2010;58:1013–20.
3. Paulsen R. Noise Exposure in Kindergartens. In CFA/DAGA'04 30 Jahrestagung für Akustik - Europäische Akustik-Ausstellung Akustik DGf ed., vol. I. pp. 573–574. Straßburg; 2004:573–574.
4. Sjodin F, Kjellberg A, Knutsson A, Landstrom U, Lindberg L. Noise and stress effects on preschool personnel. Noise Health. 2012;14:166–78.
5. Neitzel RL, Svensson EB, Sayler SK, Ann-Christin J. A comparison of occupational and nonoccupational noise exposures in Sweden. Noise Health. 2014;16:270–8.
6. Losch D. Lärm als Stressor in der Kindertagesstätte. Zentralblatt für Arbeitsmedizin, Arbeitsschutz und Ergonomie. 2016;66:20–8.
7. Koch P, Stranzinger J, Nienhaus A, Kozak A. Musculoskeletal Symptoms and Risk of Burnout in Child Care Workers - A Cross-Sectional Study. PLoS One. 2015;10:e0140980.
8. Truchnon-Gagnon C, Hetu R. Noise in Day-care centers for children. Noise Control Eng J. 1988;30:57–64.
9. Jungbauer J, Ehlen S. Stress and burnout risk in nursery school teachers: results from a survey. Gesundheitswesen. 2015;77:418–23.
10. Sjodin F, Kjellberg A, Knutsson A, Landstrom U, Lindberg L. Noise exposure and auditory effects on preschool personnel. Noise Health. 2012;14:72–82.
11. Sjodin F, Kjellberg A, Knutsson A, Landstrom U, Lindberg L. Measures against preschool noise and its adverse effects on the personnel: an intervention study. Int Arch Occup Environ Health. 2014;87:95–110.
12. Sodersten M, Granqvist S, Hammarberg B, Szabo A. Vocal behavior and vocal loading factors for preschool teachers at work studied with binaural DAT recordings. J Voice. 2002;16:356–71.
13. Niemitalo-Haapola E, Haapala S, Jansson-Verkasalo E, Kujala T. Background Noise Degrades Central Auditory Processing in Toddlers. Ear Hear. 2015;36:e342–51.
14. Maxwell LE, Evans GW. The effects of noise on preschool Chidren's Pre-readiing skills. Journal of Environmental Psychology. 2000;20:91–7.
15. Gerhardsson L, Nilsson E. Noise disturbances in daycare centers before and after acoustical treatment. J Environ Health. 2013;75:36–40.
16. European Union. Richtlinie 2003/10/EG des europäischen Parlaments und des Rates vom 6. Februar 2003 über Mindestvorschriften zum Schutz von Sicherheit und Gesundheit der Arbeitnehmer vor der Gefährdung durch physikalische Einwirkungen (Lärm). 2003. http://eur-lex.europa.eu/legal-content/DE/TXT/PDF/?uri=CELEX:32003L0010&rid=3 Accessed 20 Jun 2016.
17. The Federal Ministry of Justice, Germany. Verordnung zum Schutz der Beschäftigten vor Gefährdungen durch Lärm und Vibrationen. http://www.gesetze-im-internet.de/l_rmvibrationsarbschv/. Accessed 20 Jun 2016.
18. Berg RL, Pickett W, Fitz-Randolph M, Broste SK, Knobloch MJ, Wood DJ, Kirkhorn SR, Linneman JG, Marlenga B. Hearing conservation program for agricultural students: short-term outcomes from a cluster-randomized trial with planned long-term follow-up. Prev Med. 2009;49:546–52.
19. Brink LL, Talbott EO, Burks JA, Palmer CV. Changes over time in audiometric thresholds in a group of automobile stamping and assembly workers with a hearing conservation program. AIHA J. 2002;63:482–7.
20. Erlandsson B, Hakanson H, Ivarsson A, Nilsson P. The difference in protection efficiency between earplugs and earmuffs. An investigation performed at a workplace. Scand Audiol. 1980;9:215–21.
21. Heyer N, Morata TC, Pinkerton LE, Brueck SE, Stancescu D, Panaccio MP, Kim H, Sinclair JS, Waters MA, Estill CF, Franks JR. Use of historical data and a novel metric in the evaluation of the effectiveness of hearing conservation program components. Occup Environ Med. 2011;68:510–7.
22. Verbeek JH, Kateman E, Morata TC, Dreschler WA, Mischke C. Interventions to prevent occupational noise-induced hearing loss: a Cochrane systematic review. Int J Audiol. 2014;53 Suppl 2:S84–96.
23. Siegrist J. Adverse health effects of high-effort/low-reward conditions. J Occup Health Psychol. 1996;1:27–41.
24. Slesina W. FEBA: Fragebogen zur subjektiven Einschätzung der Belastungen am Arbeitsplatz. 2009 http://www.rueckenkompass.de/download_files/doc/Fragen-Slesina.pdf Accessed 20 Jun 2016.
25. Prümper J, Hartmannsgruber K, Frese M. KFZA - Kurzfragebogen zur Arbeitsanalyse. Zeitschrift für Arbeits- und Organisationspsychologie. 1995;39:125–32.
26. Niedhammer I, Siegrist J, Landre MF, Goldberg M, Leclerc A. Psychometric properties of the French version of the Effort-Reward Imbalance model. Rev Epidemiol Sante Publique. 2000;48:419–37.
27. Tsutsumi A, Ishitake T, Peter R, Siegrist J, Matoba T. The Japanese version of the effort-reward imbalance questionnaire: a study in dental technicians. Work & Stress. 2001;15:86–96.
28. Kristensen TS, Hannerz H, Hogh A, Borg V. The Copenhagen psychosocial questionnaire-a tool for the assessment and improvement of the psychosocial work environment. Scand J Work Environ Health. 2005;31:438–49.
29. Nübling M, Stößel U, Hasselhorn H-M, Michaelis M, Hofmann F. Measuring psychological stress and strain at work: Evaluation of the COPSOQ Questionnaire in Germany. GMS Psycho-Social-Medicine. 2006;3:1–14.
30. German Institute for Standardization. DIN 18041:2015–02 Hörsamkeit in Räumen- Vorgaben und Hinweise für die Planung. Beuth; 2015.

5

Hydrofluoric acid burns in the western Zhejiang Province of China: a 10-year epidemiological study

Yuanhai Zhang[1], Jianfen Zhang[1], Xinhua Jiang[1], Liangfang Ni[1], Chunjiang Ye[1], Chunmao Han[2], Komal Sharma[3] and Xingang Wang[2*]

Abstract

Background: Chemical burns caused by hydrofluoric acid (HF) frequently occur in the Western Zhejiang Province. This study aimed to investigate the epidemiological characteristics of HF burns within this region.

Methods: A 10-year retrospective analysis was conducted using data from all inpatients with HF burns. These patients were treated at the Department of Burns and Plastic Surgery at our hospital between January 2004 and December 2013. Information obtained for each patient included sex, age, occupation, burn location, burn cause, and the hazard category of the chemical which caused the burn. Data regarding wound site and size, accompanying injuries, serum electrolyte levels, operations, length of hospital stay, and mortality were also assessed.

Results: A total of 201 patients (189 males, 12 females; average age: 38.33 ± 10.57 years) were admitted due to HF burns. Over the 10-year period, the morbidity of HF burns in the past 10 years showed a gradual increase, which paralleled the development of local fluoride industries. Most HF injuries were work related and distributed in working-age patients. Aqueous HF solutions, especially highly concentrated ones, were the most common chemical cause of HF burns. Moreover, inappropriate operation, machine problems, and inadequate protection were identified as the leading causes of HF burns in the workplace. The burn area was <5% of TBSA in more than 90% of patients, and the most common burn sites were the head, neck, and upper extremities. Approximately 17% of patients underwent surgical operation. Accompanying injuries should be detected and treated correctly in a timely manner. Lastly, electrolyte imbalances, such as hypocalcaemia, hypomagnesaemia, and hypokalaemia, occurred frequently in patients with HF exposure; however, hyperkalaemia was not encountered in this study.

Conclusion: Based on the epidemiological results for HF burns in this region, the related enterprises and local authorities should be encouraged to upgrade management policies and to provide necessary occupational hazard education and safety training for high-risk occupations within high-risk working populations. Furthermore, the enhancement of hazardous chemicals management is also needed. Finally, for patients with HF exposure, early and correct pre-hospital triage, treatment and consequent in-hospital treatment and procedures should also be improved.

Background

Hydrofluoric acid (HF), an important industrial material, is used widely in chemical industries including: electronics manufacturing, glass etching, smelting, cleaning, and other industrial fields [1–3]. HF is very dangerous chemical, not only causing local tissue corrosion, but also systemic poisoning by ongoing absorption into the human body. Previous studies have shown that HF burns over small areas can even result in death [4, 5]. In some regions throughout the world, HF has been listed as the top cause of chemical burns [6, 7]. Our previous research investigated the epidemiological features of chemical burns occurring in Zhejiang Province between September 2008 and August 2009, where results showed that HF was the leading cause of chemical burns (27.4%, 135/492 patients) within the research population [8]. Thus, the hazard behind direct exposure to HF can be contributed towards the industrial structure of this region.

* Correspondence: wangxingang8157@zju.edu.cn
[2]Department of Burns & Wound Care Center, Second Affiliated Hospital of Zhejiang University College of Medicine, Hangzhou 310009, China
Full list of author information is available at the end of the article

Zhejiang Province, located in south-eastern China, is famous for its thriving chemical industries. By using its rich resources of fluorite, HF can be produced when reacted with concentrated sulphuric acid [9]. This region in China has therefore become the largest industrial producer of fluoride, with an annual HF output of 400,000 tons [10]. With this rapid development of fluoride industries and high turnover of chemical usage within the Zhejiang region, the incidence of chemical burns has increased dramatically. Events with severe casualties caused by HF have been reported [11, 12].

To clarify the epidemiological characteristics of chemical burns in western Zhejiang Province, a 10-year retrospective analysis was conducted. The analysis included data from patients with chemical burns admitted to our hospital's department of Burns and Plastic Surgery between January 2004 and December 2013. Preliminary results showed that the morbidity rate of chemical burns was as high as 18.6% (690 cases), and HF remained the leading cause of chemical injuries (201 cases, 29.13%) in this period and amongst the cases that were seen [10]. In this study, we further analysed the epidemiological features of the 201 inpatients with HF burns, with the aim of providing further evidence to support the upgrade of safety measurements and the formulation of preventive strategies within the Zhejiang Province.

Methods

A 10-year retrospective analysis including all patients with HF burns admitted to the Department of Burns and Plastic Surgery between January 2004 and December 2013 was conducted. Information obtained for each patient included sex, age, occupation, location of burn, cause of burn, and the category of chemical that caused the burn. Data regarding wound site and size, accompanying injuries, serum electrolyte levels, operations, length of hospital stay, and mortality were also assessed. All of the data mentioned above were collected and rechecked by two medical staff. The data recorded in the Excel form were further analysed by the statistician.

Results

Trends of HF burns

Figure 1 shows the number of patients admitted each year due to HF burns. It can be seen that the incidence of cases increased gradually over the 10-year period, although a slight fluctuation in this trend was observed in 2006. The overall number of patients with HF exposure has however, increased rapidly, especially in the recent years.

Age, sex, and education

Among the 201 patients, 189 were male and 12 were female (ratios of 15.75:1). The average age was 38.33 ±

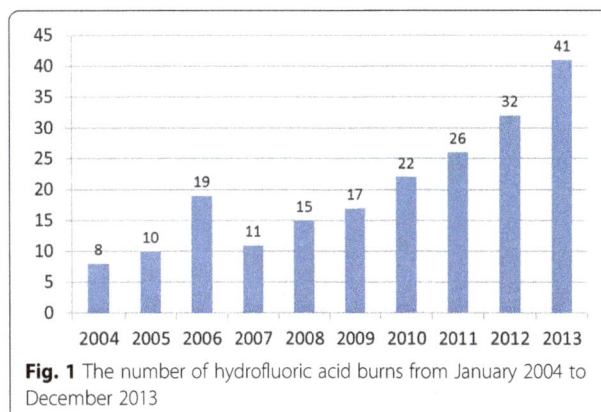

Fig. 1 The number of hydrofluoric acid burns from January 2004 to December 2013

10.57 years, with a range of 1.5–69 years. HF burns occurred most frequently in patients aged 30–39 years (33.83%), followed by those aged 40–49 years (32.84%), 20–29 years (17.41%), and 50–59 years (11.44%; Table 1).

Figure 2 shows the education levels of these patients. The majority of patients had low levels of education (illiteracy/primary school education, 21.39%; junior middle school education, 48.26%), 27.86% of patients had completed middle school / high school, and only 2.49% had tertiary education of college/university degrees or higher.

Sources of patients and causes of HF burns

Out of all the cases presented in our department, the most frequent source of HF burns was seen as work related (Table 2). More than half (109 cases, 54.23%) of these patients worked in the fluorine industry; followed by stevedoring and transportation industries (35 cases, 17.41%); the semiconductor industry (18 cases, 8.96%); metal rust removal industries (13 cases, 6.47%); glass etching industries (12 cases, 5.97%), and finally followed by waste and disposal service sectors (8 cases, 3.98%), and other sectors and industries (6 cases, 2.98%).

Furthermore, more than 95% of HF burns in this study were due to three major causes: (i) inappropriate operation (89 cases, 44.28%), (ii) inadequate protection (58 cases, 28.86%), and (iii) machine problems (44 cases,

Table 1 The age distribution of patients with HF burns

Age (Years)	Csaes	
	N	Percent (%)
<10	2	0.99
10 ~ 19	4	1.99
20 ~ 29	35	17.41
30 ~ 39	68	33.83
40 ~ 49	66	32.83
50 ~ 59	23	11.44
>60	3	1.49

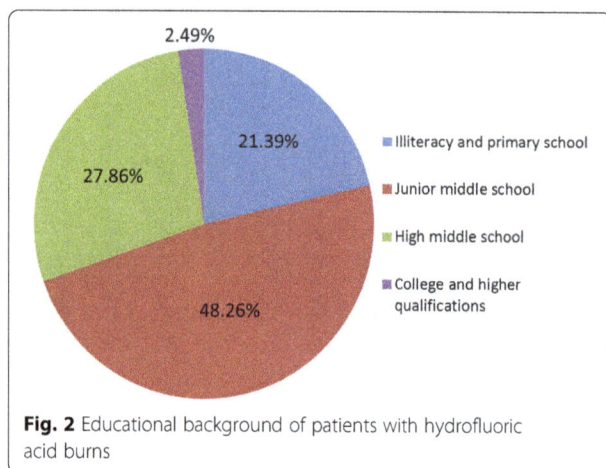

Fig. 2 Educational background of patients with hydrofluoric acid burns

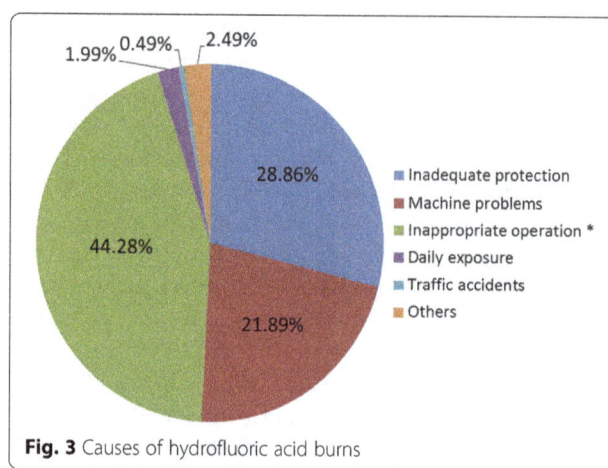

Fig. 3 Causes of hydrofluoric acid burns

21.89%). Less than 5% of cases were caused by daily exposure, traffic accidents, or other reasons (Fig. 3).

Table 3 presents the categories of chemicals that caused HF burns. The majority (177 cases, 88.06%) of HF injuries were caused by aqueous HF solutions, followed by mixtures containing HF (18 cases, 8.96%). Chemical burns caused by hydrogen fluoride accounted for the least (2.98%) of these injuries.

The concentrations of HF in the various solutions were analysed further; where the results are presented in Table 4. Aside from the 72 cases caused by unknown concentrations, high-concentration (>50%) solutions caused the majority (66 cases, 32.84%) of HF burns, followed by solutions with moderate (41 cases, 20.4%) and low (16 cases, 7.96%) concentrations of HF.

Sites and extent of HF burns
HF burns were observed at a total of 265 sites among the 201 patients (Fig. 2). The most common sites of injury were the head and neck (99 cases, 37.36%), hands (71 cases, 26.79%), legs (36 cases, 13.59%), arms (28 cases, 10.57%), foot (19 cases, 7.17%, trunk (9 cases, 3.40%), and buttocks (3 cases, 1.13%); Fig. 4).

Burn areas were calculated by estimating the sizes of first, second, and third degree burns. Table 5 shows the

burn area distribution for these patients. In all patients, burns covered <1 to 42% of the total body surface area (TBSA). One hundred and twenty-one (60.20%) patients had burns covering <1% of the TBSA, and 61 (30.35%) patients had burns covering 1–5% of the TBSA. Only 19 (9.45%) cases had burn areas of >5% TBSA.

Accompanying injuries
Injuries accompanying HF burns included ocular injuries (17 cases, 8.46%), inhalation injuries (9 cases, 4.48%), and digestive tract injuries (1 case, 0.50%).

Seasonal distribution
HF burns occurred more frequently in the summer (28.44%), autumn (26.15%), and winter seasons (25.69%) than in the spring season (19.72%; Fig. 5).

Pre-hospital treatment
In nearly 88% of cases, on-site water irrigation was immediately performed after HF burns had occurred. Amongst these cases, there were 8 patients who received immediate washing of their chemical burns by health professionals: First with Hexafluorine® solution,

Table 2 Sources of patients with HF burns

Sources	Cases	
	N	Percent (%)
Fluorine industry	109	54.23
Stevedoring and transportation	35	17.41
Semiconductor industry	18	8.96
Metal rust removing	13	6.47
Glass etching	12	5.97
Waste and disposable service	8	3.98
Others	6	2.98

Table 3 Categories of chemicals causing HF burns

Chemicals	Cases	
	N	Percent (%)
Hydrogen fluoride	6	2.98
HF solution	177	88.06
Mixture		
HF+ sulphuric acid (H_2SO_4)	10	4.98
HF+ hydrochloric acid (HCl)	2	0.99
HF + dimethylamine	1	0.49
HF + Trichloroethylene	1	0.49
HF + pentafluoropropanol	1	0.49
HF+ unknown chemicals	3	1.49

Table 4 Distribution of HF concentration

HF concentration (%)	Cases	
	N	Percent (%)
<20	16	7.96
20 ~ 50	41	20.40
>50	66	32.84
Unknown	72	35.82
Hydrogen fluoride	6	2.98

Table 5 TBSA distribution for patients with HF burns

TBSA[a] (%)	Cases	
	N	Percent (%)
<1	121	60.2
1–5	61	30.35
6–10	9	4.48
11–20	4	1.99
21–30	3	1.49
31–40	1	0.49
>40	2	0.99

[a]Calculation of TBSA refers to all the burned area involved, including the first, second and third degrees

followed by tap water. However, for all of the patients who received water irrigation treatment, the rinsing time varied greatly (Fig. 6).

Serum electrolyte levels

Results of electrolyte tests conducted within 3 days after exposure were analysed. The morbidity rates of hypocalcaemia, hypomagnesaemia, hypokalaemia, and hyperkalaemia were calculated and are listed in Table 6. Hypocalcaemia (47 cases, 23.38%) and hypomagnesaemia (28 cases, 13.93%) occurred more frequently in patients with HF burns. Only 18 (8.96%) patients had hypokalaemia, and no patient had hyperkalaemia.

Number of operations

Thirty-five (17.41%) patients underwent surgical operations. Among these, 9 cases were treated with urgent escharotomy and skin grafting. 7 cases were treated with flap transfers for wound reconstruction, and 11 cases were treated with split-thickness skin grafting for wound closure.

Length of hospital stay

The average hospital stay was 8.9 ± 10.7 days, with a range of 1–50 days (Table 7).

Mortality

Two patients died of sudden cardiac arrest caused by severe fluoride poisoning. The overall mortality rate for HF burns in this study was approximately 1%.

Discussion

The morbidity of HF burns varies among regions throughout the world [13]. In some areas, HF burns occur more frequently and have become one of the most common chemical injuries [8, 10]. Our study demonstrated an increased incidence of HF burns in western Zhejiang Province between 2004 and 2013, although a small surge was also observed in 2006 (Fig. 1). HF industries and derivatives have shown explosive growth in the past decade and play a vital role in the local economy. Consequently, the incidence of chemical burns, especially those caused by HF, has increased [10, 14, 15].

As observed in this study, the majority of chemical burns were work related, which was seen in the working-age population. This demographic was seen to be affected most frequently [7, 16, 17]. More than 95% of individuals with chemical burns were between the ages of 20 and 59 years (Table 1). Furthermore, most patients had low educational levels (primary and middle school education), and only a small number of patients

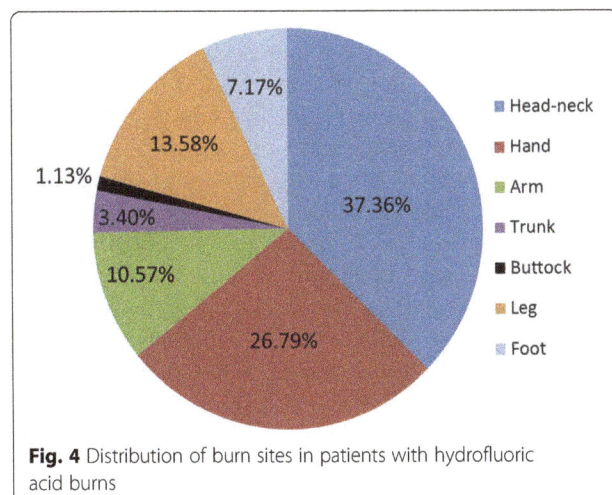

Fig. 4 Distribution of burn sites in patients with hydrofluoric acid burns

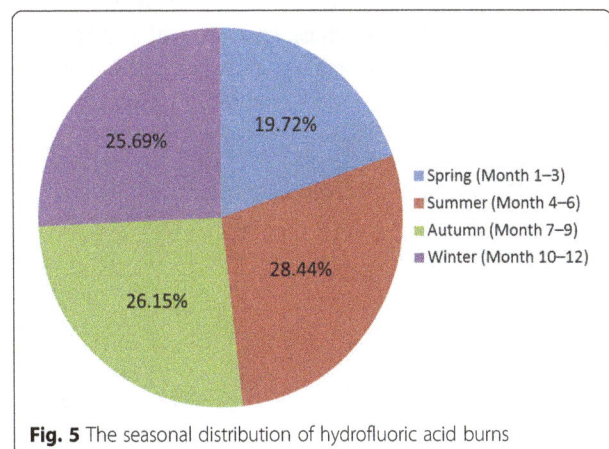

Fig. 5 The seasonal distribution of hydrofluoric acid burns

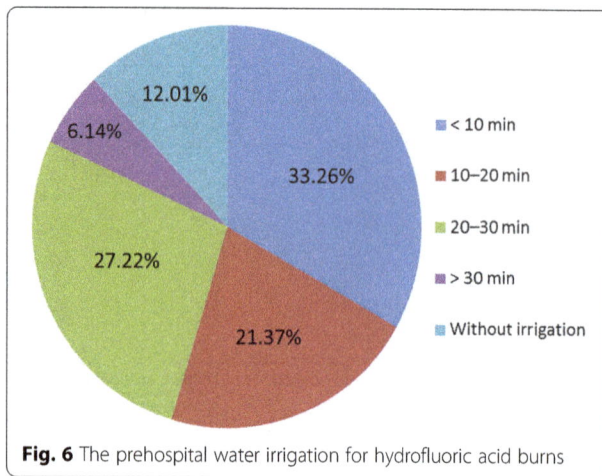

Fig. 6 The prehospital water irrigation for hydrofluoric acid burns

Table 7 Length of hospital stays for patients with HF burns

Hospital stay (days)	Cases	
	N	Percent (%)
<10	148	73.63
10–19	23	11.44
20–29	12	5.97
30–39	14	6.97
40–49	3	1.49
>50	1	0.50

had received tertiary education of college/university degrees or higher (Fig. 2). A low level of education may partly explain the higher incidence of HF burns in these patients. One case should be noted regarding two patients who were under the age of 10 years; and both of these children were victims of chemical burns in family workshops. In the past, family workshops, such as glass etching, were very popular in some regions of China. These establishments were usually contained within homes where workshops would be connected to the household private area, such as living room, allowing children easy access to dangerous chemicals and increasing the risk and likelihood of injury. In addition, more than 71% of chemical burns were work related, occurring primarily in workers in the fluoride industries, and stevedoring and transportation (Table 2). A recent study investigated acute HF exposure cases occurring in 1991–2010 using data collected from the Taiwan Poison Control Centre [18]. A total of 324 cases were identified, of which 80% were caused by occupational exposure, including those occurring in the semiconductor industry (61%), cleaning industry (15%), chemical and metal industries (13%), and other industries (11%). Some obvious differences in the occupational distribution of HF burns exist between existing data and those obtained within this study.

Workplace protection against chemical burns requires the use of personal protective equipment (PPE) and necessary professional skills and knowledge (received as

Table 6 The situations of serum electrolytes for patients with HF burns ($n = 201$)

Electroyte imbalance	Cases	
	N	Percent (%)
Hypocalcemia	47	23.38
Hypomagnesemia	28	13.93
Hypokalemia	18	8.96
Hyperkalemia	0	0

training) when operating machines or handling dangerous chemicals. More than 95% of chemical burns assessed in this study occurred in the workplace and were caused by inadequate protection, machine problems, and inappropriate machine operation (Fig. 3). Thus, shortages in occupational education and training, machine maintenance, and production management exist and can partly explain the higher incidence of HF burns in western Zhejiang.

HF, in liquid or vapour form, has the potential to cause tissue corrosion and chemical poisoning. Six patients were injured due to hydrogen fluoride exposure, and all others were burned by aqueous HF solutions (Table 3). HF burns caused by highly concentrated acid were more common, followed by moderate and low concentrations of acid (Table 4). These characteristics may correlate directly with production techniques and transportation practises in various fluoride industries. In many enterprises, highly concentrated HF solutions are produced and used, and may also be delivered to various regions if required; these processes were seen to be major causes of HF burns due to the improper handling of chemicals, as previously explained. Furthermore, HF burns may be caused by exposure to mixed compounds (Table 3); such complex situations may affect physicians' judgments and clinical decisions , leading to the incorrect management and treatment of chemical burns caused by exposure to HF [19].

Small burn areas were common in patients with HF burns (Table 5). The head and neck (37.36%) were the most common sites involved, followed by the hands (26.79%), legs (13.58%), and arms (10.57%). However, when burns involving the hands and arms were assessed together, the upper extremities (37.36%) were also the most common site of HF injury (Fig. 4), which parallels the results reported by Hatzifotis et al. [3] and Stuke et al. [17]. These authors assessed cases of patients with chemical burns, where most of the injuries involving the extremities could be prevented, once again emphasising the importance of correct occupational training, management and protection upon exposure to dangerous chemicals. In the study, by Hatzifotis et al. [3] and Stuke et al. [17], burns located on the head and neck were also usual; a result which also corresponded with the assessments of patients at our hospital department. Further analysis showed that burn injuries of this nature were caused by chemicals spilled or splashed from machines or pipes. As mentioned above, most HF burns occurred in the workplace and resulted from inadequate protection, machine problems, and inappropriate machine operation, which could explain the high frequency of HF burns affecting the head and neck. Accordingly, ocular burns were the most common accompanying injury.

In patients with fluoride poisoning, electrolyte imbalances, such as hypocalcaemia and hypomagnesaemia, occurred frequently, as fluoride ions bind to these metal ions to form insoluble salts in the body [13]. Hypocalcaemia and hypomagnesaemia can be rectified by calcium and magnesium supplementation in the clinic [20, 21]. Whether HF can cause hyperkalaemia is a matter of some controversy. Some experimental studies have shown that fluoride ions caused hyperkalaemia; when sodium fluoride was employed to investigate the effects of fluoride ions on potassium levels, hyperkalaemia was caused by inactivation of cellular sodium/potassium ATPase pumps and via the activation of sodium/calcium ion exchange [22]. However, different physiological mechanisms may be involved in patients with HF injuries. Some studies have reported that hypokalaemia occurs in patients with HF burns [22–25]. In our study, no such patient with hyperkalaemia was identified (Table 6), and this finding is paralleled in another recent epidemiological study conducted by Wu et al. [18] Hence, the exact mechanisms of HF on potassium metabolism remain unknown, and further studies are warranted. Inhibition of the ongoing absorption of fluoride ions is the key measure for the treatment of fluoride poisoning and its complications. Different methods have been developed to do so, including various decontamination methods using antidotes of calcium gluconate and others [13].

Seasonally, the distribution of HF burns remained similar in the summer, autumn, and winter; however, the number of burns decreased significantly in the spring compared with all other seasons (Fig. 5). A possible reason for this trend is the occurrence of many important holidays, such as the Chinese Spring Festival (during the spring season), which reduces the absolute working time in most fluoride enterprises.

The lengths of hospital stays and rates of surgical operation were related mainly to the severity of HF burns. Chemical burn severity is usually estimated by factors including HF concentration, exposure time, site of exposure, delay in therapy initiation, and amount of antidote delivered [2, 13, 26]. More than 90% of patients presented with small (<5% TBSA) burn areas, and most healed without surgical intervention, resulting in shorter hospital stays. Moreover, timely and correct pre-hospital

treatment is also crucial to prevent the progressive deepening and poor prognostic outcome of burn wounds. Immediate water irrigation remains the recommended decontamination method for on-site treatment of chemical burns [27, 28] as not only does it aid the removal of residual chemicals from wounds, but it also reduces the risk of developing chemical poisoning. In addition to water irrigation, other decontamination methods, including rinsing with a calcium gluconate solution and using Hexafluorine* solution have also been introduced. An increasing number of studies suggest that decontamination with Hexafluorine* solution in a very early stage post-exposure (several seconds to minutes) works well [29]. After admission, an algorithm was established in our department to treat those patients with HF exposure, which has been well documented in another review [13]. The basic strategies for HF burns were paralleled to blocking the fluoride ions from infiltrating into deep tissues by emergent decontamination [13].

As this study is part of our epidemiological survey of chemical burns, its limitations have been clarified in previously published work [10]. Briefly, one limitation is the source of the data as all our data were collected from one hospital in one area, and only inpatients were included. Hence, the estimation of morbidity based on these data may contain errors. However, the data presented here remain valuable; as Quhua Hospital is the main medical centre for the treatment of chemical burns, and it receives the majority of patients with chemical burns in western Zhejiang Province. Additionally, the epidemiological characteristics described in this study have the potential to provide valuable information to encourage the upgrading of safety measurements and formulation of preventive strategies.

Conclusions

To summarise; this epidemiological study presents characteristic findings related to HF burns in western Zhejiang Province, China. Firstly, the morbidity of HF burns in the past 10 years showed a gradual increase, which can be attributed to the development of local fluoride industries. Secondly, most HF injuries were work related and distributed in working-age patients. Thirdly, aqueous HF solutions, especially those of high concentration, were the most common chemical cause of HF burns. Furthermore, inappropriate operation of equipment, machine malfunctions, and inadequate protection were identified as the leading causes of HF burns in the workplace. The burn area was <5% of TBSA in more than 90% of patients, and the most common burn sites were the head, neck, and upper extremities. Approximately 17% of patients underwent surgical operation. Accompanying injuries should be detected and treated correctly in a timely manner. Lastly, electrolyte imbalances, such as hypocalcaemia, hypomagnesaemia, and hypokalaemia, occurred frequently in patients with HF exposure; however, hyperkalaemia was not encountered in this study. Based on these results, related enterprises and local authorities should be encouraged to upgrade their management policies and to provide the necessary occupational education and safety training to high-risk populations. The local government would benefit from the establishment of a long-term strategic plan to improve education and to enhance the management of hazardous chemicals. Moreover, strategies focusing on the production, transportation, and usage of HF should be enhanced further for labourers and professionals dealing with chemicals, including consideration of the details of injuries caused by HF and other mixtures. Early and correct pre-hospital treatment, such as water irrigation and application of antidotes should also be considered for the effective management and immediate treatment of HF burns. Thus, the education of workers to provide common emergency knowledge and skills is highly warranted.

Acknowledgements
Thanks to Dr. Ruiming Jiang, and Dr. Jia Liu, for their help in information collection and statistical analysis.

Funding
This work was financially supported by the Project of Zhejiang Science and technology (2015C37022), the Medical Health Platform Program of Zhejiang, China (2013ZD025) and the Zhejiang research project of commonweal technology (2017C33186).

Authors' contributions
YZ and XW designed this survey; JZ, XJ, LN and CY collected the data; CH conducted the statistical analysis; XW and KS prepared the manuscript. All authors have reviewed and approved the final draft.

Competing interests
The authors declare that they have no competing interests.

Author details
[1]Department of Burns & Plastic Surgery, Zhejiang Quhua Hospital, Quzhou 324004, China. [2]Department of Burns & Wound Care Center, Second Affiliated Hospital of Zhejiang University College of Medicine, Hangzhou 310009, China. [3]Zhejiang University School of Medicine, Hangzhou 310000, China.

References
1. Sheridan RL, Ryan CM, Quinby Jr WC, Blair J, Tompkins RG, Burke JF. Emergency management of major hydrofluoric acid exposures. Burns. 1995; 21(1):62–4.
2. Kirkpatrick JJ, Enion DS, Burd DA. Hydrofluoric acid burns: a review. Burns. 1995;21(7):483–93.
3. Hatzifotis M, Williams A, Muller M, Pegg S. Hydrofluoric acid burns. Burns. 2004;30(2):156–9.
4. Bertolini JC. Hydrofluoric acid: a review of toxicity. J Emerg Med. 1992;10(2):163–8.
5. Tepperman PB. Fatality due to acute systemic fluoride poisoning following a hydrofluoric acid skin burn. J Occup Med. 1980;22(10):691–2.
6. Ricketts S, Kimble FW. Chemical injuries: the Tasmanian Burns Unit experience. ANZ J Surg. 2003;73(1–2):45–8.
7. Xie Y, Tan Y, Tang S. Epidemiology of 377 patients with chemical burns in Guangdong province. Burns. 2004;30(6):569–72.
8. Zhang YH, Han CM, Chen GX, Ye CJ, Jiang RM, Liu LP, et al. Factors associated with chemical burns in Zhejiang province, China: an epidemiological study. BMC Public Health. 2011;11:746.
9. Ozcan M, Allahbeickaraghi A, Dundar M. Possible hazardous effects of hydrofluoric acid and recommendations for treatment approach: a review. Clin Oral Investig. 2012;16(1):15–23.
10. Ye C, Wang X, Zhang Y, Ni L, Jiang R, Liu L, et al. Ten-year epidemiology of chemical burns in Western Zhejiang Province of China. Burns. 2016;42(3):668–74.
11. Zhang Y, Wang X, Sharma K, Mao X, Qiu X, Ni L, et al. Injuries following a serious hydrofluoric acid leak: first aid and lessons. Burns. 2015;41(7):1593–8.
12. Qiu X, Han C, Wang Y, Wang Q, Zhan W, Lu Z, et al. Hydrofluoric acid burns of 48 cases in batches. Chin J Emerg Med. 2010;10(4):422–3.
13. Wang X, Zhang Y, Ni L, You C, Ye C, Jiang R, et al. A review of treatment strategies for hydrofluoric acid burns: current status and future prospects. Burns. 2014;40(8):1447–57.
14. Zhang Y, Wang X, Ye C, Liu L, Jiang R, Ni L, et al. The clinical effectiveness of the intravenous infusion of calcium gluconate for treatment of hydrofluoric acid burn of distal limbs. Burns. 2014;40(4):e26–30.
15. Yuanhai Z, Liangfang N, Xingang W, Ruiming J, Liping L, Chunjiang Y, et al. Clinical arterial infusion of calcium gluconate: the preferred method for treating hydrofluoric acid burns of distal human limbs. Int J Occup Med Environ Health. 2014;27(1):104–13.
16. Pitkanen J, Al-Qattan MM. Epidemiology of domestic chemical burns in Saudi Arabia. Burns. 2001;27(4):376–8.
17. Stuke LE, Arnoldo BD, Hunt JL, Purdue GF. Hydrofluoric acid burns: a 15-year experience. J Burn Care Res. 2008;29(6):893–6.
18. Wu ML, Yang CC, Ger J, Tsai WJ, Deng JF. Acute hydrofluoric acid exposure reported to Taiwan Poison Control Center, 1991–2010. Hum Exp Toxicol. 2014; 33(5):449-454.
19. Zhang Y, Ni L, Ye C, Zhang J, Wang X. A rare case of chemical burns caused by a mixture of sulphuric acid and hydrofluoric acid. Clin Toxicol. 2015;53(7):785.
20. Burkhart KK, Brent J, Kirk MA, Baker DC, Kulig KW. Comparison of topical magnesium and calcium treatment for dermal hydrofluoric acid burns. Ann Emerg Med. 1994;24(1):9–13.
21. Dowbak G, Rose K, Rohrich RJ. A biochemical and histologic rationale for the treatment of hydrofluoric acid burns with calcium gluconate. J Burn Care Rehabil. 1994;15(4):323–7.
22. Wu ML, Deng JF, Fan JS. Survival after hypocalcemia, hypomagnesemia, hypokalemia and cardiac arrest following mild hydrofluoric acid burn. Clin Toxicol. 2010;48(9):953–5.
23. Dalamaga M, Karmaniolas K, Nikolaidou A, Papadavid E. Hypocalcemia, hypomagnesemia, and hypokalemia following hydrofluoric acid chemical injury. J Burn Care Res. 2008;29(3):541–3.
24. Gallerani M, Bettoli V, Peron L, Manfredini R. Systemic and topical effects of intradermal hydrofluoric acid. Am J Emerg Med. 1998;16(5):521–2.
25. Greco RJ, Hartford CE, Haith Jr LR, Patton ML. Hydrofluoric acid-induced hypocalcemia. J Trauma. 1988;28(11):1593–6.
26. Graudins A, Burns MJ, Aaron CK. Regional intravenous infusion of calcium gluconate for hydrofluoric acid burns of the upper extremity. Ann Emerg Med. 1997;30(5):604–7.
27. Brent J. Water-based solutions are the best decontaminating fluids for dermal corrosive exposures: a mini review. Clin Toxicol. 2013;51(8):731–6.
28. Wang X, Han C. Re-emphasizing the role of copious water irrigation in the first aid treatment of chemical burns. Burns. 2014;40(4):779–80.
29. Soderberg K, Kuusinen P, Mathieu L, Hall AH. An improved method for emergent decontamination of ocular and dermal hydrofluoric acid splashes. Vet Hum Toxicol. 2004;46(4):216–8.

6

Influence of the Kinaesthetics care conception during patient handling on the development of musculoskeletal complaints and diseases

Alice Freiberg[1*], Maria Girbig[1], Ulrike Euler[1], Julia Scharfe[1], Albert Nienhaus[2,3], Sonja Freitag[2] and Andreas Seidler[1]

Abstract: The Kinaesthetics care conception is a nursing approach for patient handling which aims to prevent work-related complaints and diseases. The evidence about the influence of Kinaesthetics on musculoskeletal disorders among persons who handle patients is unclear to date. The purposes of the scoping review are to gain insight into the current state of research regarding the clinical effectiveness of Kinaesthetics (in terms of perceived exertion and musculoskeletal complaints) among persons who handle patients and to identify potential research gaps. A scoping review was conducted. The search strategy comprised a systematic search in electronic databases (MEDLINE, EMBASE, AMED, CINAHL), a hand search, a fast forward search (Web of Science) and a Google scholar-search. The review process was carried out independently by two reviewers. Methodological quality was assessed for all studies using three methodological main categories (reporting quality, internal validity, external validity). Thirteen studies with different study designs were included. Seven studies investigated musculoskeletal complaints and nine studies the perceived exertion of nursing staff. Most studies were of very low methodology. Most studies reported a decrease of musculoskeletal complaints and perceived exertion due to Kinaesthetics. In conclusion, there is only little evidence of very low quality about the effectiveness of Kinaesthetics. Out of the studies it could be assumed that Kinaesthetics may decrease the patient handling related perceived exertion and musculoskeletal pain of persons who handle patients. But an overestimation of these results is likely, due to inadequate methodology of included studies. As a result, no clear recommendations about the effectiveness of the Kinaesthetics care conception can be made yet. Since a research gap was shown, further high quality intervention studies are necessary for clarifying the effectiveness of Kinaesthetics.

PROSPERO registry number: CRD42015015811

Keywords: Kinaesthetics, Musculoskeletal, Patient handling, Scoping review

Background

The Kinaesthetics care conception (in the following called "Kinaesthetics") is an approach for patient handling which enables nursing staff to interact with patients in a way that shall protect themselves from injuries and that shall support their own as well as their patient's health development [1]. Kinaesthetics is the study of the perception of human movements which are necessary

─────────────────────────────

* Correspondence: alice.freiberg@tu-dresden.de
[1]Institute and Policlinic of Occupational and Social Medicine, Medical Faculty Carl Gustav Carus, Technische Universität Dresden, Fetscherstr. 74, Dresden 01307, Germany
Full list of author information is available at the end of the article

for the execution of activities of daily life [1, 2]. The endeavor of Kinaesthetics is to divide all human action in its parts, which are called concepts: Interaction, functional anatomy, human movement, exertion, human functions and environment [1]. Patients shall be moved with spiral, not with parallel movements, because these require less effort [1]. In the theory of Kinaesthetics the human body consists of masses (bones) and spaces (muscles) [1]. If a handling person contacts the masses and moves them in a row, handling of a patient should be easier [1]. The theoretical framework of Kinaesthetics is based on the principles of behavioral cybernetics [1]. The concept was developed in the 1980s by Frank White

Hatch and Linda Sue Maietta [2]. Training in Kinaesthetics is offered to nursing staff for about twenty years now [2]. It is applied in nursing [2], in infant handling (www.kinaesthetics.de), in palliative care [3], in education [2] and also in training of caregiving relatives [4]. There are several providers of Kinaesthetics which differ a lot in regard to quality, duration, qualification or curriculum of the training [5]. For example, in Germany the biggest and most known associations are the "European Kinaesthetics Association" and "MH Kinaesthetics Deutschland" [5].

Nursing staff has an increased risk for musculoskeletal disorders [6, 7]. A recently published review reported that musculoskeletal pain among nurses and nursing aids was highest in the lower back, followed by the shoulder joints and the neck (mean 12-month prevalence each: 55, 44, 42 %) [8]. Relative risk among nurses compared to clerks to suffer from low back pain is increased (point prevalence: 1.47 (95 % CI: 1.37–1.59)) [6]. Patient handling seems to be one of the risk factors for musculoskeletal disorders among nursing staff [9, 10]. One of the propagated effects of Kinaesthetics is the prevention of such physical complaints [2]. But the scientific evidence about the influence of Kinaesthetics on prevention of musculoskeletal complaints and diseases among persons who handle patients is unclear to date.

Review
Methods
Step 1—Identifying the research question
Since Kinaesthetics has not been studied much and it is a relatively new nursing intervention, a scoping review was conducted. The purposes of the scoping review are to gain insight into the current state of research regarding the clinical effectiveness of Kinaesthetics (in terms of perceived exertion and musculoskeletal complaints) among persons who handle patients and to identify possible research gaps. On the basis of these, the following research question arose:

"What is the scientific evidence about the influence of Kinaesthetics on the development of musculoskeletal complaints and diseases among persons who handle patients and is there a specific research gap?"

A general definition of scoping reviews does not exist [11, 12]. The purposes of scoping reviews are to map and to summarize the evidence of a certain research field and to identify research gaps [13]. On the basis of the results of a scoping review a systematic review can be conducted and recommendations for further research can be made [13]. In contrast to systematic reviews, scoping reviews are not restricted to certain study designs [13]. Furthermore, a critical appraisal of included studies is not intended [13], but its usefulness has been discussed in later

methodology papers [12, 14]. Nevertheless, a transparent procedure is required to allow other researchers replication of study results [13, 15]. The results of a scoping review are summarized tabularly and descriptively [11].

This scoping review was conducted and structured based on methodological frameworks proposed by Arksey and O'Malley [13], and modified by Levac et al. [12] and Daudt et al. [14]. For checking if all relevant sections/topics of a review are reported, the PRISMA statement (Preferred Reporting Items for Systematic Reviews and Meta-Analyses) was used, since there is no specific reporting guideline for scoping reviews and most steps of this scoping review resemble the procedures of a systematic review [16]. The study protocol of this scoping review was published on the "International Register of systematic reviews" (PROSPERO) prior to study conduct (PROSPERO registry number: CRD42015015811) [17].

Step 2—Identifying relevant studies
A broad and sensitive search strategy was developed to identify as much relevant studies as possible. The following electronic databases were searched systematically:

- MEDLINE (via PubMed, from 1946 up to February 2nd 2016)
- EMBASE (via Ovid, from 1974 up to February 2nd 2016)
- AMED (via Ovid, from 1985 up to February 2nd 2016)
- CINAHL (via EBSCOhost, from 1982 up to February 2nd 2016)

The search strategy comprised terms for the population and the intervention. The individual terms of both categories were interconnected via the Boolean Operator "AND". Search terms for the categories "outcome" and "study design" were not considered due to the aforementioned criteria of a scoping review [11]. The search string was first developed for MEDLINE and then adapted to the particular requirements of the other databases. Table 1 shows the search string for MEDLINE.

Furthermore, a fast forward search was carried out via the Web of Science with the "Cited Reference Search"-

Table 1 Search string for MEDLINE

1	Nurses [All Fields] OR nurses[mh] OR nurse [All Fields] OR Allied Health Personnel [mh] OR Health Personnel [mh] OR physiotherapy* OR physical therap* OR therapist* OR occupational therap* OR family [mh] OR family [All Fields] OR relative [All Fields] OR "caregiving volunteer" [All Fields]
2	Kinaesthetics OR kinesthetics OR kinaesthetic OR kinesthetic OR kinesthesia OR kinaesthesia
3	#1 AND #2

function. For this purpose the references of all full texts that were included after title and abstract screening were used. In addition, a hand search for eligible studies was executed in the reference lists of full texts that were included after the title and abstract screening process and in the reference lists of topic related key articles and reviews.

In the later course of research it was decided to search Google scholar additionally, because it was assumed that further relevant studies could be retrieved. The search was conducted on September 27th 2015 using two terms ("Kinästhetik", "kinaesthetics") separately from each other. The first 500 hits each were screened by one reviewer (AF). If a reference seemed to be relevant, full text was retrieved and two reviewers (AF, MG/JS) decided about inclusion or exclusion.

The search results were organized with the electronic literature management program EndNote.

Step 3—Study selection
The PICOS-criteria (population, intervention, comparison, outcome, study design) were used to define the inclusion and exclusion criteria of this scoping review [16]. Healthcare workers as well as caregiving volunteers and family members who conduct patient handling activities on a regular basis, aged 15 to 70 years, working in all kinds of facilities where patient handling takes place, regardless of their qualification, were included. Kinaesthetics as individual measure or as part of a multimodal program was considered as intervention. No specification was made regarding the comparison. Relevant outcomes were all parameters that refer to musculoskeletal complaints and diseases, including the perceived exertion during or after patient handling. Initially it was planned to include patient parameters if they were also reported in the studies, but for better comprehensibility and structuring of the research project it was decided to exclude them. Since the scope of the review were clinical outcomes only, biomechanical studies were not considered. Editorials, commentaries, expert opinions and abstracts were excluded. No language restrictions were applied.

Title and abstract screening and full text screening were done independently by two reviewers (AF, UE/MG) in accordance with the inclusion and exclusion criteria. Disagreements were discussed and in case of a lack of agreement a third reviewer (AS) was consulted [12]. The title and abstract screening was tested in a pilot phase. All excluded studies of the full text screening were documented tabularly with reasons for exclusion. The proportion of observed agreement and Cohen's Kappa were calculated to assess the agreement between the two reviewers [18].

Step 4—Charting the data
Data from included studies were extracted independently by two reviewers (AF, UE/MG) and discussed subsequently

[11]. The process was piloted beforehand [12]. Relevant study information was documented in a standardized data extraction sheet. According to the iterative procedure of scoping reviews, the data extraction sheet was adapted to the identified data material in consultation with the reviewers.

Step 5—Collating, summarizing and reporting the data
Methodological quality assessment As aforementioned, critical appraisal of included studies is still a subject of debate in methodology papers about scoping reviews [12–14]. To identify possible research gaps regarding the methodology of studies about Kinaesthetics and to give suggestions for methodological improvements for future research, it was decided to assess methodology of included studies in this scoping review. Due to the plethora of study designs methodological comparability of included studies seems hardly possible by using various appraisal tools for the appropriate study designs. According to the author's knowledge one comprehensive checklist for several different study designs is missing. Thus, it was determined to evaluate three main categories (reporting quality, internal validity, external validity) for each study by two reviewers (AF, MG/JS) adjusted to each study type guided by categories/questions of the "Downs and Black checklist" [19] (for intervention studies) and the checklists of the "Critical Appraisal Skills Programmes" (CASP) [20] (for reviews and qualitative studies), to obtain a methodological overview. Each main category is judged with "low risk of bias", "high risk of bias" or "unclear risk of bias". According to the Cochrane Handbook for Systematic Reviews of Interventions a bias is "a systematic error, or deviation from the truth, in results or inferences" [21]. "Low risk of bias" means that there is low risk of such a bias to occur in one of the main categories. "High risk of bias" means that the risk of such a bias is high. If information for judging a main category was reported insufficiently, the category was of "unclear risk of bias".

Important key points for the assessment of the main category "Reporting quality" were sufficient information about study purpose, population, intervention, comparison, outcomes, results, etc. If these key points were not or poorly reported, this category was judged as "high risk of bias".

According to the glossary of the German Network for Evidence-based Medicine (DNEbM) "Internal validity" refers to the extent to which the results of a study reflect the "true" effect of an intervention, i.e. are free of systematic bias and it is based on an optimal study planning, study conduct and study analysis [22]. For the main category "internal validity" study design specific key points (for intervention studies, qualitative studies or reviews) were given additionally. These key points were created after the designs of included studies were known (a posteriori).

The main category "External validity" is the degree to which the results of an observation withstand under other circumstances (e.g. population, setting) [23]. The basis for decision-making concerning the external validity of intervention studies were questions 11–13 of the "Downs and Black checklist" [19]. For the external validity of reviews question "8" of the CASP-review-checklist served as decision basis for judgement ("Can the results be applied to the local population?") [20]. The following hints are given for answering the question: "The patients covered by the review could be sufficiently different to your population to cause concern."; "Your local setting is likely to differ much from that of the review" [20]. Even though generalisation (and external validity) is considered important for qualitative research [24], this main category was not judged for qualitative studies, since appropriate reporting and appraisal checklists do not comprise suitable decision criteria [20, 25].

Data analysis

Retrieved data were analyzed for two main topics: study characteristics and study results. Study characteristics of interest were organizational data like year of publication, study language, place of study or setting; and research-related data concerning the PICOS-criteria [16]. Study results were distinguished between musculoskeletal complaints and perceived exertion of persons who handle patients. Data were summarized descriptively and tabularly.

Step 6—Consultation exercise

Since this step is optional, a consultation with experts and stakeholders was not undertaken.

Results

Study selection

The systematic database search yielded 1104 hits. After duplicate cleansing the titles and abstracts of 765 search results of the database search were screened. Of these, 736 studies were excluded and 29 studies were retrieved for screening the full texts. Twenty-five full texts were excluded due to an inadequate topic and/or article design (n = 18) [3–5, 26–38] or outcome (n = 7) [39–44]. Four studies were included in the scoping review [45–48]. Other search sources yielded additional nine hits. Via the fast forward search no further studies were identified. By checking the reference lists of included studies after full text screening and of topic related key articles six studies were found [49–54]. The Google scholar- search yielded three relevant studies [55–57]. Two studies of the hand search that seemed appropriate for inclusion according to their title and abstract were not deliverable via the Saxon State and University Library Dresden (SLUB) [58, 59]. For the title abstract screening of the database search an observed agreement of 0.98 and a Cohen's kappa of 0.72 (Strength of agreement after Landis & Koch [60]: substantial) was calculated. The observed agreement for the full text screening process was 0.97 and the Cohen's Kappa 0.87 (Strength of agreement after Landis & Koch [60]: almost perfect).

The results of the study selection are summarized with the PRISMA flow chart in Fig. 1. Please note that the number of hits for duplicate cleansing, title and abstract and full text screening contain additional records identified through other sources (in contrast to aforementioned numbers presented descriptively for database search only).

Study characteristics

Thirteen studies were appropriate for the qualitative analysis: Two randomized controlled trials [47, 51], one cross-over study [48], one controlled before-after study [57], three uncontrolled before-after studies [46, 49, 52], three evaluation studies [45, 50, 53], one qualitative study [55] and two reviews [54, 56]. The difference between the before-after studies and the evaluation studies was that outcomes in the evaluation studies were only measured once (at the end of the project), whereas the outcomes of the before-after studies were measured at baseline and at follow-up. Data from the cross-over-study of Tamminen-Peter were only obtained from the first study part, to avoid a carry-over effect and hence the study can be considered as a non-randomized controlled trial [48]. Twelve studies were written in German and one in Finnish [48]. The author of the Finnish study, Leena Tamminen-Peter, provided additional documents for data extraction, which were translated by a professional translator. All studies were conducted in Europe, of these six in Germany, four in Austria, two in Switzerland and one in Finland. The study setting of nine studies was a hospital, one study took place in a retirement home and one in the homely environment of caregiving family members. One of the reviews included studies with hospitals and nursing homes as study setting [56], the other review did not define the setting of interest [54]. All studies were published after 2000, four of these after 2010. Nursing staff was the population of interest in all studies but one, which investigated caregiving family members [55]. Physical therapists were examined additionally in one study [50]. Only three studies provided patient characteristics [47, 48, 51]. Four studies examined a basic course of Kinaesthetics and three studies a comprehensive implementation of Kinaesthetics as intervention. None of these seven studies but one involved a comparison group. Another three studies investigated a specific patient handling task conducted with Kinaesthetics compared to the conventional handling method respectively the Durewall method (a nursing approach that uses jiu-jitsu principles). One study investigated

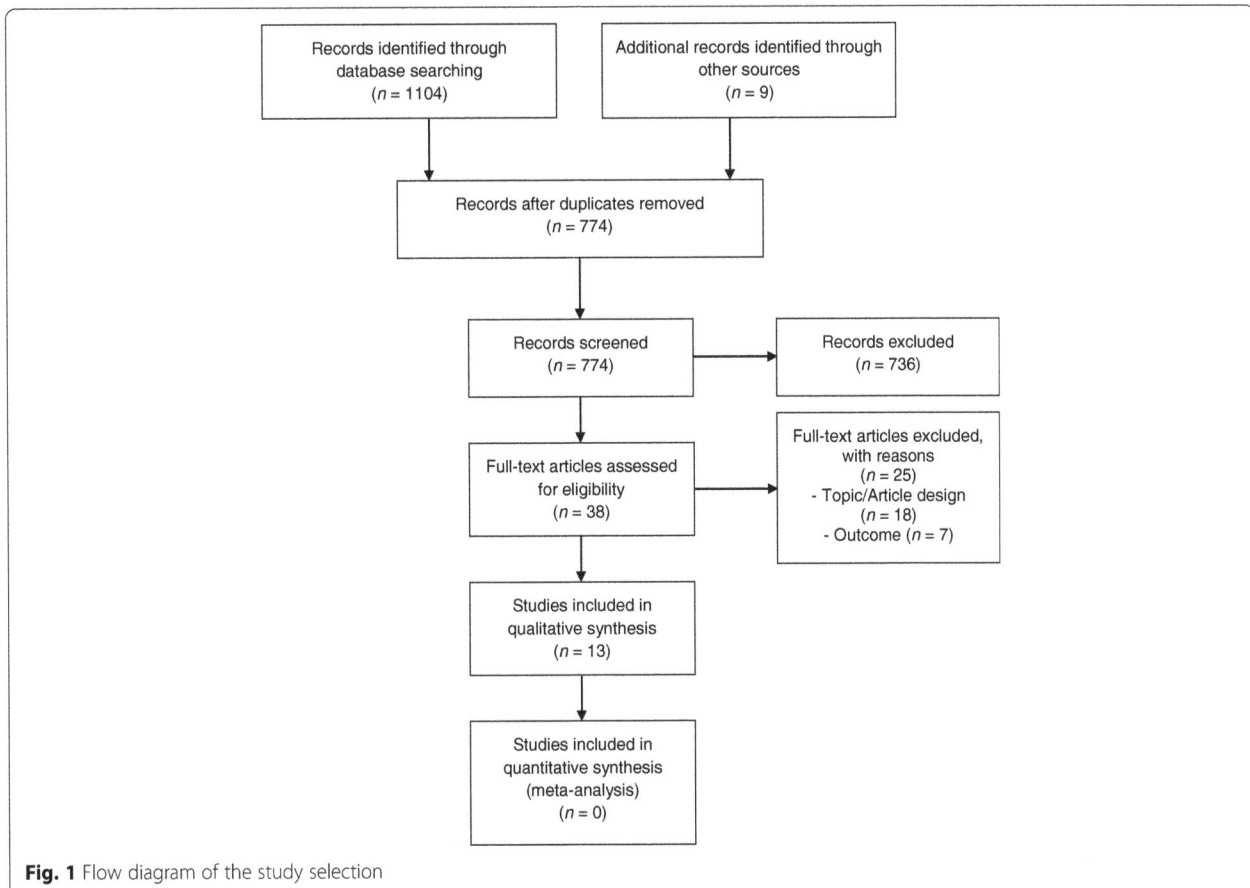

Fig. 1 Flow diagram of the study selection

the course "Kinaesthetics for caregiving family members". The two reviews considered the concept "Kinaesthetics" in general without further confinements. For further information of study characteristics see Table 2.

Methodological quality assessment

Details of methodological quality assessment of each study can be seen in Table 3.

The studies of Buge and Mahler and Huth et al. were the only two out of all included studies that were judged with "low risk of bias" in two categories each, Buge and Mahler for "Reporting quality" and "External validity" and Huth et al. for "Reporting quality" and "Internal validity" [50, 55]. Five studies received a "high risk of bias" in all three categories [45, 49, 51, 52, 53].

"Reporting quality" was at "low risk of bias" in three studies [50, 55, 57]. For three studies judgment of that category was unclear [46, 48, 56]. Although much important information in the systematic review of Sedlak-Emperer was reported (purpose, population, intervention, outcome, appraisal tools, study results), others were missing (study protocol, amount of reviewers, procedure of title-abstract- and full text screening) [56]. The same applies for the study of Christen et al [46]. Due to the Finnish language in

the study of Tamminen-Peter (and a resulting language barrier), assessment of this category was "unclear" [48]. The remaining seven studies were evaluated with "high risk of bias" for "Reporting quality", since too much important information (like population, setting, intervention, outcome measurements, statistical methods) was not or poorly reported. None of the studies did provide any information about a study protocol.

Only the qualitative study of Huth et al. was of "low risk of bias" in regard to "Internal validity" [55]. The category "Internal validity" was judged as "high risk of bias" for most of the studies ($n = 11$). In the evaluation studies a control group and a follow-up were missing [45, 50, 53]. As its name implies, a control group was missing in the uncontrolled before-after studies [46, 49, 52]. No randomization and no blinding were conducted in the non-randomized controlled trial of Tamminen-Peter and in the controlled before-after study of Hock-Rummelhardt [48, 57]. The randomized controlled trial of Lenker used an unconcealed allocation method [51]. In none of the two reviews a second reviewer was used [54, 56] and Steinwidder and Lohrmann did not appraise the methodology of included studies [54]. "Internal validity" of the randomized controlled trial of Eisenschink et al. is of "unclear risk of bias" due to

Table 2 Summary of study characteristics

Study (Language)	Study Design	Setting, Place	Time frame/Duration	Population — Persons who handle patients	Population — Patients	Intervention	Comparison	Outcome of interest
Betschon et al., 2014 (German) [45]	Evaluation Study	Nursing home, Meggen/Switzerland	Frame of the project: 2009–2012 Data collection: 2012	Nursing staff, Questionnaires n = 59 (Response: 75.0 %) Observations n = 17	NA	Basic course Kinaesthetics	NA	Physical Complaints, Perceived exertion immediately after mobilization[a]
Buge & Mahler, 2004 (German) [50]	Evaluation study	Nursing service, University Hospital, Heidelberg/Germany	Frame of the project: 2000–2003 Data collection: 2003	Nursing staff, n = 109; Physical therapists, n = 2 (Response: 33.7 %)	NA	Implementation of Kinaesthetics	NA	Feeling of physical relief (due to Kinaesthetics)[a]
Christen et al., 2002 (German) [46]	Uncontrolled before-after study	Hospital for nuclear medicine/radiotherapy, Zurich/Switzerland	Data collection: 1999 Follow-up: 6 month	Nursing staff, T0: n = 23 (Response: 92.0 %) T1: n = 20 (Response: 87.0 %) Data basis: n = 18	NA	Basic course Kinaesthetics	NA	Physical demands compared to subjective performance capacity[b]
Eisenschink et al., 2003 (German) [47]	Randomized controlled trial	Coronary care unit, University hospital, Ulm/Germany	Data collection: 1999–2000	Nursing staff, no further information	Patients after aortocoronary bypass surgery with sternotomy, I: n = 52 C: n = 50	Mobilisation of a patient with Kinaesthetics	Mobilisation of a patient with the standard mobilisation	Perceived exertion during first and second patient transfer[b]
Friess-Ott & Müller, 2006 (German) [53]	Evaluation study	University hospital, Heidelberg/Germany	Frame of the project: 1998–2003	Nursing staff, n = 159 (Response: 51.9 %)	NA	Basic course Kinaesthetics	NA	Pain, Physical relief, Effects on well-being[a]
Hock-Rummelhardt, 2013 (German) [57]	Controlled before-after study	Hospital, Vienna/Austria	Frame of the project: 2010–2012 Follow-up: 20 month	Nursing staff, I: n = 15 C: n = 27[c] (Response: 17 %)	NA	Basic course Kinaesthetics, Practical guidance	No training in Kinaesthetics	Pain during/after nursing, Perceived exertion during work[a]
Huth et al., 2013 (German) [55]	Qualitative study (Interviews)	Homely environment, Witten/Germany	Data collection: 7 weeks	Caregiving family members, n = 10	NA	Course "Kinaes-thetics for caregiving family members"	NA	Musculo-skeletal complaints, Physical work load[a]
Lenker, 2008 (German) [51]	Randomized controlled trial	Intensive care unit, hospital, Ludwigsburg-Bietigheim/Germany	Data collection: 2002–2004	NM	Patients after abdominal laparotomy, I: n = 36 C: n = 38	Mobilisation of a patient to the edge of the bed based on Kinaesthetics principles	Mobilisation of a patient to the edge of the bed with conventional methods	Back pain during patient handling, Perceived exertion during patient handling[b]
Maietta & Resch-Kröll, 2009 (German) [49]	Uncontrolled before-after study	State hospital, Hörgas/Austria	Frame of the project: nearly 24 month	Nursing staff, T0: n = 92 T1: Response: 42.7 %	NA	Implementation of Kinaesthetics	NA	Perceived exertion during patient handling[a]
Rettenberger & Schoenemeier, 2005 (German) [52]	Uncontrolled before-after study	Hospital, Heidenheim/Germany	Frame of the project: 1999–2000 Follow-up: 14 month	Nursing staff, n = 43	NA	Implementation of Kinaesthetics	NA	Back complaints during daily patient handling, Sick leave due to low back or sciatic complaints[a]

Table 2 Summary of study characteristics (Continued)

						Kinaesthetics	Conventional nursing	
Sedlak-Emperer, 2012 (German) [56]	Systematic review	Hospital, Nursing home, Austria	Search period: June 2009–March 2010 Applied publication period: 1990 – March 2010	Nursing staff from 18 years of age	Patients from 18 years of age	Kinaesthetics	Conventional nursing	Spinal complaints, Spinal loading[a]
Steinwidder & Lohmann, 2008 (German) [54]	Narrative review	Setting: NM, Austria	Search period: July–September 2007 Applied publication period: NM	Nursing staff from 18 years of age	Patients from 18 years of age	Kinaesthetics	NM	Physical loading[b]
Tamminen-Peter, 2006 (Finnish) [48]	Non-randomized controlled trial	City hospital; I: Neurological rehabilitation C: Orthopaedic rehabilitation, Turku/ Finland	Frame of the study: 2001–2002 Follow-up: 1 month	Nursing staff, I = 6 C = 6	Elderly, compliant, partially weight-bearing patients with little muscle strength and low ability to move, n = 18	Mobilisation of a patient from a wheelchair to bed with Kinaesthetics	Mobilisation of a patient from a wheelchair to bed with the Durewall method	Decrease of perceived strain of the lower back; Decrease of perceived strain of the shoulder joints[a]

Abbreviations: C control group, I intervention group, n number of participants, NA not applicable, NM not mentioned, T0 start of the trial, T1 end of the trial
[a]The outcome of interest was also a primary outcome in the study
[b]The outcome of interest was a secondary outcome in the study and only mentioned casually
[c]The paper contains different data about number of participants in the intervention and control group

Table 3 Methodological assessment of included studies

Study	Reporting quality	Internal validity	External validity
Betschon et al., 2014 [45]	HR	HR	HR
Buge & Mahler, 2004 [50]	LR	HR	LR
Christen et al., 2002 [46]	UR	HR	HR
Eisenschink et al., 2003 [47]	HR	UR	HR
Friess-Ott & Müller, 2006 [53]	HR	HR	HR
Hock-Rummelhardt, 2013 [57]	LR	HR	HR
Huth et al., 2013 [55]	LR	LR	NA
Lenker, 2008 [51]	HR	HR	HR
Maietta & Resch-Kröll, 2009 [49]	HR	HR	HR
Rettenberger & Schoenemeier, 2005 [52]	HR	HR	HR
Sedlak-Emperer, 2012 [56]	UR	HR	LR
Steinwidder & Lohrmann, 2008 [54]	HR	HR	UR
Tamminen-Peter, 2006 [48]	UR	HR	HR

General questions for each category
Reporting quality—Were important key points reported?
Internal validity—Are study results valid?
External validity—Are study results generalizable?
Abbreviations: *HR* high risk of bias, *LR* low risk of bias, *NA* not applicable, *UR* unclear risk of bias

missing or insufficient information regarding random sequence generation, allocation concealment and blinding of outcome assessment [47]. Most intervention studies recruited participants with a convenience sampling. Sample size was low in all included intervention studies (from $n = 6$ to $n = 159$). Most outcomes were obtained from subjective, self-reported data.

Two studies were evaluated as "low risk of bias" for the category "External validity" [50, 56]. The "External validity" of nine studies was judged as "high risk of bias", because generalizability in terms of population and/or setting was questionable and as "unclear risk of bias" in one study due to insufficient information [54]. "External validity" in the qualitative study of Huth et al. was not judged [55].

Overall, the methodology of most included studies is of very low quality regarding reporting quality, internal validity and external validity.

Study results

Detailed study results of the intervention studies are shown in Table 4. For each study, original (translated) terms are used. Details about measuring methods are shown in parenthesis. In the descriptive results part, results of intervention studies, the qualitative study and reviews are reported separately. Study results were not synthesized due to heterogeneity of included studies in many aspects (study design, outcome measures, intervention, etc.). Most results should be interpreted with

caution due to very low methodological quality of included studies.

a) Musculoskeletal complaints

Five intervention studies, one qualitative study and one review asked for musculoskeletal complaints of the nursing staff [45, 51–53, 55–57].

Musculoskeletal complaints—Intervention studies

The randomized controlled trial of Lenker reported a statistically significant difference (no p-value provided) for a more frequent occurrence of back pain during patient handling in the control group in comparison to the intervention group [51]. Hock-Rummelhardt found no statistically significant difference, neither between the intervention group and the control group at follow-up ($p = 0.974$), nor in the intervention group over time ($p = 0.308$) for pain during/after nursing [57]. In the study of Rettenberger and Schoenemeier back complaints during patient handling decreased from 49 to 30 % over time (no absolute numbers and p-value provided) [52]. Furthermore, sick leave due to low back or sciatic pain declined from start to end of the trial. Of those with back complaints during patient handling, 44 % took sick leave at the start of the trial, but only 4.4 % at follow-up. Betschon et al. reported that nursing staff that participated in a basic course of Kinaesthetics mainly felt physical complaints of the lower back/back (39 %), the neck (37 %) and the legs (27 %) immediately after patient handling (no absolute

Table 4 Study results

Study (design, intervention)	Musculoskeletal complaints	Perceived exertion/physical loads
Betschon et al., 2014 [45]	Physical complaints: (% of surveyed nursing staff)	Perceived exertion immediately after mobilisation: (% of surveyed nursing staff)
(Evaluation study, Basic course Kinaesthetics)	- lower back/back: 39	- exhausting: 53
	- neck: 37	- very exhausting: 13
	- legs: 27	
Buge & Mahler, 2004 [50]	NA	Feeling of physical relief (due to Kinaesthetics)
(Evaluation study, Implementation of Kinaesthetics)		(Scale: 1–10, 1: Min; Measure: M, Mdn (SD))
		- cervical spine: 4.84, 5.00 (2.65)
		- arm/shoulder: 5.65, 6.00 (2.52)
		- elbow/wrist: 4.72, 5.00 (2.49)
		- thoracic spine: 6.00, 6.00 (2.42)
		- hip: 5.64, 6.00 (2.56)
		- knee: 5.26, 5.00 (2.73)
		- lumbar spine: 6.83, 8.00 (2.46)
Christen et al., 2002 [46]	NA	Physical demands compared to subjective capacity are…: ($N = 18$)
(Uncontrolled before-after study, Basic course Kinaesthetics)		…relatively tolerable:
		- never mentioned (T0, T1): $n = 1$
		- only mentioned at T0: $n = 2$
		- only mentioned at T1: $n = 6$
		- mentioned at T0 and T1: $n = 9$
		…(rather) too high:
		- never mentioned (T0, T1): $n = 6$
		- only mentioned at T0: $n = 8$
		- only mentioned at T1: $n = 3$
		- mentioned at T0 and T1: $n = 1$
Eisenschink et al., 2003 [47]	NA	Perceived exertion…: (Scale: 0–100, 100: not exhausting; Measure: Mdn)
(Randomized controlled trial, Mobilisation of a patient with Kinaesthetics)		…during first patient transfer:
		- I: 82.5
		- C: 37.0[a] ($p = 0.132$)
		…during second patient transfer:
		- I: 84.5
		- C: 36.0[b] ($p = 0.0176$)
Friess-Ott & Müller, 2006 [53]	Pain relief due to Kinaesthetics: (% of surveyed nursing staff)	NA
(Evaluation study, Basic course Kinaesthetics)	Full agreement:	
	- back: 38	
	- neck: 25	
	Partial agreement:	
	- neck, back, knee or legs: 23–36	
	No agreement:	
	- back: 16	
	- legs: 34	

Table 4 Study results (Continued)

Hock-Rummelhardt, 2013 [57]	Pain during/after nursing…: (Scale: 1–6, 1: no pain; Measure: M (SD))	Perceived exertion during work: (Scale: 1–6, 1: not exhausting; Measure: M (SD))
(Controlled before-after study, Basic course Kinaesthetics, practical guidance)	…at T0:	…at T0:
	- I: 2.36 (0.96)	- I: 4.07 (1.34)
	- C: 2.12 (1.04)[a] (p = 0.615)	- C: 4.37 (1.25)[a,c]
	…at T1:	…at T1:
	- I: 2.05 (1.12)	- I: 4.27 (1.49)
	- C: 2.04 (0.90)[a] (p = 0.974)	- C: 4.48 (1.48)[a] (p = 0.505)
Lenker, 2008[d] [51]	Back pain during patient handling (defined as pulling sensation): (N = 69)	Perceived exertion during patient handling: (N = 70)
(Randomized controlled trial, Mobilisation of a patient with Kinaesthetics)	- yes: I: n = 0; C: n = 9	- little: I: n = 33; C: n = 25
	- no: I: n = 33; C: n = 27[b,c]	- much: I: n = 0; C: n = 12[b,c]
Maietta & Resch-Kröll, 2009 [49]	NA	Perceived exertion during patient handling of…: (Scale: 1–6, 1: great effort; Measure: M)
(Uncontrolled before-after study, Implemen-tation of Kinaesthetics)		…care-dependent patients:
		- T0: 3.10
		- T1: 3.70 (Change: −19.4 %)[c]
		…obese patients:
		- T0: 2.05
		- T1: 3.15 (Change: −53.7 %)[c]
		…patients with high body tension:
		- T0: 2.28
		- T1: 2.91 (Change: −27.6 %)[c]
Rettenberger & Schoenemeier, 2005 [52]	Back complaints during daily patient handling: (% of surveyed nursing staff)	NA
(Uncontrolled before-after study, Implementation of Kinaesthetics)	- T0: 49	
	- T1: 30[c]	
Tamminen-Peter, 2006[d] [48]	NA	Decrease of perceived exertion at T1 for…: (% of surveyed nursing staff)
(Non-randomized controlled trial, Mobilisation of a patient from wheelchair to bed with Kinaesthetics)		…lower back:
		- I: 71
		- C: 28[b] (p < 0.01)
		…shoulder joints:
		- I: 53
		- C: 49[a,c]

Abbreviation: C control group, I intervention group, M mean, Mdn median, Min minimum, N total sample size, n sub-sample size, NA not applicable, p p-value, SD standard deviation, T0 start of the trial, T1 end of the trial
[a]No statistically significant difference between groups
[b]Statistically significant difference between groups
[c]No p-value provided
[d]Data were obtained from the author of the study

numbers provided) [45]. It is unclear, whether these numerical data are a sign for symptom improvement or for adverse effects of Kinaesthetics since no comparative values (before-after or of a control group) were reported. In the study of Friess-Ott and Müller, after attending a basic course of Kinaesthetics, 38 % respectively 25 % of the nursing staff fully agreed, that they had less pain than before the course in the

back respectively the neck; 23 % to 36 % felt partial pain relief of the neck, back, knees or legs; and 16 % respectively 34 % felt no pain relief in the back respectively the legs (no absolute numbers provided) [53]. In summary, most intervention studies reported an improvement of musculoskeletal complaints (between groups and/or over time) in nursing staff due to Kinaesthetics. No adverse effects were reported.

Musculoskeletal complaints—Qualitative study

Participants in the qualitative study of Huth et al. reported a reduction of pain and muscular tension and acknowledged the preventive character of Kinaesthetics (related to musculoskeletal complaints) [55].

Musculoskeletal complaints—Review

Regarding musculoskeletal complaints the systematic review of Sedlak-Emperer reported about two studies that emphasized the preventive and rehabilitative character of Kinaesthetics (concerning spinal complaints) [52, 56].

b) Perceived exertion/physical loads

Eight intervention studies, one qualitative study and two reviews described the perceived exertion or physical loads of the nursing staff [45–51, 54–57].

Perceived exertion/physical loads—Intervention studies

In the randomized controlled trial of Eisenschink et al. the perceived exertion during a specific patient handling task with Kinaesthetics after an aortocoronary bypass surgery was rated lower than handling with the standard mobilisation [47]. During second patient transfer this difference was statistically significant ($p = 0.0176$), but not during first patient transfer ($p = 0.132$). It should be noted critically that the intervention group comprised more patients with movement restrictions than the control group (37 % versus 15 %). Similar results were seen in the randomized controlled trial of Lenker [51]. Hock-Rummelhardt observed no statistically significant difference of the perceived exertion during work between groups at follow-up ($p = 0.505$) or in the intervention group from start to end of the trial ($p = 0.490$) due to Kinaesthetics [57]. For perceived exertion of the lower spine during a specific patient handling task a statistically significant higher reduction was reported with application of Kinaesthetics in comparison with the Durewall method in the non-randomized control trial of Tamminen-Peter ($p < 0.01$) (no absolute numbers provided) [48]. Such a difference between the intervention and the control group was not seen for the reduction of perceived exertion of the shoulder joints. In a before-after study of Christen et al. physical demands of work were described mainly as too high at baseline and as relatively tolerable especially at follow-up [46]. In another before-after study, Maietta and Resch-Kröll reported the reduction of the perceived exertion during patient handling for different kinds of patients (care-dependent patients, obese patients, patients with high body tension) from baseline to follow-up (no p-values provided) [49]. Betschon et al. reported that 53 % of respondents felt exhausted immediately after mobilisation and 13 % felt very exhausted after attending a basic course of Kinaesthetics (no absolute numbers provided) [45]. As aforementioned no comparative values were available, so that an interpretation of these results is difficult. After an implementation of Kinaesthetics, 52.8 % of the participants stated a high degree of physical relief for the lumbar spine (a value of 8 to 10 on a 10-point-scale with "1" meaning no "physical relief") in the evaluation study of Buge and Mahler [50]. Overall, in all but two intervention studies a reduction of perceived exertion due to Kinaesthetics was observed [45, 57].

Perceived exertion/physical loads—Qualitative study

Participating family members in the qualitative study of Huth et al. noticed a reduction of physical work load due to Kinaesthetics [55]. They also mentioned that due to handling of a family member with Kinaesthetics, lifting and carrying can be avoided.

Perceived exertion/physical loads—Reviews

The systematic review of Sedlak-Emperer included six studies that suggest the spine-gentle aspects of Kinasthetics [56] and the included studies in the review of Steinwidder and Lohrmann showed a lowered physical load due to Kinaesthetics (especially of the spine) [54].

Discussion

To date, only little evidence about the influence of Kinaesthetics of very low quality exists. Based on the results of included studies, it might be assumed that Kinaesthetics could reduce the perceived exertion during patient handling especially for the lower back and could decrease musculoskeletal pain in general and during patient handling activities in persons who handle patients. An overestimation of the results is likely due to the inadequate methodology of studies. A selection bias is existent in most intervention studies, since convenience sampling occurred. Possibly more participants that had a positive attitude towards Kinaesthetics attended. Further, the power of all included intervention studies is questionable due to low sample sizes.

The systematic review of Sedlak-Emperer comprised seven of the ten intervention studies that were included in this scoping review [46–52]. Most of these studies dealt with the outcome of perceived exertion of nursing staff and were also included in this review, but only two studies dealt with musculoskeletal complaints of nursing staff [52, 58], of which one could not be retrieved for this scoping review [58]. Results of this systematic review are in line with the results of this scoping review concerning the decrease of perceived exertion and the musculoskeletal pain of nursing personnel due to Kinaesthetics [56]. Of the included studies in the narrative review of Steinwidder and Lohrmann [54] only one study met the inclusion criteria of this scoping review and hence was included [48].

Kinaesthetics shall also impact patients, not only persons who handle patients. But this was not the focus of this scoping review. Some of the included studies also evaluated parameters of patients [47, 49–52], but reported only few effects due to Kinaesthetics.

Concerning the methodological quality of included studies, most studies were judged as "high risk of bias" in regard to "Reporting quality", "Internal validity" and "External validity". "Reporting quality" was insufficient in seven studies, because important study information such as details about the population, intervention or outcome measures was not provided. Most studies had bias (or systematic error) in regard to study conduct and study analysis, thus were of "high risk of bias" for "Internal validity". Important methodological aspects were not fulfilled in the intervention studies (e.g. randomisation, concealed allocation, blinding) and reviews (e.g. use of a second reviewer). Most of the results of included studies seem not to endure under other circumstances (e.g. population, setting) than applied in the individual studies and were therefore rated as "high risk of bias" for "External validity". Even though results of the qualitative study of Huth et al. could eventually be transferred to care situations of other caregiving family members, it was decided not to assess "External validity" of this study design due to aforementioned reasons.

Only six of the 13 identified studies were indexed in the searched electronic databases (of which four were found with the electronic literature search). Further nine studies were found by hand search ($n = 6$) and via Google scholar ($n = 3$).

Only studies from Europe, mainly from German speaking countries, were included. It seems that the use of this nursing intervention is distributed primarily in these countries, since literature and training courses about Kinaesthetics are widely spread in Germany [32] and the European Kinaesthetics association comprises amongst few others the country organizations of Germany, Switzerland and Austria [2].

The comparability between the included studies is questionable, since different kinds of interventions (basic course of Kinaesthetics, implementation of Kinaesthetics, and execution of specific patient handling tasks with Kinaesthetics) different study designs, different types of patients and different outcome measures were applied.

It should be noted critically that a standardization of such an individual nursing method like Kinaesthetics is very difficult to ensure [61]. Further, the concept is a complex intervention [62], and not just a simple transfer and lifting technique [5].

One influencing factor of the effectiveness of Kinaesthetics in daily practice is its challenging implementation into the clinical setting [40]. Thus, various supporting respectively inhibiting factors should be taken into account, such as a good team that is willing and motivated to implement the concept, the conduct of case discussions, workshops and practical guidance or evident success respectively lack of time, rejection of the concept or fear of innovation [5, 40, 62, 63]. Training of Kinaesthetics is furthermore of little benefit if it isn't integrated into the organizational framework of a healthcare facility [5, 28], since focusing exclusively on knowledge transfer does not meet the complexity of the implementation process [63].

Based on the findings of this scoping review, the conduct of a subsequent systematic review for our research question is not indicated, since finding further relevant studies is not expected (due to the excessive search strategy of this scoping review).

One resulting research gap is the lack of high-quality research about the clinical effectiveness of Kinaesthetics in preventing musculoskeletal disorders among persons who handle patients. Thus, high-quality intervention studies, in form of cluster-randomized trials or randomized controlled trials in different settings with different health care workers, are needed to fill this research gap.

Strengths and weaknesses of the review

This is the first comprehensive overview of evidence (conducted as a scoping review) about the influence of Kinaesthetics on persons who handle patients with the same systematic and rigorous methodology used in systematic reviews that used two independent reviewers during the whole review procedure and included qualitative studies as well as reviews, in contrast to the reviews of Sedlak-Emperer [56] or Steinwidder and Lohrmann [54].

The extensive and sensitive search strategy using various sources was useful in identifying many grey literature studies about the influence of Kinaesthetics on persons who handle patients (especially hand search and Google scholar search).

Despite the heterogeneity of study designs, three main categories of methodology (reporting quality, internal validity, external validity) of each study (design) were evaluated independently by two reviewers, to ensure comparability of methodological quality of all included studies. Since this approach was utilized for the first time, no validity and reliability values are available. Even though, critical appraisal of included studies in scoping reviews was initially not intended [12, 13], later methodology papers recommend it [14, 64]. But, none of these methodology papers addressed the problem of appraisal and simultaneous comparison of different kinds of study designs.

Synthesis of study results was not possible due to heterogeneity of included studies. In general, study results of included studies are not synthesized, but summarized descriptively in scoping reviews [12–14].

Influence of the Kinaesthetics care conception during patient handling on the development...

49

Conclusions

The propagated positive effects of Kinaesthetics can only be assumed according to the findings of this scoping review. Kinaesthetics seems to decrease the perceived exertion and musculoskeletal pain of persons who handle patients. But since most included studies are of poor methodological quality an overestimation of these effects is likely. As a result, no clear recommendations about the effectiveness of Kinaesthetics on persons who handle patients can be made yet. Since a research gap was shown for the effectiveness of Kinaesthetics on persons who handle patients, further high quality intervention studies are necessary for clarifying this issue.

Abbreviations

AF: Alice Freiberg; AN: Albert Nienhaus; AS: Andreas Seidler; AMED: The Allied and Complementary Medicine Database; CASP: Critical Appraisal Skills Programmes; CINAHL: Cumulative Index to Nursing and Allied Health Literature; DNEbM: German Network for Evidence-based Medicine; e.g.: exempli gratia; EMBASE: Excerpta Medica Database; et al.: et alii; etc.: et cetera; i.e.: id est; JS: Julia Scharfe; MEDLINE: Medical Literature Analysis and Retrieval System Online; MG: Maria Girbig; n: number; p: p-value; PICOS: population, intervention, comparison, outcome, study design; PRISMA: Preferred Reporting Items for Systematic Reviews and Meta-Analyses; PROSPERO: International Register of systematic reviews; SF: Sonja Freitag; SLUB: Saxon State and University Library Dresden; UE: Ulrike Euler; 95%CI: 95 % confidence interval.

Competing interests

The authors declare that they have no competing interests.

Authors' contribution

Development of study design and conduct: AF, MG, UE, AS. Participation in study design and conduct: AN, SF. Coordination of study conduct: AF. Title-/ abstract screening: AF, UE. Full text screening and data extraction: AF, MG, UE. Quality appraisal: AF, MG, JS. Data analysis and interpretation: AF, MG, UE. Support in data analysis and interpretation: JS, AN, SF, AS. Draft of the manuscript: AF. Support in draft of the manuscript: MG, UE, JS, AN, SF, AS. All authors read and approved the final manuscript.

Acknowledgements

We acknowledge support by the German Research Foundation and the Open Access Publication Funds of the TU Dresden.

Funding

This study was funded by the German Social Accident Insurance Institution for the Health and Welfare Services (BGW).

Author details

[1]Institute and Policlinic of Occupational and Social Medicine, Medical Faculty Carl Gustav Carus, Technische Universität Dresden, Fetscherstr. 74, Dresden 01307, Germany. [2]Department of Occupational Health Research, German Social Accident Insurance Institution for the Health and Welfare Service, Pappelallee 33-37, Hamburg 22089, Germany. [3]Institute for Health Service Research in Dermatology and Nursing, University Clinics Hamburg Eppendorf, Martinistr. 52, Hamburg 20246, Germany.

References

1. Hatch F, Maietta L. Kinaesthetics. Health development and human activity [German]. 2nd ed. München: Urban & Fischer; 2003.
2. EKA: What is Kinaesthetics? [German]. Linz, Austria: European Kinaesthetics Association; 2008.
3. Schlegel R. Kinesthesia in palliative care. Better quality of life at the end of life. Krankenpfl Soins Infirm. 2012;105(4):15–7.
4. Moltmann E, Witt M. Counseling and guidance exemplified by kinesthetic mobilization: knowledge fosters safety. Pflege Z. 2005;58(7):430–1.
5. Enke A. Aspects of introduction of kinesthetics in organizations: "maintaining movement". Pflege Z. 2009;62(9):534–7.
6. Hofmann F, Stossel U, Michaelis M, Nubling M, Siegel A. Low back pain and lumbago-sciatica in nurses and a reference group of clerks: results of a comparative prevalence study in Germany. Int Arch Occup Environ Health. 2002;75(7):484–90.
7. Schneider S, Lipinski S, Schiltenwolf M. Occupations associated with a high risk of self-reported back pain: representative outcomes of a back pain prevalence study in the Federal Republic of Germany. Eur Spine J. 2006;15(6):821–33.
8. Davis KG, Kotowski SE. Prevalence of musculoskeletal disorders for nurses in hospitals, long-term care facilities, and home health care: a comprehensive review. Hum Factors. 2015;57(5):754–92.
9. Menzel NN, Brooks SM, Bernard TE, Nelson A. The physical workload of nursing personnel: association with musculoskeletal discomfort. Int J Nurs Stud. 2004;41(8):859–67.
10. Yassi A, Lockhart K. Work-relatedness of low back pain in nursing personnel: a systematic review. Int J Occup Environ Health. 2013;19(3):223–44.
11. Schmucker C, Motschall E, Antes G, Meerpohl JJ. Methods of evidence mapping [German]. Bundesgesundheitsbl Gesundheitsforsch Gesundheitsschutz. 2013;56(10):1390–7.
12. Levac D, Colquhoun H, O'Brien KK. Scoping studies: advancing the methodology. Implement Sci. 2010;5:69.
13. Arksey H, O'Malley L. Scoping studies: towards a methodological framework. Int J Soc Res Methodol. 2005;8(1):19–32.
14. Daudt HM, van Mossel C, Scott SJ. Enhancing the scoping study methodology: a large, inter-professional team's experience with Arksey and O'Malley's framework. BMC Med Res Methodol. 2013;13:48.
15. Armstrong R, Hall BJ, Doyle J, Waters E. Cochrane Update. 'Scoping the scope' of a cochrane review. J Public Health (Oxf). 2011;33(1):147–50.
16. Moher D, Liberati A, Tetzlaff J, Altman DG. Preferred reporting items for systematic reviews and meta-analyses: the PRISMA statement. Ann Intern Med. 2009;151(4):264–9.
17. Freiberg A, Euler U, Girbig M, Nienhaus A, Freitag S, Seidler A. Influence of the kinaesthetics care conception on the development of musculoskeletal complaints and diseases among persons who regularly conduct patient handling activities. PROSPERO. 2015. CRD42015015811. http://www.crd.york.ac.uk/PROSPERO/display_record.asp?ID=CRD42015015811.
18. Cohen J. A coefficient of agreement for nominal scales. Educ Psychol Meas. 1960;20(1):37–46.
19. Downs SH, Black N. The feasibility of creating a checklist for the assessment of the methodological quality both of randomised and non-randomised studies of health care interventions. J Epidemiol Community Health. 1998;52(6):377–84.
20. CASP (2014): CASP Checklists. Critical Appraisal Skills Programm (CASP). Oxford. [http://www.casp-uk.net/]
21. Higgins JPT, Green S. Cochrane Handbook for Systematic Reviews of Interventions Version 5.1.0 [updated March 2011]. The Cochrane Collaboration. 2011.
22. DNEbM (2011): Glossary about Evidence-based Medicine [German]. German Network for Evidence-based Medicine. [http://www.ebm-netzwerk.de/was-ist-ebm/images/dnebm-glossar-2011.pdf]
23. Fletcher RH, Fletcher SW, Wagner EH, Haerting J. Clinical Epidemiology: Principles and applications [German]. Wiesbaden: Ullstein Medical; 1999.
24. Mayring P. On Generalization in Qualitative Research. Forum Social Research. 2007;8(3). http://www.qualitative-research.net/index.php/fqs/article/view/291/639.
25. Tong A, Sainsbury P, Craig J. Consolidated criteria for reporting qualitative research (COREQ): a 32-item checklist for interviews and focus groups. International J Qual Health Care. 2007;19(6):349–57.
26. N.N. Part one: A description of patient/client management. Chapter 2. Sensory integrity (including proprioception and kinesthesia). Phys Ther. 1997;77(11):1211.
27. Asmussen-Clausen M, Knobel S. Versatility can be learned. Krankenpfl Soins Infirm. 2010;103(3):18–9.
28. Betschon E. With better health a longer career. Krankenpfl Soins Infirm. 2012;105(10):24–6.
29. Betschon E, Brach M, Hantikainen V. Studying feasibility and effects of a two-stage nursing staff training in residential geriatric care using a 30 month mixed-methods design [ISRCTN24344776]. BMC Nurs. 2011;10(1):10.

30. Darmann I. Movement as interaction–systemic-constructivist approach to movement and consequences for nursing care. Pflege. 2002;15(5):181–6.

31. Hantikainen V. Kinaesthetics: understanding human movement processes and their effective use in care practice contribute to rehabilitative approach [Finnish]. Sairaanhoitaja. 2007;80(11):27–30.

32. Heyn M. Back sparing job performance using kinesthetic principles. Tilting, pushing, pulling. Pflege Z. 2012;65(12):734–7.

33. Kirchner E. Promoting physical activity in nursing: recognizing and using the health potentials of patients. Pflege Z. 2007;60(8):430–3.

34. Leufgen M. Discovering physical action possibilities. Kinesthesia in routine nursing. Pflege Z. 2011;64(2):89–93.

35. Mensdorf B. Mobilization of an immobile patient: kinesthetics activates patient resources and spares the nurses. Pflege Z. 1999;52(7):487–91.

36. Mensdorf B. Step by step to nursing care competence-8: patient mobilization: with as little effort as possible to achieve the goal. Pflege Z. 2007;60(12):691–4.

37. Schiller B. Kinesthesis: a basic course, especially for parents with bodily impaired children and pediatric nurses. Kinderkrankenschwester. 2002;21(8): 351–2.

38. Schmidt S. What is kinesthetics in nursing? Krankenpflege (Frankf). 1990; 44(3):145–8.

39. Christen L, Scheidegger J, Grossenbacher G, Christen S, Oehninger R. Experiences and results from standardised observations of conventional and kinaesthetic nursing in a nuclear and radio-therapeutic ward [German]. Pflege. 2005;18(1):25–37.

40. Fringer A, Huth M, Hantikainen V. Nurses' experiences with the implementation of the Kinaesthetics movement competence training into elderly nursing care: a qualitative focus group study. Scand J Caring Sci. 2014;28(4):757–66.

41. Kean S. Effects on oxygen saturation levels of handling premature infants within the concepts of kinaesthetic infant handling: pilot study. Intensive Crit Care Nurs. 1999;15(4):214–25.

42. Muller K, Schwesig R, Leuchte S, Riede D. Coordinative treatment and quality of life - a randomised trial of nurses with back pain. Gesundheitswesen. 2001;63(10):609–18.

43. Rudiger D. Early mobilization of patients with increased intracranial pressure: kinesthetics for the benefit of patients and nurses. Pflege Z. 2005;58(4):214–6.

44. Hantikainen V, Tamminen-Peter L, Stenholm S, Arve S. Does the nurses' skills in Kinaesthetics influence to the physical strain on the nurses? Preliminary results. J Anästh Intensiv Behandlung. 2005;1:150–3.

45. Betschon E, Weber H, Lehmann G, Hantikainen V. At the pace of the residents. Krankenpfl Soins Infirm. 2014;107(10):13–5.

46. Christen L, Scheidegger J, Grossenbacher G, Christen S, Oehninger R. Qualitative and quantitative comparison of physical and mental state during nursing before and after a basic introduction into kinesthetic nursing in a nuclear and radio-therapeutic clinic [German]. Pflege. 2002;15(3):103–11.

47. Eisenschink AM, Kirchner E, Bauder-Mißbach H, Loy S, Kron M. The effect of kinaesthetic mobilization compared to standard mobilization on respiratory function with post-op patients after aortal coronary bypass surgery. Pflege. 2003;16(4):205–15.

48. Tamminen-Peter L. New patient transfer methods better for nurses and patients. Sairaanhoitaja. 2006;79(6-7):18–20.

49. Maietta L, Resch-Kröll U. MH-Kinaesthetics promotes employees' health [German]. Die Schwester Der Pfleger. 2009;48(4):1–5.

50. Buge R, Mahler C. Evaluation report - Evaluation of the survey about the Kinaesthetics project. Heidelberg: University Hospital Heidelberg; 2004.

51. Lenker M. Result of the pilot study Kinaesthetics – Less pain during handling of "critically ill patients" [German]. Intensiv. 2008;16(02):95–101.

52. Rettenberger K, Schoenemeier T. Healthy living–and the working world of the clinic. Pflege Aktuell. 2005;59:154–7.

53. Friess-Ott G, Muller UM. Kinesthetics–an economical nursing concept? Colleagues evaluate the introduction positively. Pflege Z. 2006;59(2):110–3.

54. Steinwidder G. The support of movements with Kinaesthetics by nursing staff for adult patients with movement restrictions [German]. Osterr Pflegezeitschrift. 2008;05/06:10–4.

55. Huth M. The benefit of Kinaesthetics training for handling the caregiving situation at home – The perspective of family members [German]. Pflegewissenschaft. 2013;15(11):586–99.

56. Sedlak-Emperer M: The effect of Kinaesthetics on nursing staff, patients and hospital organisation. A systematic literature analysis. Diploma thesis. Vienna, Austria: Universität Wien; 2012.

57. Hock-Rummelhardt C: Effect and efficacy of a Kinaesthetics program on nursing staff. Diploma thesis. Vienna, Austria: Universität Wien; 2013.

58. Burns E, Sailer G: Efficiency and health development in nursing with Kinaesthetics: Project at the hospital Hietzing with neurologic centre Rosenhügel of the city Vienna [German]. Pressbaum; 2007.

59. Scheidegger J: Systematic application of health promoting and health maintaining care measures - Final report hospital Witikon [German]. Edited by Oehninger R, Wettstein A. Zürich: Krankenpflegeschule Zürich; 1999.

60. Landis JR, Koch GG. The measurement of observer agreement for categorical data. Biometrics. 1977;33(1):159–74.

61. Haasenritter J, Eisenschink AM, Kirchner E, Bauder-Mißbach H, Brach M, Veith J, Sander S, Panfil E-M. Effects of a preoperative movement training program with the for kinaesthic mobilisation composed Viv-Arte-learning model on mobility, pain and postoperative dwell time in patients with elective median laparotomy [German]. Pflege. 2009;22(1):19–28.

62. Behncke A, Balzer K, Köpke S: Scientific monitoring of the implementation of Kinaesthetics [German]. In 15th Annual meeting of the German Network for Evidence-based Medicine: 2014; Haale (Saale). 2014.

63. Arnold D. But to put it into practice is difficult: A qualitative study of the theory-practice-transfer in nursing using the example of Kinaesthetics [German]. Pflege. 2000;13(1):53–63.

64. Davis K, Drey N, Gould D. What are scoping studies? A review of the nursing literature. Int J Nurs Stud. 2009;46(10):1386–400.

7

An etiologic prediction model incorporating biomarkers to predict the bladder cancer risk associated with occupational exposure to aromatic amines

Giuseppe Mastrangelo[1], Angela Carta[2,3], Cecilia Arici[2,3], Sofia Pavanello[1*] and Stefano Porru[3,4]

Abstract

Background: No etiological prediction model incorporating biomarkers is available to predict bladder cancer risk associated with occupational exposure to aromatic amines.

Methods: Cases were 199 bladder cancer patients. Clinical, laboratory and genetic data were predictors in logistic regression models (full and short) in which the dependent variable was 1 for 15 patients with aromatic amines related bladder cancer and 0 otherwise. The receiver operating characteristics approach was adopted; the area under the curve was used to evaluate discriminatory ability of models.

Results: Area under the curve was 0.93 for the full model (including age, smoking and coffee habits, DNA adducts, 12 genotypes) and 0.86 for the short model (including smoking, DNA adducts, 3 genotypes). Using the "best cut-off" of predicted probability of a positive outcome, percentage of cases correctly classified was 92% (full model) against 75% (short model). Cancers classified as "positive outcome" are those to be referred for evaluation by an occupational physician for etiological diagnosis; these patients were 28 (full model) or 60 (short model). Using 3 genotypes instead of 12 can double the number of patients with suspect of aromatic amine related cancer, thus increasing costs of etiologic appraisal.

Conclusions: Integrating clinical, laboratory and genetic factors, we developed the first etiologic prediction model for aromatic amine related bladder cancer. Discriminatory ability was excellent, particularly for the full model, allowing individualized predictions. Validation of our model in external populations is essential for practical use in the clinical setting.

Keywords: Urinary bladder neoplasms, Occupational exposure, Risk, Logistic models, ROC curve

Background

Bladder cancer (BC) accounts for 5–10% of all malignancies among males in Europe and USA [1]. The most important risk factors are smoking, genetic susceptibility and occupational exposure [2].

An excess BC risk was identified since the early 1950s in the rubber industry and was associated to the use of b-naphthylamine [3]. Small excesses of BC risk have continued to be observed even in more recent studies of rubber workers published in the 1980s and 1990s [4]. Other aromatic amines (AAs) have been shown to be carcinogenic [5]. Nonetheless, occupational exposure to AAs has continued due to their industrial and commercial value [6]. AAs exposure can occur at lower extent in many other occupational settings. A systematic review of Italian studies estimated that 4 to 24% of BCs are attributable to occupational exposure [7]. BC cases effectively compensated by INAIL were 440 from 2000 to 2006, on average 63 per year [8]. Because in Italy incident cases of BC in 2006 were about 17,000/ year in males [9], the expected cases of occupational

* Correspondence: sofia.pavanello@unipd.it
[1]Department of Cardiac, Thoracic, and Vascular Sciences, Unit of Occupational Medicine, University of Padova, Via Giustiniani 2 -, 35128 Padova, Italy
Full list of author information is available at the end of the article

disease should be between 680 (17,000×0.04) and 4080 (17,000×0.24), and underreporting between 91% ((63/680) -1) and 98% ((63/4080) -1).

There is a strong genotoxic mechanism for carcinogenicity of several AAs, and multiple metabolic pathways as well as many polymorphic genes have been found to be implicated in the activation of AAs into DNA-reactive intermediates [10]. Over the last 20 years, numerous biomarkers have been investigated in workers exposed to AAs [6]. A key biomarker are the DNA adducts which are considered as the 'biologically effective dose' because they represent an integrated measure of carcinogen exposure, absorption, distribution, metabolism and DNA repair [11].

Few studies have combined clinical factors with blood and urinary biomarkers into risk profiles that can be used to predict the likelihood of etiological diagnosis of BC [12–16]. To the best of our knowledge, no study has tried to use biomarkers to predict the etiological diagnosis of occupational BC. The causal attribution to occupation usually relies on thorough occupational history collection, pertinent and documented risk assessment, availability of industrial hygiene measurements, appraisal and reference to evidence based literature data; to reach etiological diagnosis, the likely best option is to refer patients to occupational health specialists. An etiologic prediction model tool divides an initial population of BC cases into a smaller fraction of 'positives' that should be referred to an occupational health specialist for etiologic assessments, and a larger portion of 'negatives' that should no longer be considered. To be effective, an algorithm should increase the number of single BC cases receiving an etiologic ascertainment cases, therefore leading to a decrease of underreporting and undercompensation; eventually, such actions are beneficial for the individual, as well as for public health.

The aim of the present study was therefore to find a biomarker profile enabling to discriminate AA-related BC from non-AA-related BC and evaluate the algorithm with the approach of Receiver Operator Characteristic (ROC) curves, within the framework of a well-established case-control study on BC.

Methods

Study design and population

The present study includes the "cases" arm stemming from of an earlier hospital-based case-control study fully described in previous publications [17–20]. Inclusion criteria were being male, aged 20–80, Italian. Cases were all 199 newly diagnosed, histologically confirmed BC patients, admitted to the Urology Departments of two large hospitals from 1997 to 2000. Controls were all 214 non-neoplastic urological patients matched to cases by age (±5 years), period and hospital of admission. A

written informed consent was obtained from each subject; the local Ethical Committee approved the study.

Data collection

Peripheral blood lymphocytes (PBLs) were collected and automated DNA extraction was performed according to Extragen kit (Extragen BC by TALENT) [17]. Genotyping of glutathione S-transferase M1 (GSTM1) null, GSTT1 null, GSTP1 I105V, N-acetyltransferase 1 (NAT1) fast, NAT2 slow, cytochrome P450 1B1 (CYP1B1) V432 L, sulfotransferase 1A1 (SULT1A1) R213H, myeloperoxidase (MPO) G-463A, catechol-O-methyltransferase (COMT) V108 M, manganese superoxide dismutase (MnSOD) A-9 V, NAD(P)H:quinone oxidoreductase (NQO1) P187S, X-ray repair cross-complementing group 1 (XRCC1) R399Q, XRCC3 T241 M, and xeroderma pigmentosum complementation group (XPD) K751Q polymorphisms was assessed using Amplification Refractory Mutation System assay [17]. Bulky-DNA adducts were detected by 32P–postlabeling after Nuclease P1 enrichment and labelled adducts resolution on Thin Layer Chromatography (TLC) [20]. DNA adducts levels were measured as relative adduct level per 10^8 nucleotides. A trained interviewer collected information on demographic variables, lifetime smoking history, coffee and other liquid consumption, dietary habits, lifetime occupation history by questionnaire. Job titles and individual activities, as well as occupational exposures to AAs, were blindly coded by an occupational physician according to methodology described in previous publication [21]. Occupations involving exposure to AAs were attributed to 11 International Standard Classification of Occupations (ISCO, International Labour Office, 1968) codes for job tasks (1–61.30: Painter, Artist; 3–70.20: Mail Sorting Clerk; 5–70.30: Barber-Hairdresser; 7–41.40: Mixing- and Blending-Machine Operator, Chemical and Related Processes; 8–01.10: Shoemaker, General; 8–11.20: Cabinetmaker; 8–73.70: Vehicle Sheet-Metal Worker; 9–01.35: Rubber Moulding-Press Operator; 9–31.20: Building Painter; 9–39.20: Brush-Painter, except Construction; 9–39.30: Spray-Painter, except Construction) and 11 International Standard Industrial Classification of all Economic Activities (ISIC, United Nations, 1968) codes for industrial activities (3240: Manufacture of footwear, except vulcanized or moulded rubber or plastic footwear; 3320: Manufacture of furniture and fixtures, except primarily of metal; 3521: Manufacture of paints, varnishes and lacquers; 3559: Manufacture of rubber products not elsewhere classified; 3819: Manufacture of fabricated metal products except machinery and equipment not elsewhere classified; 3824: Manufacture of special industrial machinery and equipment except metal- and wood-working machinery; 3843: Manufacture of motor vehicles; 5000: Construction; 9415: Authors, music composers and other independent artists not elsewhere classified; 9513: Repair of motor vehicles and motorcycles; 9591: Barber and beauty shops).

Best-case definition

We investigated exposure to AA in all jobs held during lifetime, carefully assessing the level and the temporal aspects of such exposure according to standardized procedures [21]. Then, in order to achieve an optimal case definition [22], the critical values for time since first exposure (TSFE) and time since last exposure (TSLE) were chosen based on literature findings. In a cohort of Italian dyestuff workers [23], the risk of BC mortality decreased with increasing TSLE and became non-significant at ≥30 years since last exposure. Out of 19 BC patients observed in a Japanese dyestuff-plant, 17 showed a TSFE ≥20 years and 18 a TSLE ≤35 years [24]. Thus, the criteria for best-case definition were: TSFE higher than 20 years; TSLE lower than 35 years; length of exposure of at least 1 year; any value of cumulative exposure to AAs. The 15 BC cases complying with the above criteria were considered AA-related bladder cancer.

Variables and statistical analyses

Smoking was a categorical variable with three levels: nonsmokers; former smokers from >20 years; current smokers and former smokers from less than 20 years. Life-long time-weighted average of cups/day of coffee and age at diagnosis were broken down in four classes according to the tertiles. DNA adducts were transformed in logarithm, and all values >1 were coded as 1 and otherwise as 0. Genetic biomarkers were coded as 0/1 variables as follows: GSTM1 ("NULL" variant =1, otherwise = 0); GSTP1 ("1A/1A" = 0, otherwise = 1); GSTT1 ("NULL" = 1); NAT1 ("S" = 1); NAT2 ("S" = 1); MPO ("A/A" = 1); COMT ("WW" = 1); MnSOD ("WW" = 1); NQO1 ("MM" = 1); CYP1B1 ("WW" = 0); XRCC1 ("G/G" = 0); XRCC3 ("C/C" = 0); XPD ("A/A" = 0). All the above variables became the predictors in a model of logistic regression in which the dependent variable was 1 for the 15 patients (cases) with AA-related BC (see above) and 0 for the other 184 BC patients (controls). A stepwise selection of independent variables was made using 0.10 as "p-to-enter" and 0.15 as "p-to-remove". Therefore, from the same sample of 199 cases of BC, two algorithms were obtained (full model and short model) reporting for each regressor the OR with 95% CI and p-value. The best fitting model was chosen with measures of predictive power (R-square and area under the ROC curve) and GOF statistics (Pearson chi-square and Hosmer-Lemeshow test). The criterion

was "the higher the better" for the former, and "p-value above 0.05" for the latter. The graphical outputs of the ROC curves were obtained and the AUC was interpreted according to the classification proposed: 0.5 (not informative test); 0.5–0.70 (inaccurate test); 0.7–0.9 (moderately accurate test); 0.9–1.0 (highly accurate test); 1 (perfect diagnostic test) [25]. A statistical test comparing the equality of AUCs was also calculated. Lastly, using the prediction equation we obtained a new variable containing the model-predicted probability of a positive outcome; the same computer program provided the "best cut-off" of predicted probability [26] that maximized the difference between BC patients with or without AA-related disease in both models. Using such value we built the classification table (true positive, false positive, true negative and false negative) from which we calculated sensitivity, specificity, positive and negative predictive values and diagnostic accuracy of each model. Purely statistical measures for comparing two risk prediction models have, however, limited use for medical decision making because they do not incorporate harms and benefits related to treatment decisions arising from the risk prediction model [27]. To evaluate whether clinical use of prediction models, diagnostic tests, and molecular markers would do more good than harm, a simple type of decision analysis (net benefit, NB, approach) has been used [28]. The NB depends on the benefit B, the cost C, the prevalence P of the outcome, and the risk threshold, R, which expresses the model's classification accuracy, that is the ability of the risk model to assign high risks to cases and low risks to controls. The key quantity is R, which is a function of the harms and benefits of the possible outcomes without detailed specification of harms and benefits [29]. Therefore, the NB to the population of using the risk model is:

$$NB_R = (TPR_R \times P) - \left(\left(\frac{R}{1-R} \right) \times FPR_R \times (1-P) \right)$$

where:

TPR_R = true positive rate, also called sensitivity;

FPR_R = false positive rate, also called one minus specificity;

P = probability of diseases at a given time, also called prevalence;

R = risk threshold, also called model-predicted probability of a positive outcome.

Net benefit can be plotted against a range of R, in what is called a "decision curve". Decision curves are now widely used in the literature [28]. In the present study, however, wider effects on NB were observed with variations of P rather than of R.

Sample size

In the present one-sample study, the sample size was estimated based on Fisher's z test assuming a correlation 0.28 (that between DNA adducts and the 0/1 variable "presence/absence of occupational AA-related BC") and a significance level of 0.05. For a two-sided hypothesis test, the estimated sample size was 98 or 130 patients setting the power at 0.80 or 0.90, respectively [30]. The actual number of BC patients was 199. All statistical analyses were performed with STATA 13.

Results

Table 1 shows the main characteristics of BC patients and their distribution by genotypes (only patients with value set at 1 according to the above definitions). Those with disease related to AAs showed higher level of

Table 1 Occupational AA-related BC cases and other BC cases by DNA adducts, age, smoking categories, pack-years, coffee consumption and genotypes

Variables		15 AA-related BC cases		184 other BC cases	
		Mean (SD)	Number (%)	Mean (SD)	Number (%)
DNA adducts×10^8 nucleotides (ln)		1.40 (1.5)		0.76 (1.2)	
	≥1		11 (73.3)		69 (37.5)
Age (years)		60.0 (10.4)		63.4 (11.2)	
	≤ 56.9 years		7 (46.7)		43 (23.4)
	57–65.9 years		3 (20.0)		50 (27.2)
	66–70.9 years		3 (20.0)		44 (23.9)
	≥ 71 years		2 (13.3)		47 (25.5)
Smoking (categories)					
	Non Smokers & Ex Smokers quitting >20 years		2 (13.3)		35 (19.0)
	Ex Smokers quitting <20 years		1 (6.7)		60 (32.6)
	Current smokers		12 (75.0)		87 (47.3)
Pack years (cigarettes smoked lifetime)		31.5 (12.3)		35.6 (26.2)	
	≤ 18.9		1 (6.7)		46 (25.1)
	19–32.9		8 (53.3)		45 (24.6)
	33–46.9		4 (26.7)		46 (24.6)
	≥ 47		2 (13.3)		47 (25.7)
Coffee consumption (weighted mean)		2.1 (1.7)		2.4 (2.4)	
	≤ 1 cup/day		6 (40.0)		71 (38.8)
	2 cups/day		4 (26.7)		36 (19.7)
	3 caps/day		3 (20.0)		32 (17.5)
	≥ 4 cups/day		2 (13.3)		44 (24.0)
Genotypes (legend below)	GSTM1		12 (80.0)		117 (63.9)
	GSTT1		3 (20.0)		38 (20.8)
	GSTP		5 (33.3)		92 (50.3)
	NAT1		4 (26.7)		60 (32.8)
	NAT2		10 (66.7)		111 (60.7)
	MPO		1 (6.7)		6 (3.3)
	COMT		7 (46.7)		132 (72.1)
	MnSOD		4 (26.7)		63 (34.4)
	CYP1B1		12 (80.0)		156 (82.3)
	XRCC1		7 (46.7)		98 (53.4)
	XRCC3		6 (40.0)		103 (56.3)
	XPD		7 (46.7)		113 (61.8)

GSTM1 Glutathione S-transferase M1, GSTT1 Glutathione S-transferase T1, GSTP1 Glutathione S-transferase P1, NAT1 N-acetyltransferase isozymes 1, NAT2 N-acetyltransferase isozymes 2, MPO Myeloperoxidase, MnSOD Manganese Superoxide Dismutase, COMT Catechol-O-methyltransferase, CYP1B1 Cytochrome p450 1B1, XRCC1 X-ray repair cross-complementing protein 1, XRCC3 X-ray repair cross-complementing protein 3, XPD xeroderma pigmentosum group D

adducts, lower mean age (with higher percentage of youngest subjects) and higher number of smokers. Except for *COMT, GSTM1* and *GSTP1* other differences were insignificant.

Table 2 shows the logistic regression analysis obtained with the full and short models (with the subset of predictors chosen by the stepwise selection procedure). As expected from distribution of BC cases, significant ORs were few (DNA adducts and *COMT*) in both models. Nonetheless, measures of predictive power (R-squares and AUCs) were elevated. The full model seemed more performing, although both models passed the test and were correctly specified.

Figure 1 shows the ROC curves obtained for the full and short model; the AUC and its standard error is also reported. A chi-square test comparing the two AUCs gave a value of 4.0438, with $p = 0.0443$, suggesting that including more variables (algorithm 1) could significantly improve the prediction (e.g. probabilities of occupational AA-related BC). The ROC area of model 1 (= 0.931) fell in the category of highly accurate tests; however, the cost of such high diagnostic accuracy was entering the algorithm 12 genotypes together with DNA adducts and some clinical factors.

Table 3 shows the 15 AA-related BC cases and 184 non-AA-related BC cases, classified as positive and

Table 2 Logistic regression (full and short models)

Variables	Classes	Full model			Short model		
		OR	95% CI	p-value	OR	95% CI	p-value
Age (years)[a]	57–65.9	0.12	0.01–0.98	0.048			
	66–70.9	0.29	0.04–2.25	0.239			
	≥ 71	0.10	0.01–1.07	0.056			
Smoking[b]	Ex-smokers	0.05	0.00–1.47	0.083	0.11	0.01–1.49	0.096
	Smokers	1.16	0.16–8.60	0.887	1.56	0.31–7.94	0.589
Coffee consumption[c]	2	0.63	0.09–4.64	0.654			
	3	1.96	0.27–14.24	0.505			
	≥4	0.05	0.00–0.86	0.039			
DNA adducts[d]	≥1	19.20	2.52–146.	0.004	6.02	1.66–21.8	0.006
Genotypes[e]	*GSTM1*	3.01	0.51–17.7	0.223			
	GSTT1	0.29	0.04–1.92	0.198			
	GSTP1	0.19	0.03–1.08	0.061	0.41	0.12–1.38	0.150
	NAT1	0.27	0.05–1.52	0.139			
	NAT2	2.55	0.52–12.6	0.25			
	MPO	1.38	0.03–65.1	0.871			
	COMT	0.05	0.01–0.39	0.005	0.21	0.06–0.72	0.014
	MnSOD	0.30	0.06–1.49	0.142			
	CYP1B1	0.27	0.03–2.42	0.24			
	XRCC1	0.97	0.22–4.22	0.966			
	XRCC3	0.38	0.09–1.68	0.203	0.40	0.12–1.34	0.139
	XPD	0.31	0.05–1.81	0.195			
Constant term		5.95	0.06–545.	0.439	0.18	0.03–1.30	0.09

Reference groups: [a]patients with ≤56.9 years; [b]non smokers and ex-smokers from >20 years; [c]patients with consumption of ≤1 cup/day; [d]patients with <1 (logarithm values) of DNA adducts×10^8 nucleotides; [e]patients with genotype values set at 0 (see text for definition).

Measures of fit for logistic regression		Full model	Short model
R-square		0.389	0.228
Area under the ROC curve		0.931	0.856
Pearson chi-square test:	p-value	0.087	0.826
	no. covariates	197	44
Hosmer-Lemeshow test:	p-value	0.130	0.942
	no. groups	10	10

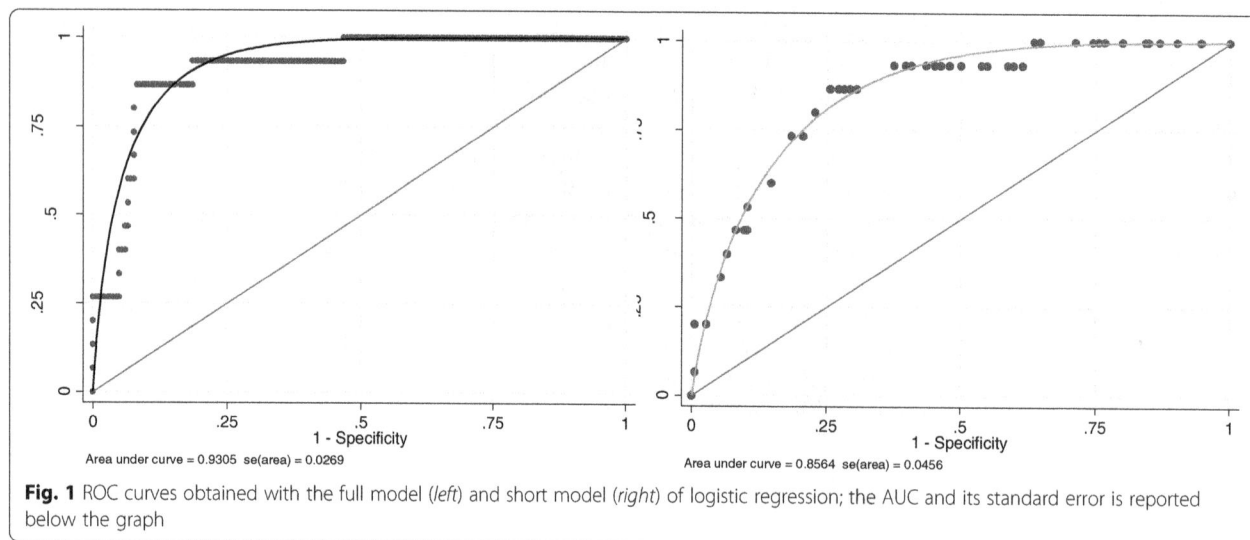

Fig. 1 ROC curves obtained with the full model (*left*) and short model (*right*) of logistic regression; the AUC and its standard error is reported below the graph

negative according to the full or short model, always using the "best cut-off" of predicted probability provided by computer program to maximize the difference between BC patients with or without AA-related disease. With respect to the full model, the short one reduced the percentage of cases correctly classified (150/ 199 = 75% against 182/199 = 92%) by decreasing specificity (137/184 = 75% versus 169/184 = 92%). BC cases classified as 'positive' are those to be referred for evaluation by an occupational physician for etiological diagnosis; these patients were 28 (full model) or 60 (short model). Therefore, using 3 instead of 12 genotypes can double the number of patients to be referred for etiologic diagnosis. BC cases classified as 'negative' should be leaved out from etiologic workup. Since the negative predictive value was about 99% (169/171 according to the full model and 137/139 according to the short model), the model may be used to identify patients who can carefully avoid further evaluation. The other

side of the coin was that two out of 15 true AA-related BC patients were classified as 'false negative' cases, which like the 'true negatives' should not undergo etiologic assessment of their disease. The NB per 100 patients was +4.9 and +4.1 in the left and right panel, respectively, when using panel-specific sensitivity, one minus specificity and the risk threshold R, along with the prevalence of AA-related BC, which was always 0.0754 (= 15/199). Comparing the left and right panel, values of NB were close in spite of divergent values of R.

Table 4 shows the results of a different strategy in which we purposely reduced the "best cut-off" of predicted probability supplied by computer program in order to reduce the false negatives (1 in place of 2). The cost balancing the benefit (decrease of false negatives and increase of true positives) was a higher number of positives (from 28 to 48 with full algorithm; from 60 to 87 with short algorithm) requiring referral to an occupational physician. The NB per 100

Table 3 Classification of 15 AA-related BC cases (D) and 184 other BC cases (−D) according to the full model (left panel) or short model (right panel) of logistic regression

Classified	True		Total	Classified	True		Total
	D	−D			D	−D	
Positive	13	15	28	Positive	13	47	60
Negative	2	169	171	Negative	2	137	139
Total	15	184	199	Total	15	184	199
Sensitivity			86.7%	Sensitivity			86.7%
Specificity			91.9%	Specificity			74.5%
Positive predictive value			46.4%	Positive predictive value			21.7%
Negative predictive value			98.8%	Negative predictive value			98.6%
Correctly classified			91.5%	Correctly classified			75.4%
Net Benefit per 100 patients			+4.9	Net Benefit per 100 patients			+ 4.1

The risk threshold R (optimal cut-off point of predicted probability provided by the program) was 0.181 and 0.093 in the left and right panel, respectively. Net Benefit per 100 patients calculated from the above values

Table 4 Classification of 15 AA-related BC cases (D) and 184 other BC cases (–D) according to the full model (left panel) or short model (right panel) of logistic regression

Classified	True		Total	Classified	True		Total
	D	–D			D	–D	
Positive	14	34	48	Positive	14	73	87
Negative	1	150	151	Negative	1	111	112
Total	15	184	199	Total	15	184	199
Sensitivity			93.3%	Sensitivity			93.3%
Specificity			81.5%	Specificity			60.3%
Positive predictive value			29.2%	Positive predictive value			16.1%
Negative predictive value			99.3%	Negative predictive value			99.1%
Correctly classified			82.4%	Correctly classified			62.8%
Net Benefit per 100 patients			+ 5.3	Net Benefit per 100 patients			+ 5.1

The risk threshold R (purposely chosen cut-off point of predicted probability) was 0.09 and 0.05 in the left and right panel, respectively. Net Benefit per 100 patients calculated from the above values

patients was +5.3 and +5.1 in the left and right panel, respectively, when using panel-specific sensitivity, one minus specificity and the risk threshold R, along with the prevalence of AA-related BC, which was always 0.0754 (= 15/199). Comparing the left and right panel, values of NB were close in spite of the divergent values of R.

The little effect on NB with variations of R is also shown in Fig. 2, which depicts NBs as squares and hollow squares (corresponding to R values of 0.181 and 0.093, respectively, see Table 3), or as circles and hollow circles (corresponding to R values of 0.090 and 0.050, respectively, see Table 4). By contrast wider differences and a steep increasing trend of NBs were found with prevalence of AA-related BC going from 0.0 to about 0.14. When prevalence approaches to 0.0, the sign of NBs became negative indicating costs that overwhelm benefits.

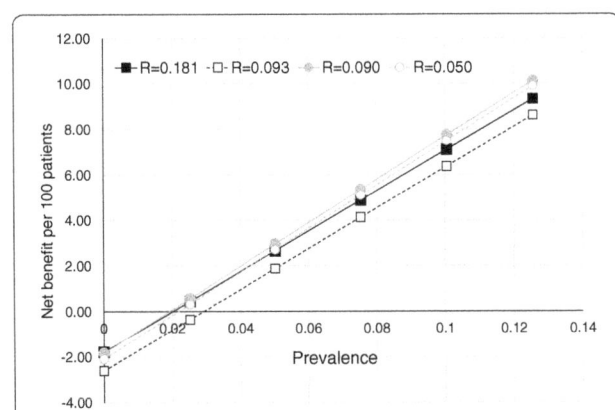

Fig. 2 Decision curves of Net Benefit per 100 patients against different values of prevalence of AA-related BC, separately according to different values of risk threshold (R), i.e. cut-off point of predicted probability

Discussion

With the aim of finding a biomarker profile enabling to discriminate AA-related BC from non-AA-related BC, an etiologic prediction model was developed integrating 12 genotypes, DNA adducts, age, smoking and coffee consumption, while using 15 AA-related BC cases. The procedure classified the whole 199 BC patients in 28 positives and 171 negatives. The latter could be leaved out from etiologic workup, the former are those to be referred for etiological diagnosis. The cases correctly classified were 92% (182/199) and the discriminatory ability was excellent (AUC = 0.93). Examining 3 rather than 12 genotypes the cost of etiologic assessment increased because 60 (instead of 28) positives should receive a further testing (see Table 3, left and right panel). Nevertheless, there were two false negative cases. To overcome this detrimental outcome we used a second strategy (a lower risk threshold) that involved 1 false negative in place of 2 but increased the cost of diagnostic workup since the positives became 48 (instead of 28) or 87 (instead of 60) according to the full or short model, respectively (see Table 4, left and right panel). With the second strategy, despite the lower percentage of cases correctly classified and regardless of AUC reduction to values (0.7 to 0.9) indicating a moderately accurate test, the benefits were higher than the costs, as it can be seen by comparing the values of NB reported in the Tables 3 and 4.

In our earlier study [20], occupational AAs exposure was found to be positively associated with both BC risk ($p = 0.041$) and DNA adducts ($p = 0.028$). Since they were not associated with BC risk, DNA adducts were likely biomarkers of exposure. However, the responsible electrophilic substance could not be identified because adducts detected by the nuclease P1 method of 32P–post-labeling are not specific.

As shown in Table 2, many genotypes have given partial regression coefficients (namely, logarithms of ORs) that are not statistically significant. Each could be eliminated without significantly affecting the measures of fit for logistic regression, while the suppression of the whole set had a major effect. In fact, AUC of 0.931 for the full model reduced to 0.69 by entering DNA adducts as single predictor in the logistic regression. This occurs when the variables are strongly related to one another; if one is eliminated the other variables of the group act as substitutes. If, however, the entire group is removed do not remain other variables to compensate the lack of them [31]. In view of the above, we considered all regressors to obtain the predicted probability of a positive outcome, even though it can become difficult to attribute a meaning to each partial regression coefficient.

The etiologic prediction model tool that we have elaborated, enables to divide an initial population into a smaller fraction of "positives" and a larger portion of "negatives". The former could be referred for further diagnostic assessments, the latter should be no longer considered. The "diagnosis" consists in attributing the disease to an exposure/occupational risk factor; this may happen or might be necessary in several context, such as individual case appraisal, compensation claims, litigation, health authority enquiries. Attributing the disease to an exposure/occupational risk factor may result in several advantages from clinical, epidemiological, individual and public health standpoints. Unfortunately, underreporting to health authorities and under compensation of occupational cancers are well known facts [32–34]. The latter evidence strengthens the need to adopt the second strategy aimed at increase as much as possible the identification of AA-related BC cases.

All BC patients are hospitalized at some point in time. Hospital physicians might then face two alternatives when dealing with a tumor, such as BC, with significant incidence and prevalence and with relevant attributable fraction of occupational risk factors: seeking for advice by an occupational health specialist for the patients or manage the case by themselves. A non-selective application of etiologic workup and appraisal would however results in a great loss of clinical and preventive opportunities. In addition to traditional methodology of etiological diagnosis, a reliable option could therefore be the tool described in this paper that enables discrimination of BC patients with high probability of occupational BC. However, attention should be paid to the underlying risk factors of AA-related bladder cancer. The greater the local degree of industrial development, the higher the chance of occurrence of an occupational disease, and the better the net benefit of using the tool that we have elaborated to ascertain this disease (see Fig. 2).

Validation of model in an external population is an essential next step towards practical use in the clinical setting. External validation requires a multicenter cohort and a prospective collection of data. At the end of the study, the individual characteristics of the validation cohort are multiplied by the regression coefficients of the corresponding variables (those obtained in the internal population) and the products are added to the constant term of the logistic regression. This value quantifies the individual predicted probability of having an AA-related BC. Subsequently, calibration plots are used to graphically explore the association between predicted probabilities and observed proportions: the points should be centered along a 45-degree line in the graph [12].

Conclusions

BC cases with occupational AA-related disease can be individually assessed and stratified based on a predefined molecular biomarker profile. This tool can help ranking BC patients for referrals to an occupational physician for etiologic workup and appraisal. However, practical use in the clinical setting requires validation of the model in another population.

Abbreviations
Aas: Aromatic Amines; BC: Bladder Cancer; COMT: Catechol-O-Methyltransferase; CYP1B1: Cytochrome P450 1B1; FPR_R: False positive rate, also called one minus specificity; GSTM1: Glutathione S-Transferase M1 Null; GSTP1: Glutathione S-Transferase P1; GSTT1: Glutathione S-Transferase T1 Null; INAIL: Istituto Nazionale Assicurazione Infortuni Sul Lavoro; ISCO: International Standard Classification Of Occupations; Mnsod: Manganese Superoxide Dismutase; MPO: Myeloperoxidase; NAT1: N-Acetyltransferase 1; NB: Net Benefit; NQO1: NAD(P)H:Quinone Oxidoreductase; P: Probability of diseases at a given time, also called prevalence; Pbls: Peripheral Blood Lymphocytes; R: Risk threshold, also called model-predicted probability of a positive outcome; ROC: Receiver Operator Characteristic; SULT1A1: Sulfotransferase 1A1; TLC: Thin Layer Chromatography; TPR_R: True positive rate, also called sensitivity; TSFE: Time Since First Exposure; TSLE: Time Since Last Exposure; XPD: Xeroderma Pigmentosum Complementation Group; XRCC1: X-Ray Repair Cross-Complementing Group 1; XRCC3: X-Ray Repair Cross-Complementing Group 3

Acknowledgements
None.

Funding
None.

Authors' contributions
All authors have a substantial contributions to the conception or design of the work; or the acquisition, analysis, or interpretation of data for the work; Drafting the work or revising it critically for important intellectual content; Final approval of the version to be published; Agreement to be accountable for all aspects of the work in ensuring that questions related to the accuracy or integrity of any part of the work are appropriately investigated and resolved. Moreover, SP, AC and CA have a substantial contributions in subject enrollment, physical examination, interview with structured questionnaires, Ethics Committee application. SP and GM in Laboratory analysis and stastistics. All authors read and approved the final manuscript.

Competing interests

The Authors declare that they have no conflict of interest.

Author details

[1]Department of Cardiac, Thoracic, and Vascular Sciences, Unit of Occupational Medicine, University of Padova, Via Giustiniani 2 -, 35128 Padova, Italy. [2]Department of Medical and Surgical Specialties, Radiological Sciences and Public Health, Section of Public Health and Human Sciences, University of Brescia, Brescia, Italy. [3]University Research Center "Integrated Models for Prevention and Protection in Environmental and Occupational Health", University of Brescia, Brescia, Italy. [4]Department of Diagnostics and Public Health, Section of Occupational Health, University of Verona, Verona, Italy.

References

1. Ferlay J, Parkin DM, Steliarova-Foucher E. Estimates of cancer incidence and mortality in Europe in 2008. Eur J Cancer. 2010;46:765–81.
2. Burger M, Catto JW, Dalbagni G, Grossman HB, Herr H, Karakiewicz P, Kassouf W, Kiemeney LA, La Vecchia C, Shariat S, Lotan Y. Epidemiology and risk factors of urothelial bladder cancer. Eur Urol. 2013;63:234–41.
3. IARC monographs on the evaluation of carcinogenic risk of chemicals to humans. The rubber industry. IARC Monogr Eval Carcinog Risk Chem Hum. 1982;28. http://monographs.iarc.fr/ENG/Monographs/vol1-42/mono28.pdf. Accessed 3 Nov 2015.
4. Kogevinas M, Sala M, Boffetta P, Kazerouni N, Kromhout H, Hoar-Zahm S. Cancer risk in the rubber industry: a review of the recent epidemiological evidence. Occup Environ Med. 1998;55:1–12.
5. Baan R, Straif K, Grosse Y, Secretan B, El Ghissassi F, Bouvard V, Benbrahim-Tallaa L, Cogliano V. WHO International Agency for Research on Cancer monograph working group, carcinogenicity of some aromatic amines, organic dyes, and related exposures. Lancet Oncol. 2008;9:322–3.
6. Talaska G. Aromatic amines and human urinary bladder cancer: exposure sources and epidemiology. J Environ Sci Health C Environ Carcinog Ecotoxicol Rev. 2003;21:29–43.
7. Barone-Adesi F, Richiardi L, Merletti F. Population attributable risk for occupational cancer in Italy. Int J Occup Environ Health. 2005;11:23–31.
8. Scarselli A, Scano P, Marinaccio A, Iavicoli S. Occupational cancer in Italy: evaluating the extent of compensated cases in the period 1994-2006. Am J Ind Med. 2009;52:859–67.
9. AIRT Working Group. Italian cancer figures – report 2006: 1. Incidence, mortality and estimates. Epidemiol Prev. 2006;30(1 Suppl 2):8–10.
10. IARC monographs on the evaluation of carcinogenic risks to humans. Chemical agents and related occupations. IARC Monogr Eval Carcinog Risks Hum. 2012; 100F. http://monographs.iarc.fr/ENG/Monographs/vol100F/mono100F.pdf. Accessed .3 Nov 2015.
11. Pavanello S, Pulliero A, Clonfero E. Influence of *GSTM1 null* and low repair *XPC PAT* + on anti-B[a]PDE-DNA adduct in mononuclear white blood cells of subjects low exposed to PAHs through smoking and diet. Mutat Res. 2008;638:195–204.
12. Lotan Y, Svatek RS, Krabbe LM, Xylinas E, Klatte T, Shariat SF. Prospective external validation of a bladder cancer detection model. J Urol. 2014;192:1343–8.
13. Kluth LA, Black PC, Bochner BH, Catto J, Lerner SP, Stenzl A, Sylvester R, Vickers AJ, Xylinas E, Shariat SF. Prognostic and prediction tools in bladder cancer: a comprehensive review of the literature. Eur Urol. 2015;68:238–53.
14. Terracciano D, Ferro M, Terreri S, Lucarelli G, D'Elia C, Musi G, de Cobelli O, Mirone V, Cimmino A. Urinary long noncoding RNAs in nonmuscle-invasive bladder cancer: new architects in cancer prognostic biomarkers. Transl Res. 2017;184:108–17.
15. Terreri S, Durso M, Colonna V, Romanelli A, Terracciano D, Ferro M, Perdonà S, Castaldo L, Febbraio F, de Nigris F, Cimmino A. New Cross-Talk Layer between Ultraconserved Non-Coding RNAs, MicroRNAs and Polycomb Protein YY1 in Bladder Cancer. Genes (Basel). 2016;7:127.
16. Olivieri M, Ferro M, Terreri S, Durso M, Romanelli A, Avitabile C, De Cobelli O, Messere A, Bruzzese D, Vannini I, Marinelli L, Novellino E, Zhang W, Incoronato M, Ilardi G, Staibano S, Marra L, Franco R, Perdonà S, Terracciano D, Czerniak B, Liguori GL, Colonna V, Fabbri M, Febbraio F, Calin GA, Cimmino A. Long non-coding RNA containing ultraconserved genomic region 8 promotes bladder cancer tumorigenesis. Oncotarget. 2016;7:20636–54.
17. Shen M, Hung RJ, Brennan P, Malaveille C, Donato F, Placidi D, Carta A, Hautefeuille A, Boffetta P, Porru S. Polymorphisms of the DNA repair genes *XRCC1, XRCC3, XPD*, interaction with environmental exposures, and bladder cancer risk in a case–control study in northern Italy. Cancer Epidemiol Biomark Prev. 2003;12:1234–40.
18. Covolo L, Placidi D, Gelatti U, Carta A, Scotto Di Carlo A, Lodetti P, Piccichè A, Orizio G, Campagna M, Arici C, Porru S. Bladder cancer, GSTs, NAT1, NAT2, SULT1A1, XRCC1, *XRCC3, XPD* genetic polymorphisms and coffee consumption: a case-control study. Eur J Epidemiol. 2008;23:355–62.
19. Pavanello S, Mastrangelo G, Placidi D, Campagna M, Pulliero A, Carta A, Arici C, Porru S. CYP1A2 polymorphisms, occupational and environmental exposures and risk of bladder cancer. Eur J Epidemiol. 2010;25:491–500.
20. Porru S, Pavanello S, Carta A, Arici C, Simeone C, Izzotti A, Mastrangelo G. Complex relationships between occupation, environment, DNA adducts, genetic polymorphisms and bladder cancer in a case-control study using a structural equation modeling. PLoS One. 2014;9(4):e94566.
21. Porru S, Placidi D, Carta A, Gelatti U, Ribero ML, Tagger A, Boffetta P, Donato F. Primary liver cancer and occupation in men: a case-control study in high-incidence area in northern Italy. Int J Cancer. 2001;94:878–83.
22. Coggon D, Martyn C, Palmer KT, Evanoff B. Assessing case definitions in the absence of a diagnostic gold standard. Int J Epidemiol. 2005;34:949–52.
23. Pira E, Piolatto G, Negri E, Romano C, Boffetta P, Lipworth L, McLaughlin JK, La Vecchia C. Bladder cancer mortality of workers exposed to aromatic amines: a 58-year follow-up. J Natl Cancer Inst. 2010;102:1096–9.
24. Miyakawa M, Tachibana M, Miyakawa A, Yoshida K, Shimada N, Murai M, Kondo T. Re-evaluation of the latent period of bladder cancer in dyestuff-plant workers in Japan. Int J Urol. 2001;8:423–30.
25. Swets JA. Measuring the accuracy of diagnostic systems. Science. 1998;240:1285–93.
26. Youden WJ. Index for rating diagnostic tests. Cancer. 1950;3:32–5.
27. Baker SG. Putting risk prediction in perspective: relative utility curves. J Natl Cancer Inst. 2009;101:1538–42.
28. Vickers AJ, Calster BV, Steyerberg EW. Net benefit approaches to the evaluation of prediction models, molecular markers, and diagnostic tests. BMJ. 2016;352:i6.
29. Kerr KF, Brown MD, Zhu K, Janes H. Assessing the clinical impact of risk prediction models with decision curves: guidance for correct interpretation and appropriate use. J Clin Oncol. 2016;34:2534–40.
30. Demidenko E. Sample size and optimal design for logistic regression with binary interaction. Stat Med. 2008;27:36–46.
31. Armitage P. Statistical methods in medical research. 1st ed. Oxford: Blackwell Science; 1971.
32. Fan ZJ, Bonauto DK, Foley MP, Silverstein BA. Underreporting of work-related injury or illness to workers' compensation: individual and industry factors. J Occup Environ Med. 2006;48:914–22.
33. Straif K. The burden of occupational cancer. Occup Environ Med. 2008;65:787–8.
34. Eurogip. Reporting of occupational diseases: issues and good practices in five European countries. Ref. Eurogip-102/E February 2015. http://www.eurogip.fr/images/publications/2015/Report_DeclarationMP_EUROGIP_102EN.pdf. Accessed 3 Nov 2015.

8

Prevalence and predictors of musculoskeletal pain among Danish fishermen

Gabriele Berg-Beckhoff[1*], Helle Østergaard[2] and Jørgen Riis Jepsen[2]

Abstract

Background: Fishermen work in a physically challenging work environment. The aim of this analysis was to estimate the prevalence and predictors of musculoskeletal pain among Danish fishermen.

Method: A cross-sectional survey in a random sample of Danish fishermen was done with application of the Nordic questionnaire regarding musculoskeletal pain considering lower back, shoulders, hand neck, knee, upper back elbow, hip and feet. In total, 270 fishermen participated in the study (response rate: 28%). Workload, vessel type, skipper, duration of work, sideline occupation, days/weeks of fishing at sea, age, BMI and education were used as predictors for the overall musculoskeletal pain score (multiple linear regression) and for each single pain site (multinomial logistic regression).

Results: The prevalence of pain was high for all musculoskeletal locations. Overall, more than 80% of the responding Danish fishermen reported low back pain, which in 37% lasted for a minimum of 30 days during the past year. In the multiple linear regression analysis, middle workload was associated with a 32% (95% CI: 19-46%) and high workload with 60% (95% CI: 46-73%) increased musculoskeletal pain score compared to low work load. Multinomial logistic regression models showed that workload was the only predictor for all pain sites, in particular regarding upper and lower limb pain.

Conclusion: Although changes were implemented to improve the fishermen's work environment, the work continues to be physically demanding and impacting their musculoskeletal pain. Potential explanation for this unexpected result like increased work pressure and reduced financial attractiveness in small scale commercial fishery needs to be confirmed in future research.

Keywords: Fishermen, Musculoskeletal pain, Work load, Cross-sectional study

What this article adds

Fishermen work in a challenging physical work environment and therefore have a high prevalence of musculoskeletal pain. However, during the last 10 to 20 years, several positive structural changes for the physical work environment took place, but it does not lead to a decreased musculoskeletal pain in fishermen's. The only stringent predictor for this pain is still the workload.

* Correspondence: gbergbeckhoff@health.sdu.dk
[1]Unit for Health Promotion Research, University of Southern Denmark, Niels Bohrs Vej 9, 6700 Esbjerg, Denmark
Full list of author information is available at the end of the article

Background

Physical workload of commercial fishing has been highly reduced in contemporary fishing in countries like Denmark, but may still be excessive at times depending on the type of fishing and the applied gear. Not only do fishermen work in challenging settings, their work has little routine and is dictated by various external factors such as weather and waves [1, 2]. Fishery is regarded as a dangerous occupation as demonstrated by a high rate of occupational fatalities [3] and of hospitalisation for various diseases [4–6]. Furthermore, though the work environment may still include physical demands, little is known about the current prevalence of musculoskeletal pain in fishermen [7]. During the last two decades, many new safety measures in Danish fisheries have been developed and applied, and consequently positive structural changes for the physical work environment in fisheries have taken place. There has been development in the used equipment, and it has facilitated the ergonomic loads, new vessels with better technique have been developed and introduced, and information of correct moving and carrying heavy loads has been implemented [8, 9]. However, the most cited publication on the prevalence of low back pain in fishermen derives from an old cross-sectional study of 1642 Swedish deep-sea fishermen in which approximately 50% experienced low back symptoms, their most common impairment, during the last 12 months [10]. In a cohort study started in 1999 on 215 fishermen in North Carolina, USA, low back pain was also the most frequent symptom with a prevalence of 52% [11]. Seven percent of 210 fishermen in a British cross-sectional study from 2007 had visited a doctor because of low back pain during the past year [12]. A survey in Turkish Aegean small scale fishermen reports that, between 2009 and 2010, 84% of respondents had musculoskeletal disorders leading to physician visits within one year [13]. Finally, a recent cross sectional study from Sri Lanka done in 2011 revealed a prevalence of musculoskeletal symptoms of 61%; prevalence of low back pain was 37.6% [14]. In a comprehensive literature research further recent studies estimating musculoskeletal pain in fishermen were not found. None of the studies discussed the population based approach to omit selection bias about potential job related pain.

Predictors for musculoskeletal pain in fishermen are rarely studied. In the North-Carolina cohort study [1, 11], the following predictors for low back pain were tested: age, smoking year's length of time in occupation, type of fishing and gear, job title, and fishing part time, years of fishing experience, or working more than one job. Significant increased risks for low back pain could be shown for young age (18–29) and history of low back pain. The authors additionally stated that job characteristics for low back pain are undetermined [1, 11].

Therefore the aim of this analysis is to estimate prevalence and predictors of musculoskeletal pain in Danish fishermen considering a population based approach. Due to the structural changes that have taken place in the trade and the reduced workload in contemporary fishery, our expectation was a reduced prevalence of musculoskeletal pain.

Method

This cross-sectional survey took place between February and April 2015 and addressed 2500 randomly selected active fishermen registered with the Danish AgriFish Agency [15]. The study was promoted through a leaflet and press release and questionnaires were mailed out to potential respondents. To increase participation rate, the questionnaire could be completed either online (SurveyXact), or on paper and returned by mail, and an additional reminder was sent to non-respondents. Developed procedures were guided by the STROBE statement [16]. Informed consent was obtained from participants and this study has been approved by the Danish data Protection Agency (Jnr. 2014-41-3245).

Of the selected fishermen, 251 had an unknown address and 13 had died. Out of the remaining 2,236 fishermen, 637 answered the questionnaire resulting in a response rate of 28%. However, out of the responding fishermen, 355 were no longer full time active fishermen. Two fishermen were additionally deleted due to many missing answers. Finally, 270 fishermen were used for analyses. The questionnaire collected general health data and socio-demographic information as well as work-related information (see Fig. 1).

Based on the Nordic musculoskeletal questionnaire [17], questions on *musculoskeletal pain* during the past 12 months were posed for the following anatomical sites: Neck, shoulder, elbow, hand, upper back, lower back, hip, knee, and foot. Potential categories for the Danish version was 0 days, 1–7 days, 8 to 30 days, 31 to 90 days, more than 90 days, and every day [18]. For descriptive purposes, pain lasting for a minimum of 30 days was presented. For an additional pain score summing up the pain in all nine anatomic sites, a conditional missing imputation was used with answers missing for up to four questions. Missing answers were calculated out of the mean value of the remaining answers from the relevant person. To estimate the consistency of the overall score given the 9 different musculoskeletal pain sites, Cronbach alpha was used. It was 0.91 indicating a very good internal consistency of the scale [19].

The *physical workload* was estimated by questions developed during the FINALE project [20] addressing the frequency of seven tasks: standing, pushing and pulling, carrying and lifting, lifting with hands above shoulders, bending forwards with the back, twisting and bending, and heavy work with fingers. Participants answers were coded (5) full time; (4) ¾ of time; (3) half of time; (2) a quarter of time; (1) rarely; and (0) never. For analysis, a score was developed by the sum of all seven questions. A conditional missing imputation was used with up to two missing answers. Missing answers were calculated out of the mean value of the remaining answers from the relevant person. Cronbach alpha was 0.81 indicating a good internal consistency of the scale [18]. For categorical purposes, tertils were built described as low, middle, or high workload.

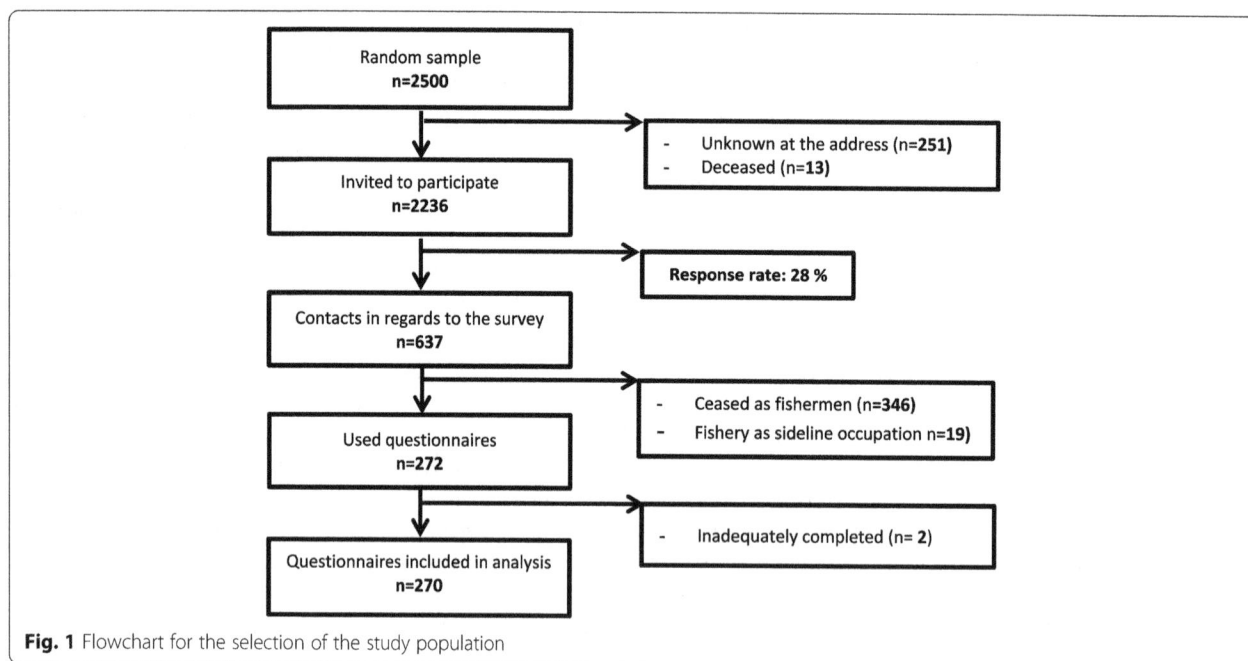

Fig. 1 Flowchart for the selection of the study population

Questions about work-related information reflected differences between *skipper* and *deckhands* for the analysis. In order not to omit missings ($n = 19$), we regarded these persons as deckhands, because skippers would always know their tasks while deckhands might have difficulties in defining their jobs. For the question about the *type of vessel* used, we considered the most frequently used type of vessel. The following types of vessels were presented: trawlers, Danish seiners, netters, liners, potters, and "others". The relevant missing answers ($n = 5$) were rated as "others". Information on days/weeks of fishing *at sea* was categorised into "1 day", "up to one week", and "more than one week". More specific categorisation for longer stay at sea wasn't feasible due to the small numbers of fishermen sailing longer time. The *duration of work* (in years) and *side line occupation* (yes or no) were also reported.

Demographic variables included the fishermen's *age* and *education* (basic, skilled, and advanced). Based on self-reported weight (kg) and height (m), body mass index (*BMI*) was calculated (kg/m^2) and categorized as normal (<25 kg/m^2), overweight ($25 - 30$ kg/m^2) and obese (>30 kg/m^2) [21].

Time to response was applied for checking potential selection bias with regard to pain. The completed questionnaires were collected time-dependently. For the internet version, the time for completion of the questionnaire was automatically saved while for the printed version, the date of receipt was used. The fastest completed questionnaire was received one day after distribution while the latest arrived 70 days later. For analysis

purposes, this time-variable was split into tertiles (early, middle, and late responders).

Statistical analyses were conducted in SAS Version 9.4 ($P < 0.05$). The prevalence of pain at different locations was presented overall and stratified for early, middle, and late responders to check for a potential selection bias related to musculoskeletal pain (data not shown). The association between workload (as score) and pain (low, middle and high workload) was analyzed by multiple linear regression. Considered predictors were work task, boat type, years of fishing, duration of work experience, days/weeks fishing at sea, sideline occupation, education, and BMI. Model assumptions were graphically tested and fulfilled after log transformation of the pain score.

A multinomial logistic regression model compared different pain locations within pain duration of 1 to 30 days, of more than 30 days, and no pain, given the last group as reference group. The proportional OR was used derived using a multinomial logistic regression model. We expect that a logistic regression gives trustful estimates and standard errors compared for example to the log binomial model. Estimates or standard errors do not differ between the models when high outcome prevalence's are considered [22]. In contrast to the conditional imputation for musculoskeletal pain score, in categorical variables such a procedure is not feasible any more. Instead, an additional category "missing" was considered in the multinomial logistic regression to keep persons with missing values in the analysis. The models were adjusted for workload, vessel type, years of fishing, duration of work experience, days/weeks fishing at sea, sideline occupation, education, and BMI.

Results

Table 1 shows the work characteristics and demographics of the study population. All responding fishermen were males and most were skippers and worked on trawlers. Fishing voyages were mostly short with half of the fishermen at sea for one day only. Most fishermen had a basic education, were overweight, and above 50 years of age.

The prevalence of musculoskeletal pain at different locations distributed is presented in Table 2. Pain lasting less than 30 days during the last year and more than 30 days per year was chosen to explore weak and more prolonged musculoskeletal pain, respectively. Overall, any low back and shoulder pain were most common and experienced by 4/5 of the fishermen during the last year (pain ≤ 30 days per year and pain > 30 days per year together). Hand and neck pain was secondly most frequent with a pain prevalence of around 2/3. Prolonged

Table 1 Work characteristics and socio demographic variable cross sectional survey of the 270 Fishermen in 2015

	Number	Percent	Missing
Skipper	167	66.53	0[a]
Boat			
Trawler	118	43.70	0[b]
Danish seiners	14	5.19	
Netters and liners	75	27.28	
Potters	28	10.37	
Other type	35	12.96	
Days/weeks of fishing on sea			
1 day	124	48.06	12
>1 to 7 days	90	34.88	
More than 7 days	44	17.05	
Education			
Basic education	137	54.80	8
Skilled worker	63	25.20	
Advanced education	50	20.00	
BMI			
Normal weight (<25 kg/m^2)	55	21.57	3
Overweight (25 – 30 kg/m^2)	119	46.67	
Obese (≥30 kg/m^2)	81	31.76	
Age			
<30 years	20	7.81	3
30-40 years	21	8.20	
40-50 years	52	20.31	
50-60 years	82	32.03	
≥ 60 years	81	31.64	
Total	270	100.00	

[a] $n = 19$; included in deckhands
[b] $n = 5$; included in other type

low back, shoulder and hand pain was also common and present in about 1/3 of the fishermen. The pain prevalence in all musculoskeletal locations did not differ between early, medium and late respondents (data not shown).

Multiple linear regression analyses of predictors for the overall pain score showed that fishermen categorized with middle workload had a 32% increased musculoskeletal pain score compared to the fishermen with low of workload, whereas fishermen with high workload had a 60% increased pain score compared to workers with low work load. These associations were highly significant and showed a positive trend. Having a sideline occupation was associated with a 15% significantly reduced musculoskeletal pain score. All other considered variables such as skipper, boat type, days/weeks fishing at sea, education, BMI, and duration of work had no effect on pain after additional adjustment for workload (Table 3).

Table 4 shows the multinomial logistic regression models for the different pain locations using the same predictors as in the multiple linear model. The only constant predictor for all pain sites was workload which indicated that all locations of prolonged musculoskeletal pain were highly significantly associated with high workload displaying odds ratios mostly exceeding 10. High workload was particularly associated with prolonged pain in hands and feet (odds ratios around 20 and more). High workload was already consistently and significantly associated with pain of less than 30 days of duration in elbow, hand and upper back. However, the concrete estimates need to be interpret with caution due to the wide confidence intervals particular for the group with musculoskeletal pain for more than 30 days per year. There were two additional predictors; sideline occupation was associated with less shoulder pain, and work duration of more than 30 days per year was a risk factor for hip pain.

Discussion

In this cross sectional study about fishermen the prevalence of musculoskeletal pain is high and the main predictor of musculoskeletal pain is the workload of fishermen which continues to be physically demanding in Danish fishermen even though structural changes took place. With more than 80% of the Danish fishermen reporting only low back pain during the past year and 37% reporting low back pain for at least 30 days during the past year, the prevalence of low back pain among Danish fishermen is high. A more recent survey among Turkish Aegean small-scale fishermen (2009–2010) found a similarly high prevalence of musculoskeletal disorders of 84%, even though the prevalence is based on physician visits within one year and combined

Table 2 Prevalence of less and more than 30 day per year pain in different areas of the body; cross sectional survey in 270 fishermen 2015

	Number	Percent
Lower Back		
No pain	42	17.9
Pain ≤30 days/year	104	44.3
Pain >30 days/year	89	37.9
missing	35	
Hand		
No pain	80	34.9
Pain ≤30 days/year	87	38.0
Pain >30 days/year	62	27.1
missing	41	
Knee		
No pain	86	39.6
Pain ≤30 days/year	88	40.6
Pain >30 days/year	43	19.8
missing	53	
Hip		
No pain	144	56.9
Pain ≤30 days/year	74	29.3
Pain >30 days/year	35	13.8
missing	17	
Elbow		
No pain	131	53.0
Pain ≤30 days/year	85	34.4
Pain >30 days/year	31	12.6
missing	23	
Shoulder		
No pain	48	21.4
Pain ≤30 days/year	104	46.4
Pain >30 days/year	72	32.1
missing	46	
Neck		
No pain	89	33.6
Pain ≤30 days/year	112	42.3
Pain >30 days/year	64	24.2
missing	5	
Upper back		
No pain	102	41.6
Pain ≤30 days/year	95	38.8
Pain >30 days/year	48	19.6
missing	25	

Table 2 Prevalence of less and more than 30 day per year pain in different areas of the body; cross sectional survey in 270 fishermen 2015 *(Continued)*

	Number	Percent
Feet		
No pain	147	61.8
Pain ≤30 days/year	59	24.8
Pain >30 days/year	32	13.5
missing	32	

different forms of musculoskeletal disorders [13]. Older surveys using the same questionnaire in Sweden (10, 1988) and USA (11, 1999) showed 50% and 51% of respondents claiming low back pain during the last year, respectively, which are both lower than the prevalence found in this current survey. However, direct comparison with these surveys is hampered as the Danish version of this questionnaire uses one additional category (the category of 30 to 90 days of pain) [18]. A greater choice of options for answers with more categories may

Table 3 Multiple linear regression model on predictors on the overall musculoskeletal pain score. Cross sectional survey in 270 fishermen, 2015

	Musculoskeletal pain score	
	Beta[a]	95% CI
Workload:		
Low workload	**Ref.**	
Middle workload	**0.32**	**0.19-0.46**
High workload	**0.60**	**0.46-0.73**
BMI [in kg/m^2]	−0.00	−0.01; 0.01
Duration of work experience [in years]	0.00	−0.00; 0.00
Sideline occupation		
Yes	**−0.15**	**−0.28; −0.02**
No	ref.	
Occupation:		
Captain	0.05	−0.06; 0.17
Other than captain	Ref.	
Vessel type		
Trawler	0.03	−0.09 ;0.15
Other than trawler	Ref.	
Education		
More than basic education	0.06	−0.19; 0.03
Basic education or less	Ref.	
Days/weeks of fishing at sea		
1 day	Ref.	
1 to 7 days	0.06	−0.06;0.19
More than 7 days	0.07	−0.09;0.24

[a]bold estimates are significant

Table 4 Multinomial logistic regression[a] of predictors on musculoskeletal pain sites – only significant results are shown; Cross sectional survey in 270 fishermen, 2015

	No pain[b] OR	Pain less than 30 days/years OR[c] (95% CI)	Pain more than 30 days/years OR[c] (95% CI)	Missing OR[c] (95% CI)
Model 1: Lower back				
Workload				
Low workload	1 (ref)			
Middle workload		0.91 (0.34-2.48)	**4.64 (1.48-14.57)**	0.85 (0.24-3.03)
High workload		0.99 (0.33-2.99)	**12.46 (3.70-41.99)**	1.40 (0.37-5.23)
Model 2: Shoulder				
Workload				
Low workload	1 (ref)			
Middle workload		1.13 (0.45-2.87)	2.88 (0.94-8.80)	0.90 (0.31-2.67)
High workload		2.66 (0.89-7.96)	**11.99 (3.41-42.06)**	1.40 (0.39-5.01)
Sideline occupation				
No	1 (ref)			
Yes		1.32 (0.51-3.43)	**0.28 (0.08-0.96)**	1.13 (0.37-3.45)
Model 3: Hand				
Workload				
Low workload	1 (ref)			
Middle workload		**3.06 (1.28-7.30)**	**6.70 (2.12-21.17)**	1.09 (0.38-3.08)
High workload		**4.06 (1.61-10.25)**	**19.82 (6.26-62.79)**	0.86 (0.25-2.94)
Model 4: Neck				
Workload				
Low workload	1 (ref)			
Middle workload		1.09 (0.51-2.35)	**3.87 (1.37-10.90)**	nn.
High workload		1.89 (0.82-4.22)	**10.18 (3.52-29.40)**	0.69 (0.03-18.57)
Model 5: Knee				
Workload				
Low workload	1 (ref)			
Middle workload		2.01 (0.87-4.66)	**4.24 (1.26-14.33)**	0.76 (0.29-2.01)
High workload		**4.46 (1.85-10.73)**	**10.99 (3.18-38.02)**	1.46 (0.53-4.01)
Model 6: Upper back				
Workload				
Low workload	1 (ref)			
Middle workload		**2.83 (1.28-6.25)**	**37.35 (4.20-332.10)**	3.01 (0.81; 11.19)
High workload		**5.16 (2.14-12.46)**	n.n.	2.61 (0.58-11.78)
Model 7: Hip				
Workload				
Low workload	1 (ref)			
Middle workload		0.97 (0.43-2.22)	3.17 (0.86-11.67)	3.07 (0.63-14.96)
High workload		**2.93 (1.37-6.25)**	**9.21 (2.62-32.37)**	1.34 (0.20-8.92)
Work duration				
per year		1.01 (0.99-1.04)	**1.05 (1.01-1.09)**	1.03 (0.98-1.08)

Table 4 Multinomial logistic regression[a] of predictors on musculoskeletal pain sites – only significant results are shown; Cross sectional survey in 270 fishermen, 2015 *(Continued)*

Model 8: Feet				
Workload				
Low workload	1 (ref)			
Middle workload		2.13 (0.88-5.12)	**19.43 (2.30-164.59)**	1.64 (0.53-5.08)
High workload		**2.50 (1.04-5.97)**	**24.00 (2.90-199.01)**	1.20 (0.39-3.73)
Model 9: Elbow				
Workload				
Low workload	1 (ref)			
Middle workload		**2.23 (1.00-4.97)**	3.42 (0.88-13.26)	0.99 (0.25; 3.95)
High workload		**5.18 (2.26-11.84)**	**10.98 (2.88-41.81)**	1.18 (0.29-4.92)

[a]All models contained workload, vessel type, years of fishing, duration of work experience, sideline occupation, education, and BMI.
[b]no pain during the last year
[c]bold estimate are significant, as the 95% CI does not include 1

lead to higher rates of prevalence. Furthermore, the recent Danish fishermen had the highest mean age compared to the other studies' participants dealing with musculoskeletal pain. However, with regard to the musculoskeletal pain, no trend between age and pain could be identified which was similar to other surveys observing this association [10, 11].

Population based surveys in occupational settings may be hampered by low response rates which can additionally bias prevalence estimations. With a response rate of 75.5%, the Swedish survey is optimal and therefore the most cited, though it is the oldest [10]. Response rate in the British survey was 68% [12]. The response rate of the cross sectional survey in Sri Lanka was named to be unbelievable 100% [14]. No information on the response rate was given in the cohort study from USA [11, 23] and in the Turkish survey [13]. The response rate of 28% in the current survey is low, but this is to be expected in a population based postal survey of fishermen. To check for potential selection bias, we collected time to response and compared prevalence's between early, middle and late respondents. For such a bias the expectation was that participants with pain would answer earlier due to a higher interest in the study than participants without pain [24]. The absence of such trend suggests that pain prevalence rates from our survey are not systematically over or under presented and they might represent musculoskeletal pain of Danish fishermen. In summary, age and low response rate cannot explain the high pain prevalence in the Danish fishermen study. Conclusively, lack of decrease in musculoskeletal pain prevalence and the high rates of reported pain in Danish fishermen were unexpected.

In the present study, workload was the most important predictor for musculoskeletal pain. For all pain locations there was a consistent, significant, and pronounced association between high workload and pain exceeding

30 days in the last year even though the exact estimates should be considered carefully due to the wide confidence intervals. The association between workload and pain was most pronounced for the extremities such as hands and feet. Additionally, the overall multiple linear analyses as well as the multinomial logistic regression on shoulder pain demonstrated that sideline occupation was significantly negatively associated with pain indicating that having a sideline occupation was associated with less pain. The American survey revealed the same result even though not significant [11]. This can be explained in various ways. Firstly, fishermen with a sideline occupation may be less exposed to the physically challenging work environment as full-time fisherman and therefore experience less musculoskeletal pain. Secondly, the healthiest fishermen may have the capacity to take extra work in addition to fishing. Further research is necessary to clarify underlying causal pathways.

When adjusting for workload neither occupational tasks, boat type, education, BMI, work experience nor time on sea were associated with musculoskeletal pain. Similar findings were reported in the American survey in which, with the exception of gender, there was no significant association between low back pain and age, BMI, fishing full time or having an additional job [11].

A number of health and safety measures on board the vessels have been developed and introduced, and structural changes in the trade have taken place in recent years [8, 9]. In spite of this there is no trend of improved musculoskeletal health in the studied sample of fishermen. What are the potential reasons for this? Firstly, globalisation, overcapacity and reduced fish prices has reduced the number of fishing vessels as well as fishermen in Western countries including Denmark [8, 25]. Fishing quota and season limit days restricts the catch, the volume of which commercial fishery is highly dependent. Therefore the fishermen strive to fish as much as possible within the limits indicated by increasing the workload and work pace at sea. A further explanation might be the reduced job satisfaction over time compared with the high work satisfaction of fishermen, which has been discussed as reasons for former potential underreporting of musculoskeletal symptoms in Swedish fishermen [2, 10, 26]. Furthermore, it is shown recently that job-dissatisfaction increase in Danish fishermen nowadays [27]. Current structural changes in Western fishery with high competition, overcapacity, and job uncertainty might lead to dissatisfaction, unhealthy behaviour and decreased health. Fishermen were previously satisfied with their job; they are now under pressure, particularly with regard to the consequences of globalisation, the highly regulated trade, and the reduced financial attractiveness of small scale commercial fisheries. Unfortunately, no similar survey was done in Denmark before structural changes took place, and therefore direct comparisons are hampered and suggestions are still speculative. Future research should focus on the health outcome of the potentially enhancing effect of occupational stress on tremendous workload in fishermen. Finally, the age structure is changing. Job uncertainty and unclear future occupational perspectives result in concerns of young workers to start a career as fishermen. Consequently, the majority of fishermen are quite old.

The very good internal consistency of the scale with a Cronbach alpha of 0.91 showed that all locations of pain are highly inter-correlated. A fisherman reporting hand pain is likely to also report pain in other locations. However, as shown, workload is the best predictor for pain, particularly in extremities, like hands and feet, which should therefore be addressed in further research. This can be confirmed by recommendations of the fishermen who were asked for suggestions relating to workplace improvements on board. Sixteen fishermen provided their ideas relating to standing (more space, rubber mats, better footwear, and chairs), as well as monotony and lifting (cutting table, lifting equipment, conveyor, and other mechanical equipment to reduce manual loads).

The cross-sectional study design causes some limitations. The direction of the association between the predictor and pain cannot be ascertained. Although the questions regarding exposure addressed the current circumstances, it cannot be ruled out tha t previous exposures explain a proportion of the reported pain. Additionally fishermen suffering from pain may experience more pain with certain current exposures such as workload, which may therefore be overrated. Furthermore, a healthy worker selection may cause bias because fishermen with pain are more likely to have left the trade rather than fishermen without pain and consequently those who remain in the occupation are healthier [28]. These limitations are innate in the cross-sectional design

and cannot be overcome. While most studies undertaken in this context have used the same design, future research should apply longitudinal designs to allow a better estimation of a causal pathway of the relevant associations. The low response rate (28%) is a well-known limitation in representative occupational surveys. It was shown that a potential selection bias due to low response rate with regard to musculoskeletal pain was not likely. Another limitation is the missing values in pain-related questions, some of which were due to an error in the questionnaire construction. Missing values were considered through conditional missing imputation in the pain score and for the single pain sites, no such imputation was done. However, an additional category for missing values was considered to see if missing by itself has an effect on the outcome. Overall, the odds ratios for missing categories were small and far from significance. These stringent results in all analyses suggest that missing values do not dramatically bias the overall analyses.

Conclusion

In conclusion, the prevalence of musculoskeletal pain is high in the studied sample of Danish fishermen and pain in all considered locations is related to the perceived workload. Future research should focus more on the causes for such a high prevalence. To consider healthy worker bias and to follow up with the overall life time occupation in fishermen, a cohort design would allow for consideration of the relative importance in the development of musculoskeletal pain of various exposures as well as different reasons for working full-time, part-time, or quitting the job. Further interventions should particularly focus on the effect of workload on pain in hands and feet.

The work as a fisherman remains physically demanding although much less than it has been prior to the implementation of structural changes. The potential effect of working under pressure due to consequences of globalisation, the highly regulated trade, and the reduced financial attractiveness of small scale commercial fisheries require future research that focus on the health outcome of the potentially enhancing effect of occupational stress on tremendous workload in fishermen.

Acknowledgements
Not applicable.

Funding
This work was supported by The European fisheries fund (journal. no. 33010-13-k-0264).

Authors' contributions

JRJ is originator of the study. HØ and GB-B were responsible for the conduct of the study. HØ was responsible for the survey and the data collection. GB-B suggested the research question for the article and it was clarified together with HØ and JRJ. GB-B conducted the analyses and prepared the first draft of the manuscript which was finalized jointly by all authors. She is the guarantor of the work. All authors read and approved the final manuscript.

Competing interests

The authors declare that they have no competing interests.

Author details

[1]Unit for Health Promotion Research, University of Southern Denmark, Niels Bohrs Vej 9, 6700 Esbjerg, Denmark. [2]Centre of Maritime Health and Society, University of Southern Denmark, Niels Bohrs Vej 9, Esbjerg 6700, Denmark.

References

1. Kucera KL, Loomis D, Lipscomb HJ, Marshall SW, Mirka GA, Daniels JL. Ergonomic risk factors for low back pain in North Carolina crab pot and gill net commercial fishermen. Amer J Ind Med. 2009;52(4):311–21.
2. Törner M, Alsmström C, Karlsson R, Kadefors R. Working on a moving surface –a biomechanical analysis of musculo-skeletal load due to ship motions in combination with work. Ergonomics. 1994;37(2):345–62.
3. Laursen LH, Hansen HL, Jensen OC. Fatal occupational accidents in Danish fishing vessels 1989–2005. Int J Inf Contr Saf Promot. 2008;15(2):109–17.
4. Kaerlev L, Jensen A, Hannerz H. Surveillance of hospital contacts among Danish seafarers and fishermen with focus on skin and infectious diseases-a population-based cohort study. Int J Environ Res Public Health. 2014; 11(11):11931–49.
5. Kaerlev L, Jensen A, Nielsen PS, Olsen J, Hannerz H, Tüchsen F. Hospital contacts for injuries and musculoskeletal diseases among seamen and fishermen: a population-based cohort study. BMC Musculoskelet Disord. 2008;23(9):8.
6. Kaerlev L, Dahl S, Nielsen PS, Olsen J, Hannerz H, Jensen A, Tüchsen F. Hospital contacts for chronic diseases among Danish seafarers and fishermen: a population-based cohort study. Scand J Public Health. 2007;35(5):481–9.
7. Østergaard H, Poulsen TR, Nørregaard Remmen L, Berg-Beckhoff G. Ergonomisk arbejdsmiljø, fysisk belastning og fatigue på danske fiskefartøjer. Esbjerg: Syddansk Universitet. Center for Maritime Sundhed og Samfund; 2015.
8. Poulsen TR, Burr H, Hansen HL, Jepsen JR. Health of Danish seafarers and fishermen 1970–2010: What have register-based studies found? Scand J Public Health. 2014;42(6):534–45.
9. Grøn S, Rasmussen HB, Poulsen TR, Christensen FN. Safety in the Danish fishing industry. Esbjerg: Center for Maritim Sundhed og Samfund, SDU, Syddansk Universitetsforlag; 2014.
10. Törner M, Blide G, Eriksson H, Kadefors R, Karlsson R, Petersen I. Musculo-skeletal symptoms as related to working conditions among Swedish professional fisherman. Appl Ergon. 1988;19(3):191–201.
11. Lipscomb HJ, Loomis D, McDonald MA, Kucera K, Marshall S, Li L. Musculoskeletal symptoms among commercial fishers in North Carolina. Appl Ergon. 2004;35(5):417–26.
12. Grimsmo-Powney H, Harris EC, Reading I, Coggon D. Occupational health needs of commercial fishermen in South West England. Occup Med (Lond). 2010;60(1):49–53.
13. Percin F, Akyol O, Davas A, Saygi H. Occupational health of Turkish Aegean small-scale fishermen. Occup Med (Lond). 2012;62(2):148–51.
14. Harshani SRAP, Abeysena HTCS. Musculoskeletal symptoms, skin disorders and visual impairment among fishermen in the Divisional Secretariat Division of Kalpitiya. Ceylon Med J. 2015;60:90–4.
15. Østergaard H, Jepsen JR, Berg-Beckhoff G. The workload of fishermen: a cross sectional survey among Danish commercial fishermen. Int Marit Health. 2016;67(2):97–103.
16. Vandenbroucke JP, von Elm E, Altman DG, Gøtzsche PC, Mulrow CD, Pocock SJ, et al. STROBE Initiative. Strengthening the Reporting of Observational Studies in Epidemiology (STROBE): explanation and elaboration. PLoS Med. 2007;4(10):e297.
17. Kuorinka I, Jonsson B, Kilbom A, Vinterberg H, Biering-Sørensen F, Andersson G, et al. Standardized Nordic questionnaires for the analysis of musculoskeletal symptoms. Appl Ergon. 1987;18:233–7.
18. Christensen JR, Overgaard K, Carneiro IG, Holtermann A, Søgaard K. Weight loss among female health care workers a 1-year workplace based randomized controlled trial in the FINALE-health study. BMC Public Health. 2012;12:625.
19. Santos RA. Cronbach's Alpha: A Tool for Assessing the Reliability of Scales. J Extension. 1999;37(2):e.2ToT3.
20. Holtermann A, Jorgensen MB, Gram B, Christensen JR, Faber A, Overgaard K, et al. Worksite interventions for preventing physical deterioration among employees in job-groups with high physical work demands: background, design and conceptual model of FINALE. BMC Public Health. 2010;10(120): 1–12.
21. WHO. Obesity: Preventing, and managing the global epidemic. Geneva: World Health Organization; 2000.
22. Skov T, Deddens J, Petersen MR, Endahl L. Prevalence proportion ratio: estimation and hypothesis testing. Int J Epidemiol. 1998;27:91–5.
23. Moe CL, Turf E, Oldach D, Bell P, Hutton S, Savitz D, et al. Cohort studies of health effects among people exposed to estuarine waters: North Carolina, Virginia, and Maryland. Environ Health Perspect. 2001;109(S5):781–6.
24. Kowall B, Breckenkamp J, Heyer K, Berg-Beckhoff G. German wide cross sectional survey on health impacts of electromagnetic fields in the view of general practitioners. Intern J Public Health. 2010;55(5):507–12.
25. Holm P. Verdensmarkedet for fisk – Internationalisering og globalisering 1880–1997. Sjæk'len 1997. Esbjerg: Fiskeri- og Søfartsmuseet; 1998. p. 29–42.
26. Törner M, Zetterberg C, Anden U, Hansson T, Lindell V. Workload and musculoskeletal problems: a comparison between welders and office clerks (with reference also to fishermen). Ergonomics. 1991;34(9):1179–96.
27. Christiansen JM. Carlsbæk AB. Fiskerne der forsvandt - hvorfor ophører fiskerne i fiskerierhvervet, og hvor går de hen? [Fishermen that disappeared – why stopped fishermen fishery and where do they go?]. Denmark: Center for Maritim Sundhed og Samfund, Syddansk Universitetsforlag Esbjerg; 2015.
28. Punnett L. Adjusting for healthy worker selection effect in cross sectional studies. Int J Epidemiol. 1999;25(5):1068–76.

The Portuguese long version of the Copenhagen Psychosocial Questionnaire II (COPSOQ II) – a validation study

Susel Rosário[1][*] [iD], Luís F. Azevedo[2,3,4,5], João A. Fonseca[1,2,6], Albert Nienhaus[1,7,8], Matthias Nübling[9] and José Torres da Costa[1,5,10]

Abstract

Background: Psychosocial risks are now widely recognised as one of the biggest challenges for occupational safety and health (OSH) and a major public health concern. The aim of this paper is to investigate the Portuguese long version of the Copenhagen Psychosocial Questionnaire II (COPSOQ II), in order to analyse the psychometric properties of the instrument and to validate it.

Methods: The Portuguese COPSOQ II was issued to a total of 745 Portuguese employees from both private and public organisations across several economic sectors at a baseline and then 2 weeks later. Methodological quality appraisal was based on COnsensus-based Standards for the selection of health Measurement INstruments (COSMIN) recommendations. An analysis of the psychometric properties of the long version of COPSOQ II (internal consistency, intraclass correlation coefficient, floor and ceiling effects, response rate, missing values, mean and standard deviation, exploratory factor analysis) was performed to determine the validity and reliability of the instrument.

Results: The COPSOQ II had a response rate of 60.6% (test) and a follow-up response rate of 59.5% (retest). In general, a Cronbach's alpha of the COPSOQ scales (test and retest) was above the conventional threshold of 0.70. The test-retest reliability estimated by the intraclass correlation coefficient (ICC) showed a higher reliability for most of the scales, above the conventional 0.7, except for eight scales. The proportion of the missing values was less than 1.3%, except for two scales. The average scores and standard deviations showed similar results to the original Danish study, except for eight scales. All of the scales had low floor and ceiling effects, with one exception. Overall, the exploratory factor analysis presented good results in 27 scales assuming a reflective measurement model. The hypothesized factor structure under a reflective model was not supported in 14 scales and for some but not all of these scales the explanation may be a formative measurement model.

Conclusion: The Portuguese long version of COPSOQ II is a reliable and valid instrument for assessing psychosocial risks in the workplace. Although the results are good for most of the scales, there are those that should be evaluated in greater depth in future studies. This instrument may contribute to the promotion of a healthy working environment and workforce, providing clear benefits for companies and employees.

Keywords: Psychosocial risks, Occupational health and safety, Risk assessment (89/391/EEC framework directive), Validation, Portugal

* Correspondence: skrosario@gmail.com
[1]Doctoral Programme in Occupational Safety and Health, Faculty of Engineering of the University of Porto, Rua Dr. Roberto Frias, s/n 4200-465 Porto, Portugal
Full list of author information is available at the end of the article

Background

In line with the Europe 2020 objective [1] and the European Union Strategic Framework for Health and Safety at Work 2014–2020 [2], ensuring a healthy and safe working environment contributes considerably to labour productivity and promotes economic growth, competitiveness and welfare [3]. Psychosocial risks are considered the most challenging risk factors across the European Union and a key challenge in modern occupational safety and health (OSH) management, as they are linked not only to health outcomes but also to performance-related outcomes such as absenteeism, ability to work and, in particular, job satisfaction [2, 4]. According to the Framework Directive (89/391/EEC) [5], employers have a legal responsibility to ensure the safety and health of workers in every aspect related to work, including psychosocial risks in the workplace [6].

Although the implementation of these provisions varies from one country to another, the Framework specifies that risks must be identified and assessed, and prevented and managed [7–9]. One of the most important aspects to consider is that risk assessment at work requires the use of valid and reliable methods in order to identify the risk factors in organisations [7, 9–11]. Occupational safety and health legislation therefore places a central focus of risk assessment on preventive approaches [12], which should be considered a priority for organisations [8, 13, 14].

Many measures (mainly questionnaire-based) related to working conditions have been developed, namely the Copenhagen Psychosocial Questionnaire [15, 16], Job Content Questionnaire [17, 18], Effort-Reward Imbalance Questionnaire [19, 20], Pressure Management Indicator [21], Stress Profile [22], Health and Safety Executive Indicator Tool [23], Work Environment Scale [24], General Nordic Questionnaire [25], Job Characteristics Inventory [26], Job Diagnostic Survey [27] and Stress Diagnostic Survey [28], among others, in order to support both employers and employees in the enhancement of OSH processes for prevention and management in organisations [29].

The Copenhagen Psychosocial Questionnaire (COPSOQ) is a comprehensive questionnaire that includes numerous dimensions based on an eclectic set of theories on psychosocial factors at work and on empirical research, rather than being linked to one particular theory [15, 16]. It covers a wide variety of dimensions, describing psychosocial working conditions, and is considered an instrument for research and psychosocial risk prevention in the workplace.

The COPSOQ is an instrument that was developed relatively recently. It was developed in 2000 by Tage S. Kristensen and Vilhelm Borg at the Danish National Research Centre for the Working Environment [15], and revised in 2010 (version II) [16]. In the second version of the

Danish COPSOQ study, the psychometric qualities of the instrument were tested in a representative sample of 3517 working Danes between 20 and 59 years of age (52% women, response rate 60.4%). COPSOQ is now one of the most widely used instruments for assessing psychosocial risks in the workplace. It has gained prominent recognition in the scientific community in several countries and has been translated into more than 25 languages, which enables comparison between countries [30, 31]. An increasing number of validation studies have been performed in several countries such as Germany [32, 33], Spain [34], China [35], France [36], Sweden [37], Chile [38] and Iran [39], among others. According to a recent publication by the International Labour Organization [29], the COPSOQ was the first monitoring model to include population-based reference values to assess the need for action and to support the decision-making process concerning preventive measures at the workplace level. Founded in 2009, the COPSOQ International Network (http://www.copsoq-network.org) promotes scientific research and risk assessment using the COPSOQ and aims to facilitate communication between multiple groups. It is therefore linked to governments, universities and research institutions, enterprises and social agents from European and other countries all over the world [40].

The aim of this paper is to present the Portuguese long version of the Copenhagen Psychosocial Questionnaire II (COPSOQ II) and to analyse the psychometric properties of the instrument.

Methods

The validation study was conducted in two phases. In 2013, the original Danish long version of the Copenhagen Psychosocial Questionnaire II (COPSOQ II) was cross-culturally validated [41, 42] and its appraisal based on COnsensus-based Standards for the selection of health Measurement INstruments (COSMIN) recommendations [43–46]. The Portuguese version showed satisfactory reliability [47, 48]. Secondly, following implementation of the Portuguese version, data was collected between April 2013 and July 2015 and tested for further psychometric quality. Appraisal was based on COSMIN recommendations concerning the psychometric properties of instruments, which are widely accepted internationally. In this validation study, the following COSMIN domains were evaluated: reliability and factorial validity [43–46]. In addition, we compared our results with the original Danish COPSOQ II study.

Content and structure of the questionnaire

The Portuguese long version of COPSOQ II is a 128-item standardised self-report measure designed for psychosocial risk assessment and prevention. This version has kept the full content and structure of the original

Danish long version, in that the 128-item questionnaire consisted of 41 scales reflecting 7 dimensions as outlined in Table 1.

Most item responses were scored on a five-point Likert scale with five options: always, often, sometimes, seldom, never/hardly ever or to a very large extent, to a large extent, somewhat, to a small extent, to a very small extent. The following items were reverse-scored: "Do you have enough time for your work tasks?", "Do you have to do the same thing over and over again?", "How often do you consider looking for work elsewhere?", "Do employees withhold information from each other?", "Do employees withhold information from the management?" and "Does the management withhold important information from employees?".

The scales were calculated as an average of the scores of the items included and transformed to a range of 0 to 100, with high values representing a high level of the concept being measured. The long version of COPSOQ II also includes questions aimed at the sociodemographic characterisation of the participant. The questionnaire takes 30 min to complete. To score the COPSOQ II scales, at least half of the items should be answered for calculating a particular scale [16]. The Portuguese questionnaire is freely available in the public domain as a PDF download from http://www.copsoq.pt/ [49].

Study sample

The study was conducted in 34 companies located in the north and centre of Portugal, between 1 April 2013 and 31 July 2015. It was approved by the Ethics Committee of the University of Porto. After being properly informed about the aim of the study, all of the participants signed the consent form prior to being issued with the questionnaire.

The sample included a total of 745 employees from both private and public organisations across several economic sectors (education, construction, wholesale and retail trade, financial and insurance, manufacturing, human health and social work, other sectors) at the baseline assessment (N = 745). A retest was conducted after two weeks (7–17 days) to assess reproducibility (N = 394). Figure 1 provides details of the participants according to the Classification of Economic Activities. For the current study, we included all workers aged 18 to 65 who were willing to participate in the study and who gave their informed consent.

The response rate was 60.6%. For test-retest validation, the response rate was 59.5%. The sample size included in this study was based not only on COSMIN recommendations (excellent sample size: ≥ 100), [44] but also on the recommendations of Comrey and Lee [50] and McCullum et al. [51], who recommend more than 640

participants for factor analysis (in this case, based on the number of subjects per item/variable: 5 * 128 = 640), as well as in accordance with the recommendations of the Ethics Committee of the University of Porto.

The sample was classified by different sectors of economic activity according to the nomenclature of the Portuguese Classification of Economic Activities (CAE) Revision 3 (CAE – Rev. 3) [52], which is harmonised with the Classification of Economic Activities in the European Union (NACE – Rev. 2) [53] and the International Standard Classification of Activities, Revision 4 (ISIC – Rev. 4) of the United Nations [54]. The classification used data from Pordata, the Data Base of Contemporary Portugal [55] (Additional file 1).

Overall, the "education" and the "human health and social work activities" sectors of economic activities in our sample are considerably higher than in the general working population. The "construction" and "financial and insurance activities" displayed values very close to the population. Furthermore, the "Other sectors" that were considered (E, J, M, N, O, R, S, T, U), despite covering nine more sectors than expected, also displayed very close values. However, the "wholesale and retail trade" and "manufacturing" sectors of our study show representative values far below those for the population in general, suggesting that they should be confirmed by an appropriate sample in future. The characteristics of the study are shown in Tables 2 and 3. The majority of the participants were female (65.6%). The average age of the respondents was 39 (SD = 9.9), with a range of between 19 and 65. The distribution of organisations between public (n = 300) and private (n = 445) sectors was nearly balanced. Professional groups were classified according to the Portuguese Classification of Occupations [56] and are shown in Table 3. The 2010 Portuguese Classification of Occupations is the most recent international framework (according to the International Standard Classification of Occupations – ISCO 2008) [57].

Study procedure

The procedure was initiated by presenting the study to organisations across several sectors of economic activity. The organisations that were contacted and were available to participate in the study formalised their interest with a signed consent. In every organisation, we tried to cover employees belonging to different hierarchical levels and in different functions in order to ensure that the sample was representative. Data collection activities were developed according to the way each institution worked and in accordance with the dates stipulated in the study.

Data collection included questionnaires available in paper format or as a digital survey. Of the 34 companies in total, digital survey data was collected in three. Before

Table 1 Domains, scales and number of items in the Portuguese long version of COPSOQ II

Domain	Scale	Number of Items
Demands at work	Quantitative demands	4
	Work pace	3
	Cognitive demands	4
	Emotional demands	4
	Demands for hiding emotions	3
Work organisation and job contents	Influence	4
	Possibilities for development	4
	Variation	2
	Meaning of work	3
	Commitment to the workplace	4
Interpersonal relations and leadership	Predictability	2
	Recognition	3
	Role clarity	3
	Role conflicts	4
	Quality of leadership	4
	Social support from colleagues	3
	Social support from supervisors	3
	Social community at work	3
Work-individual interface	Job insecurity	4
	Job satisfaction	4
	Work-family conflict	4
	Family-work conflict	3
Values in the workplace	Mutual trust between employees	3
	Trust regarding management	4
	Justice	4
	Social inclusiveness	4
Health and well-being	General health perception	1
	Burnout	4
	Stress	4
	Sleeping troubles	4
	Depressive symptoms	4
	Somatic stress	4
	Cognitive stress	4
	Self-efficacy	6
Offensive behaviour	Sexual harassment	1
	Threats of violence	1
	Physical violence	1
	Bullying	1
	Unpleasant teasing	1
	Conflicts and quarrels	1
	Gossip and slander	1
Total	Number of scales 41	
	Number of items	128

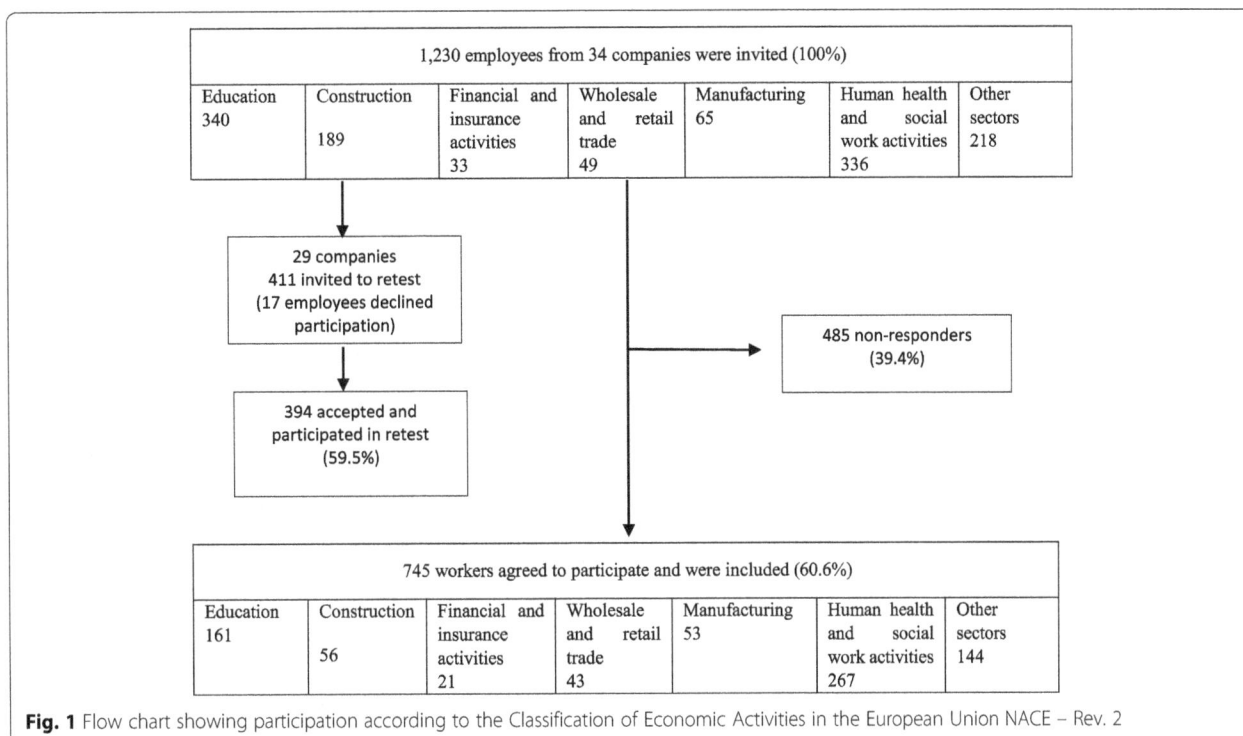

Fig. 1 Flow chart showing participation according to the Classification of Economic Activities in the European Union NACE – Rev. 2

taking part in the digital survey, participants had to meet the following criteria: aged 18 to 65, with each participant having a computer permanently assigned to them for the performance of their duties and willing to participate in the study and to give their informed consent. The COPSOQ II paper format was used and completed in convenient rooms on the organisations' own premises. The questionnaires were delivered directly to the participants who were supervised while they completed the questionnaire. In the case of the digital survey, the participants filled in an online consent form and completed the online questionnaire. The online questionnaire was made available in order to facilitate data collection, and employees received an email invitation encouraging them to fill out the form at a time and place of their choosing. Employees had 3 weeks to complete the survey and non-respondents received two email reminders during this time. For test-retest validation, similar data collection (paper format or online survey) was conducted after 2 weeks to assess reproducibility. All of the organisations have received a report with a summary of their results.

Psychometric and statistical analysis

Data analysis was performed and included descriptive statistics using mean and standard deviation (SD). The assessment of the psychometric validity of the Portuguese version of the COPSOQ II followed the COSMIN recommendations [43–46] as well as internationally recommended standards [58–61], and included:

(i) the internal consistency of the 41 scales (test and retest) through Cronbach's alpha;

(ii) test-retest reliability within two weeks was estimated by the intraclass correlation coefficient (ICC) for quantitative variables;

(iii) descriptive statistics comprising mean and standard deviation for all scales;

(iv) floor and ceiling effects;

(v) response rate (test) and follow-up response rate (retest);

(vi) missing values; and

(vii) exploratory factor analysis.

The items in COPSOQ II were analysed using explorative factor analyses within each of the seven major domains: *Demands at work; Work organisation and job content; Interpersonal relations and leadership; Work-individual interface; Values at the workplace; Health and well-being* and *Offensive behaviour.*

The assessments of internal consistency and test-retest reliability were performed according to available recommendations [58, 59]. Analysis of internal consistency was undertaken by assessing Cronbach's alpha. As recommended by Nunnally and Bernstein [60], a Cronbach's alpha of 0.70 is the threshold value for this assessment. The original Danish study [16] also considered the conventional threshold of 0.70.

For the interpretation of the magnitude of the intraclass correlation coefficient (ICC), an ICC greater than 0.70 was considered adequate [62, 63].

Table 2 Characteristics of the study population

	n	%
Total participants	745	
Gender		
Female	489	65.6
Male	256	34.4
Age distribution		
19–29	141	19.0
30–39	261	35.0
40–49	194	26.0
50–59	139	18.7
60–65	10	1.3
Marital status		
Single	241	32.3
Married	376	50.5
Cohabiting	62	8.3
Divorced	54	7.2
Widowed	12	1.6
Education		
≤ 9th year	100	13.4
10th to 12th year	177	23.8
Bachelor	20	2.7
University degree	318	42.7
Postgraduate degree	1	0.1
Master's degree	102	13.7
PhD	27	3.6
Economic activities		
Manufacturing	53	7.1
Construction	56	7.5
Wholesale and retail trade	43	5.8
Financial and insurance activities	21	2.8
Education	161	21.6
Human health and social work activities	267	35.8
Other sectors	144	19.3
Sectors		
Public	300	40.3
Private	445	59.7

Table 3 Distribution of professionals groups

Occupation CNP [a]	n	%
Management of companies and public administration	18	2.4
Technical and scientific professionals and intellectuals	341	45.8
Technical and associate professionals	113	15.2
Administrative employees	105	14.1
Workers in catering services, personnel, security, etc.	122	16.4
Skilled agricultural and fishery	0	0
Tradespeople and skilled workers in manufacturing	2	0.3
Plant and machine operators, assemblers	29	3.9
Unskilled workers	14	1.9
Missing value	1	0.1
Total	745	100

[a] Portuguese National Classification of Occupations

Exploratory factor analysis was conducted following a recommendation by the Ethics Committee of the University of Porto. Factorial validity was assessed by definition and evaluation of the factor structure of the instrument using methods of exploratory factor analysis [59, 64, 65]. Models of exploratory factor analysis were defined using principal components analysis for factor extraction [59, 64, 65]. The extraction of the main factors was performed using varimax rotation with Kaiser normalisation. Selection of the number of factors to retain took into account Kaiser's criterion (eigenvalues greater than one); graphical analysis of the scree plot; a criterion based on the total variance explained (at least greater than 50%); and the Kaiser-Meyer-Olkin (KMO). In the factor analysis, the missing items were handled by using the list-wise deletion method [66]. For all hypothesis tests, a significance level of $\alpha = 5\%$ was used. Statistical analyses were performed using the Statistical Package for the Social Sciences (SPSS) v20.0® software program.

Results

A total of 745 employees from 34 companies completed the questionnaire. The average age of the participants was 39 (SD = 9.6). The majority (65.6%) of respondents were female. The participants worked an average of 42.9 h/week (SD = 7.2) and had been in their current jobs for 9.4 years (SD = 9.5) on average. The rate of participation in the test ($N = 745$) was 60.6%, and in the retest ($N = 394$) it was 59.5%. The scale characteristics for the dimensions in COPSOQ II are shown in Table 4.

For 29 of the 41 scales, Cronbach's alpha was generally above the conventional threshold of 0.70, nine scales ranged between 0.60 and 0.70, and three scales had a reliability of less than 0.60 (*Influence at work*, *Variation* and *Predictability*). Test-retest reliability was assessed by examining the correlation of the scale score in the baseline long version of the COPSOQ II questionnaire with

A descriptive statistics (mean and standard deviation) analysis was performed for sociodemographic data and for all 41 scales.

Similar to the original Danish COPSOQ II study, floor and ceiling effects, defined as the proportion of respondents selecting the lowest (floor) and highest (ceiling) response options for all items in a scale, were determined for all scales.

The missing values considered if respondents had answered less than half of the questions in a particular scale, and was analysed for all 41 scales.

Table 4 Comparison of the reliability and summary descriptive statistics between the Portuguese (n = 745) and the original COPSOQ II Danish (n = 3517) study sample

Domain	Scale	Danish Cronbach's α n = 3517	Portuguese Cronbach's α Test n = 745	Portuguese Cronbach's α Retest n = 394	Danish Mean	Danish SD	Portuguese Mean	Portuguese SD	Danish % Floor	Danish % Ceiling	Portuguese % Floor	Portuguese % Ceiling	Danish Missing (%)	Portuguese Missing N (%)	Portuguese Test-retest reliability ICC (95% CI)
Demands at work	Quantitative demands	0.82	0.69	0.67	40.2	20.5	36.3	18.2	2.9	0.3	3.6	0.3	2.2	2 (0.3)	0.818 (0.770-0.859)
	Work pace	0.84	0.74	0.72	59.5	19.1	63.1	19.2	0.5	3.4	0.8	4.6	2.2	2 (0.3)	0.845 (0.804-0.880)
	Cognitive demands	0.74	0.63	0.71	63.9	18.7	57.0	18.4	0.3	1.1	1.1	0.9	2.2	3 (0.4)	0.778 (0.721-0.828)
	Emotional demands	0.87	0.73	0.76	40.7	24.3	54.9	20.8	5.7	0.4	1.5	0.4	2.2	2 (0.3)	0.783 (0.727-0.831)
	Demands for hiding emotions	0.57	0.60	0.62	50.6	20.8	39.7	23.3	1.5	0.9	7.0	0.8	2.3	4 (0.5)	0.719 (0.644-0.784)
Work organisation and job contents	Influence	0.73	0.53	0.68	49.8	21.2	47.2	19.0	1.6	0.5	1.2	0.5	2.2	3 (0.4)	0.629 (0.531-0.712)
	Possibilities for development	0.77	0.71	0.73	65.9	17.6	68.7	17.0	0.4	2.3	0.3	4.4	2.6	2 (0.3)	0.810 (0.761-0.852)
	Variation	0.50	0.23	0.26	60.4	21.4	50.4	19.8	2.0	4.2	2.7	1.1	2.2	3 (0.4)	0.474 (0.324-0.598)
	Meaning of work	0.74	0.70	0.70	73.8	15.8	75.9	17.7	0.1	7.3	0.1	15.6	2.8	2 (0.3)	0.779 (0.745-0.844)
	Commitment to the workplace	0.76	0.61	0.71	60.9	20.4	69.5	16.4	0.7	2.2	0.1	4.7	2.2	2 (0.3)	0.521 (0.307-0.628)
Interpersonal relations and leadership	Predictability	0.74	0.50	0.62	57.7	20.9	58.6	19.5	1.5	4.2	1.2	3.0	2.3	2 (0.3)	0.736 (0.660-0.799)
	Recognition	0.83	0.67	0.76	66.2	19.9	66.9	19.2	0.9	5.8	0.4	4.4	2.8	2 (0.3)	0.807 (0.755-0.851)
	Role clarity	0.78	0.72	0.73	73.5	16.4	60.2	14.7	0.0	7.5	0.3	0.9	2.7	2 (0.3)	0.777 (0.717-0.828)
	Role conflicts	0.67	0.70	0.67	42.0	16.6	44.2	19.0	1.3	0.2	1.8	0.5	2.6	3 (0.4)	0.785 (0.729-0.833)
	Quality of leadership	0.89	0.90	0.88	55.3	21.1	64.6	21.5	1.2	1.9	0.3	10.7	2.0	167[a] (22.4)	0.926 (0.903-0.945)
	Social support from colleagues	0.70	0.65	0.74	57.3	19.7	59.6	21.9	1.1	1.9	0.3	12.8	2.0	5 (0.7)	0.748 (0.748-0.808)
	Social support from supervisors	0.79	0.84	0.82	61.6	22.4	68.4	19.2	0.9	4.4	0.8	3.1	2.7	165[b] (22.1)	0.834 (0.780-0.878)
	Social community at work	0.85	0.81	0.77	78.7	18.9	59.3	20.3	0.2	24.4	1.9	2.6	2.6	3 (0.4)	0.832 (0.787-0.870)
Work-individual interface	Job insecurity	0.77	0.77	0.79	23.7	20.8	43.9	26.1	19.0	0.5	6.9	2.0	2.3	2 (0.3)	0.835 (0.793-0.872)
	Job satisfaction	0.82	0.72	0.80	65.3	18.2	62.5	16.0	0.7	5.1	0.3	3.0	2.8	3 (0.4)	0.864 (0.826-0.897)
	Work-family conflict	0.80	0.84	0.85	33.5	24.3	40.0	26.7	9.7	1.2	9.3	4.0	2.9	3 (0.4)	0.905 (0.880-0.927)
	Family-work conflict	0.79	0.76	0.88	7.6	15.3	10.7	16.9	74.6	0.2	65.4	0.4	2.9	2 (0.4)	0.792 (0.751-0.842)
Values at the workplace	Mutual trust between employees	0.77	0.66	0.65	68.6	16.9	69.0	16.6	0.0	5.6	0.1	4.7	3.2	10 (1.3)	0.752 (0.685-0.809)
	Trust regarding management	0.80	0.60	0.65	67.0	17.7	62.8	18.2	0.2	3.9	0.7	3.7	2.5	7 (0.9)	0.785 (0.729-0.834)
	Justice	0.83	0.81	0.83	59.2	17.7	61.8	18.3	0.4	1.6	0.4	3.0	2.6	7 (0.9)	0.878 (0.846-0.906)
	Social inclusiveness	0.63	0.65	0.64	67.5	16.3	59.0	20.7	0.1	3.8	0.7	2.2	2.8	8 (1.1)	0.685 (0.601-0.758)
Health and well-being	General health perception	-	-	-	66.0	20.9	58.3	22.8	0.8	14.8	1.3	9.8	1.2	0 (0)	0.820 (0.753-0.869)
	Burnout	0.83	0.91	0.94	34.1	18.2	32.9	22.5	1.7	0.2	10.9	0.3	0.6	1 (0.1)	0.938 (0.922-0.952)
	Stress	0.81	0.83	0.87	26.7	17.7	43.9	22.3	5.2	0.1	4.0	1.5	0.6	1 (0.1)	0.904 (0.879-0.925)
	Sleeping troubles	0.86	0.88	0.93	21.3	19.0	38.7	21.6	17.4	0.0	5.4	0.3	0.6	2 (0.3)	0.930 (0.912-0.946)
	Depressive symptoms	0.76	0.77	0.82	21.0	16.5	32.9	22.5	10.3	0.0	10.9	0.3	0.7	1 (0.1)	0.862 (0.826-0.893)
	Somatic stress	0.68	0.70	0.78	17.8	16.0	26.9	18.9	16.6	0.0	12.2	0.3	0.6	1 (0.1)	0.843 (0.802-0.878)

Table 4 Comparison of the reliability and summary descriptive statistics between the Portuguese (n = 745) and the original COPSOQ II Danish (n = 3517) study sample (Continued)

Cognitive stress	0.83	0.84	0.88	17.8	15.7	31.8	18.8	18.6	0.0	5.9	0.1	0.7	1 (0.1)	0.915 (0.893–0.934)
Self-efficacy	0.80	0.80	0.89	67.5	16.0	66.1	17.9	0.0	1.8	0.1	2.3	1.3	1 (0.1)	0.890 (0.862–0.914)
Offensive behaviour														
Sexual harassment	-	-	-	2.9%	-	0.6%	-	97.0	0.1	98.1	0.1	3.3	7 (0.9)	0.655 (0.526–0.749)
Threats of violence	-	-	-	7.8%	-	1.5%	-	92.2	0.3	95.1	0.1	3.2	8 (1.1)	0.909 (0.875–0.934)
Physical violence	-	-	-	3.9%	-	0.2%	-	96.1	0.0	99.2	0.8	3.3	8 (1.1)	0.888 (0.871–0.903)
Bullying	-	-	-	8.3%	-	1.0%	-	91.7	0.5	96.7	0.1	2.5	8 (1.1)	0.562 (0.399–0.681)
Unpleasant teasing	-	-	-	8.3%	-	5.2%	-	91.7	0.3	82.5	0.3	3.2	7 (0.9)	0.813 (0.743–0.864)
Conflicts and quarrels	-	-	-	51.2%	-	5.8%	-	48.8	1.3	79.9	0.4	2.5	7 (0.9)	0.683 (0.564–0.769)
Gossip and slander	-	-	-	38.9%	-	5.3%	-	61.1	3.5	83.6	0.8	2.6	7 (0.9)	0.658 (0.531–0.751)

a Most cases are "not applicable" rather than there being "no answers" from participants. The data results of the "non-answers" and not applicable are the following for the two scales: *Quality of leadership* [no answers n = 10; not applicable n = 157] and *Social support from supervisors* [no answers n = 9; not applicable n = 156] the COPSOQ II questionnaire scale score completed 2 weeks after the baseline assessment. According to the adopted criteria for the interpretation of the magnitude of the ICC (> 0.70), this analysis indicated an acceptable reliability for 33 out of 41 scales. For the eight scales where we had ICC values of less than 0.70, five of them had very close values and three were indicative of poor reliability.

The average scores and standard deviations showed similar results to the original Danish study [16]. However, the average scores showed moderate differences in eight scales [Demand for hiding emotions (Portugal = 39.7, Denmark = 50.6), Social support from supervisors (Portugal = 68.4, Denmark = 61.6), Social community at work (Portugal = 59.3, Denmark = 78.7), Stress (Portugal = 43.9, Denmark = 26.7), Sleeping troubles (Portugal = 38.7, Denmark = 21.3), Depressive symptoms (Portugal = 32.9, Denmark = 21.0), Somatic stress (Portugal = 26.9, Denmark = 17.8) and Cognitive stress (Portugal = 31.8, Denmark = 17.8)] and very significant differences in three scales [Job insecurity (Portugal = 43.9, Denmark = 23.7), Conflicts and quarrels (Portugal = 5.8%, Denmark = 51.2) and Gossip and slander (Portugal = 5.3%, Denmark = 38.9)]. These verified differences are positive and negative, depending on each case.

Most of the scales had low floor and ceiling effects, except *Family–work conflict*, which had a high floor effect (65.4%).

For 39 of the 41 scales in the long questionnaire, the percentage of missing values was less than 1.3% (0.1– 1.3%). Two scales had high values [*Quality of leadership* (22.4%) and *Social support from supervisors* (22.1%)] although most cases are not applicable rather than there being no answers from participants.

An exploratory factor analysis was conducted considering the seven dimensions of the long version of the COPSOQ II, and the results are summarized in Tables 5, 6, 7, 8, 9, 10, 11.

In the *Demands at work* dimension, the results support the scales (*Quantitative demands, Work pace, Emotional demands* and *Demands for hiding emotions*). However, items in the scale of *Cognitive demands* have the highest loadings on three different factors, indicating that the construct validity of this scale is not supported (Table 5).

In the *Work organisation and Job Contents* dimension, the results support the *Commitment to the workplace* scale. Items in the *Influence* scale are split into two factors (one factor concerning influence in general and concerning what you do, and one factor concerning influence on who you work with and the amount of work). In the scale concerning *Possibilities for development*, one item loads on factor 5 rather than factor 1. In the *Variation* scale, one item loads on factor 5 while the other item loads highest on factor 3, together with two items concerning *Influence*. In the *Meaning of work* scale, one

Table 5 Exploratory factor analysis of items in the *Demands at work* dimension (n = 700) of COPSOQ II (long version): loadings for each factor and each item in the scale after varimax rotation and factor extraction using principal components

Scale	Item	Factors *				
		1	2	3	4	5
Quantitative demands						
QD1	Is your workload unevenly distributed so it piles up?	0.104	**0.673**	0.198	-0.053	0.231
QD2	How often do you not have time to complete all your work tasks?	0.004	**0.577**	-0.019	**0.499**	0.017
QD3	Do you get behind with your work?	0.194	**0.743**	-0.044	0.066	-0.071
QD4	Do you have enough time for your work tasks?	0.023	**0.710**	0.197	-0.038	0.010
Work pace						
WP1	Do you have to work very fast?	0.055	0.274	**0.767**	0.085	0.030
WP2	Do you work at a high pace throughout the day?	0.268	0.123	**0.784**	0.023	0.025
WP3	Is it necessary to keep working at a high pace?	0.148	0.083	**0.635**	**0.433**	-0.015
Cognitive demands						
CD1	Do you have to keep your eyes on lots of things while you work?	0.102	0.134	0.301	**0.701**	0.061
CD2	Does your work require that you remember a lot of things?	0.199	-0.142	**0.444**	0.258	0.191
CD3	Does your work demand that you are good at coming up with new ideas?	0.259	-0.101	0.152	**0.713**	-0.101
CD4	Does your work require you to make difficult decisions?	**0.573**	0.228	0.253	0.136	0.050
Emotional demands						
ED1	Does your work put you in emotionally disturbing situations?	**0.585**	**0.437**	0.119	0.095	0.218
ED2	Do you have to relate to other people's personal problems as part of your work?	**0.639**	0.102	0.021	**0.392**	0.132
ED3	Is your work emotionally demanding?	**0.761**	0.162	0.207	0.048	0.208
ED4	Do you get emotionally involved in your work?	**0.681**	-0.100	0.103	0.063	-0.069
Demands for hiding emotions						
HE1	Are you required to treat everyone equally, even if you do not feel like it?	0.075	0.056	-0.066	0.170	**0.747**
HE2	Does your work require that you hide your feelings?	**0.348**	0.119	0.129	-0.277	**0.560**
HE3	Are you required to be kind and open towards everyone – regardless of how they behave towards you?	0.008	0.010	0.013	-0.052	**0.816**

*Five factors explaining 59% of the total variance; KMO=0.820; Bartlett's Test of Sphericity: p < 0.001. Bold values indicate factor loading of greater than 0.3. Grey shading values indicate the highest loading for each item.

*Five factors explaining 59% of the total variance; KMO = 0.820; Bartlett's Test of Sphericity: *p* < 0.001. Bold values indicate factor loading of greater than 0.3. Grey shading values indicate the highest loading for each item

Table 6 Exploratory factor analysis of items in the *Work organisation and job contents* dimension (n = 699) of COPSOQ II (long version): loadings for each factor and each item in the scale after a varimax rotation and factor extraction using principal components

Scale	Item	Factors *				
		1	**2**	**3**	**4**	**5**
Influence						
IN1	Do you have a large degree of influence concerning your work?	0.223	-0.132	**0.732**	0.226	0.076
IN2	Do you have a say in choosing who you work with?	0.041	-0.020	0.176	**0.712**	0.174
IN3	Can you influence the amount of work assigned to you?	0.000	0.069	0.081	**0.772**	-0.123
IN4	Do you have any influence on what you do at work?	0.121	0.178	**0.774**	0.021	-0.149
Possibilities for development						
PD1	Does your work require you to take the initiative?	**0.658**	-0.159	0.262	0.174	0.155
PD2	Do you have the possibility of learning new things through your work?	**0.409**	0.339	-0.002	0.049	**0.483**
PD3	Can you use your skills or expertise in your work?	**0.576**	0.316	0.209	0.138	0.130
PD4	Does your work give you the opportunity to develop your skills?	**0.514**	0.329	0.043	0.282	0.383
Variation						
VA1	Is your work varied?	-0.007	0.016	**0.578**	0.104	**0.439**
VA2	Do you have to do the same thing over and over again?	-0.052	-0.045	0.024	-0.018	**0.788**
Meaning of work						
MW1	Is your work meaningful?	**0.727**	0.141	0.183	-0.288	-0.140
MW2	Do you feel that the work you do is important?	**0.735**	0.290	-0.021	-0.076	-0.118
MW3	Do you feel motivated and involved in your work?	0.309	**0.703**	0.250	-0.156	-0.011
Commitment to the workplace						
CW1	Do you enjoy telling others about your place of work?	0.298	**0.548**	-0.002	0.188	0.133
CW2	Do you feel that your place of work is of great importance to you?	**0.553**	0.498	-0.047	0.133	0.044
CW3	Would you recommend a good friend to apply for a position at your workplace?	0.074	**0.657**	-0.186	0.230	0.144
CW4	How often do you consider looking for work elsewhere?	0.036	**0.738**	0.096	-0.209	-0.156

*Five factors explaining 60% of the total variance; KMO=0.830; Bartlett's Test of Sphericity: p < 0.001. Bold values indicate factor loading of greater than 0.3. Grey shading values indicate the highest loading for each item.

*Five factors explaining 60% of the total variance; KMO = 0.830; Bartlett's Test of Sphericity: *p* < 0.001. Bold values indicate factor loading of greater than 0.3. Grey shading values indicate the highest loading for each item

item loads highest on factor 2, together with the items on *Commitment to the workplace* (Table 6).

In the *Interpersonal relations and leadership* dimension (Table 7), the results support the *Role clarity, Role conflict, Social support from colleagues* and *Social community at work* scales. Two scales (*Quality of leadership* and *Social support from supervisors*) load on the same factor. Two other scales (*Predictability* and *Recognition*) load on several factors.

In the *Work-individual interface* dimension, the results support the hypothesised scale structure (Table 8).

In the *Values at the workplace* dimension, the results support the hypothesised scale structure for two scales (*Justice* and *Social inclusiveness*), while the other two scales are split between several factors (Table 9).

In the *Health and well-being* dimension, the results support the hypothesised scale structure for five scales (*Sleeping problems, Burnout, Somatic stress, Cognitive stress* and *Self-efficacy*). The stress scale is split into several factors. In the *Depressive symptoms* scale, DS1 loads strongest on factor 2 (Table 10).

In the *Offensive behaviour* dimension (Table 11), the results support the *Bullying, Unpleasant teasing, Conflict and quarrels* and *Gossip and slander* scales. The other three scales load on factor 2 rather than factor 1.

The results of the exploratory factor analysis showed that, from the 41 total scales, 27 support the hypothesised scale structure while the factor results differ from the scale structure for 14 scales (Cognitive demands, Influence, Possibilities for development, Variation, Meaning of work, Predictability, Recognition, Mutual trust between employees, Trust between management, Stress,

Depressive symptoms, Sexual harassment, Threats of violence and Physical violence).

Discussion

This paper described the Portuguese validation of the long version of COPSOQ II using rigorous methodology based on both psychometric and conceptual criteria.

In general, a Cronbach's alpha of the COPSOQ scales (test and retest) indicated acceptable reliability (0.7). Furthermore, the fact that Cronbach's alpha is influenced by the number of items in the scale explains the findings of lower values of alphas.

The test-retest reliability results indicate that most of the scales showed good temporal stability and reliability in the considered time interval. However, there were eight scales that showed ICC values below 0.7 (*Influence, Variation, Commitment to the workplace, Social inclusiveness, Sexual harassment, Bullying, Conflicts and quarrels* and *Gossip and slander*). Out of these eight four belonged to the offensive behaviour dimension, three to belonged to the Work organisation and job contents and the remaining one to the Values at workplace dimension.

The three scales concerning the *Variation, Commitment to the workplace* and *Bullying* showed poor ICC values. The reason for the poor test-retest reliability should be evaluated in future studies.

The test-retest design showed a good reliability for most of the scales, namely where Cronbach's alpha was low, as reported in a previous study by Thorsen and Bjorner [67]. These authors examined the reliability of the COPSOQ work environment questionnaire and have concluded that the test-retest design and intraclass correlation appears to be more appropriate than Cronbach's

Table 7 Exploratory factor analysis of items in the *Interpersonal relations and leadership* dimension ($n = 516$) of COPSOQ II (long version): loadings for each factor and each item in the scale after a varimax rotation and factor extraction using principal components

Scale	Item	Factors *					
		1	2	3	4	5	6
Predictability							
PR1	At your place of work, are you informed well in advance concerning for example important decisions, changes or plans for the future?	0.306	0.089	-0.193	0.018	0.173	**0.744**
PR2	Do you receive all the information you need in order to do your work well?	0.263	**0.716**	-0.172	0.064	0.075	0.192
Recognition							
RE1	Is your work recognised and appreciated by the management?	**0.383**	**0.366**	-0.086	0.150	0.050	**0.526**
RE2	Does the management at your workplace respect you?	**0.496**	0.289	-0.258	0.206	-0.079	0.234
RE3	Are you treated fairly at your workplace?	0.182	**0.669**	0.030	0.214	-0.006	0.020
Role clarity							
CL1	Does your work have clear objectives?	0.143	**0.769**	0.005	-0.023	0.049	0.126
CL2	Do you know exactly which areas are your responsibility?	0.114	**0.710**	0.173	0.180	-0.130	-0,256
CL3	Do you know exactly what is expected of you at work?	0.082	**0.722**	-0.056	0.017	0.042	0.086
Role conflicts							
CO1	Do you do things at work which are accepted by some people but not by others?	-0.010	0.188	**0.653**	-0.174	0.002	-0.129
CO2	Are contradictory demands placed on you at work?	-0.185	-0.089	**0.696**	-0.137	0.093	-0.093
CO3	Do you sometimes have to do things which ought to have been done in a different way?	-0.184	-0.297	**0.691**	0.051	-0.110	0.253
CO4	Do you sometimes have to do things which seem to be unnecessary?	-0.010	0.188	**0.653**	-0.174	0.002	-0.129
Quality of leadership	To what extent would you say that your immediate superior:						
QL1	– makes sure that the individual member of staff has good development opportunities?	**0.752**	0.158	-0.081	0.174	0.080	0.241
QL2	– gives high priority to job satisfaction?	**0.796**	0.136	-0.104	0.148	0.029	0.242
QL3	– is good at work planning?	**0.798**	0.062	-0.134	0.106	0.035	0.110
QL4	– is good at solving conflicts?	**0.791**	0.075	-0.157	0.127	0.013	0.152
Social support from colleagues							
SC1	How often do you get help and support from your colleagues?	0.180	0.011	-0.021	0.255	**0.671**	0.014
SC2	How often are your colleagues willing to listen to your problems at work?	0.060	0.210	0.085	0.296	**0.715**	-0.036
SC3	How often do your colleagues talk with you about how well you carry out your work?	0.160	-0.203	-0.087	0.112	**0.744**	0.247
Social support from supervisors[a]							
SS1	How often is your immediate superior willing to listen to your problems at work?	**0.764**	0.212	-0.103	0.142	0.118	-0.071
SS2	How often do you get help and support from your immediate superior?	**0.801**	0.170	-0.064	0.106	0.213	-0.069
SS3	How often does your immediate superior talk with you about how well you carry out your work?	**0.689**	0.149	-0.059	-0.119	**0.342**	0.040
Social community at work							
SW1	Is there a good atmosphere between you and your colleagues?	0.184	0.040	-0.119	**0.839**	0.183	-0.049
SW2	Is there good co-operation between the colleagues at work?	0.228	0.117	-0.111	**0.760**	0.305	0.045
SW3	Do you feel part of a community at your place of work?	0.115	0.220	-0.126	**0.703**	0.201	0.143

*Six factors explaining 65% of the total variance; KMO=0.894; Bartlett's Test of Sphericity: p < 0.001. [a] These questions were only addressed to respondents who were not supervisors themselves, and who had a supervisor. Bold values indicate factor loading of greater than 0.3. Grey shading values indicate the highest loading for each item.

*Six factors explaining 65% of the total variance; KMO = 0.894; Bartlett's Test of Sphericity: $p < 0.001$. [a] These questions were only addressed to respondents who were not supervisors themselves, and who had a supervisor. Bold values indicate factor loading of greater than 0.3. Grey shading values indicate the highest loading for each item

alpha for assessing the reliability of COPSOQ's psychosocial work environment scales.

Thorsen and Bjorner [67] specified assumptions for 26 COPSOQ scales, eight of each were assumed to exhibit a reflective model (internal consistency) and 18 were assumed to exhibit a formative model.

The exploratory factor analysis findings assumed that from the 41 total scales, 27 are based on a reflective model of effect indicators, in which all of the items are a manifestation of the same underlying construct [46, 68, 69]. The remaining 14 scales did not show a clear factor in the exploratory factor analysis. Out of these, three (Meaning of work, Stress and Depressive symptoms) cannot be assumed

to exhibit the formative model, since they had previously been assumed to exhibit a reflective measurement model, as reported by Thorsen and Bjorner [67]. Future studies should evaluate these three scales in greater depth.

The remaining 11 scales assumed to exhibit a formative model in which items are combined due to their hypothesised common effect rather than their common cause. High inter-item correlation is not a necessary criterion of construct validity and these do not need to be correlated [46, 67, 70, 71].

Following this line of thinking, as Thorsen and Bjorner [67] also state, Cronbach's alpha might not be a good measure of reliability for these scales because it might

Table 8 Exploratory factor analysis of items in the *Work-individual interface* dimension (*n* = 704) of COPSOQ II (long version): loadings for each factor and each item in the scale after a varimax rotation and factor extraction using principal components

Scale	Item	Factors *			
		1	2	3	4
Job insecurity					
JI1	Are you worried about becoming unemployed?	-0.094	**0.827**	-0.049	0.009
JI2	Are you worried about new technology making you redundant?	-0.011	**0.715**	0.150	0.035
JI3	Are you worried about it being difficult for you to find another job if you became unemployed?	-0.075	**0.798**	0.007	-0.045
JI4	Are you worried about being transferred to another job against your will?	0.074	**0.718**	0.009	0.083
Job satisfaction	Regarding your work in general, how pleased are you with:				
JS1	– your work prospects?	-0.109	-0.018	**0.776**	-0.018
JS2	– the physical working conditions?	-0.222	-0.034	**0.453**	0.115
JS3	– the way your abilities are used?	0.020	0.103	**0.823**	-0.113
JS4	– your job as a whole, everything taken into consideration?	-0.048	0.080	**0.793**	-0.089
Work-family conflict					
WF1	Do you often feel a conflict between your work and your private life, making you want to be in both places at the same time?	**0.711**	-0.032	-0.096	0.190
WF2	The next three questions concern the ways in which your work affects your private life: Do you feel that your work drains so much of your energy that it has a negative effect on your private life?	**0.842**	0.031	-0.156	0.105
WF3	Do you feel that your work takes so much of your time that it has a negative effect on your private life?	**0.863**	-0.018	-0.123	0.161
WF4	Do your friends or family tell you that you work too much?	**0.780**	-0.084	-0.007	0.073
Family-work conflict	The next two questions concern the ways in which your private life affects your work:				
FW1	Do you feel that your private life takes so much of your energy that it has a negative effect on your work?	0.215	0.083	-0.063	**0.861**
FW2	Do you feel that your private life takes so much of your time that it has a negative effect on your work?	0.210	0.007	-0.020	**0.858**

*Four factors explaining 64% of the total variance; KMO=0.750; Bartlett's Test of Sphericity: p < 0.001. Bold values indicate factor loading of greater than 0.3. Grey shading values indicate the highest loading for each item.

*Four factors explaining 64% of the total variance; KMO = 0.750; Bartlett's Test of Sphericity: *p* < 0.001. Bold values indicate factor loading of greater than 0.3. Grey shading values indicate the highest loading for each item

underestimate true reliability. In this circumstance, the internal consistency is not considered relevant for items that form a formative model [46, 70–74].

In accordance with these findings, the authors Bjorner and Pejtersen [75] argue that the traditional psychometric techniques (e.g. factor analysis and reliability through Cronbach's alpha) may not be appropriate for some COPSOQ II scales for which the items are combined based on a hypothesised common effect rather than a hypothesised common cause.

As quoted in their work [75] *"Bollen pointed out that not all questionnaires scales can be conceived as consisting of effect indicator items, being that some items must be seen as causes of the latent construct rather than effects"* [70, 71].

These insights can help to explain the apparently "inconsistent" findings that were reported in some of the results of the exploratory factor analysis.

The average scores and standard deviations showed similar results to the original Danish study, except for 11 scales, which may be explained by the context of unstable

Table 9 Exploratory factor analysis of items in the *Values at the workplace* dimension (*n* = 683) of COPSOQ II (long version): loadings for each factor and each item in the scale after a varimax rotation and factor extraction using principal components

Scale	Item	Factors *			
		1	2	3	4
Mutual trust between employees					
TE1	Do the employees withhold information from each other?	0.342	0.004	-0.003	**0.840**
TE2	Do the employees withhold information from the management?	-0.024	-0.067	**0.547**	**0.680**
TE3	Do the employees in general trust each other?	**0.564**	0.205	-0.067	0.372
Trust regarding management					
TM1	Does the management trust the employees to do their work well?	0.252	-0.022	**0.759**	-0.099
TM2	Can you trust the information that comes from the management?	**0.673**	0.028	**0.462**	-0.023
TM3	Does the management withhold important information from the employees?	0.040	0.040	**0.709**	0.374
TM4	Are the employees able to express their views and feelings?	**0.671**	0.221	0.198	0.107
Justice					
JU1	Are conflicts resolved in a fair way?	**0.749**	0.096	0.100	0.162
JU2	Are employees appreciated when they have done a good job?	**0.752**	0.041	0.014	-0.010
JU3	Are all suggestions from employees treated seriously by the management?	**0.802**	0.076	0.090	0.045
JU4	Is the work distributed fairly?	**0.710**	0.216	0.029	0.177
Social inclusiveness					
SI1	Are men and women treated equally at your workplace?	**0.365**	**0.376**	**0.355**	0.063
SI2	Is there space for employees of a different race and religion?	0.065	**0.792**	0.164	0.016
SI3	Is there space for elderly employees?	0.149	**0.633**	-0.368	-0.007
SI4	Is there space for employees with various illnesses or disabilities?	0.181	**0.806**	-0.004	-0.010

*Four factors explaining 62% of the total variance; KMO=0.861; Bartlett's Test of Sphericity: p < 0.001. Bold values indicate factor loading of greater than 0.3. Grey shading values indicate the highest loading for each item.

*Four factors explaining 62% of the total variance; KMO = 0.861; Bartlett's Test of Sphericity: *p* < 0.001. Bold values indicate factor loading of greater than 0.3. Grey shading values indicate the highest loading for each item

Table 10 Exploratory factor analysis of items in the *Health and well-being* dimension (*n* = 694) of COPSOQ II (long version): loadings for each factor and each item in the scale after a varimax rotation and factor extraction using principal components

Scale	Item	Factors *				
		1	2	3	4	5
General health perception						
GH1	In general, would you say your health is: excellent, very good, good, fair, poor?	-	-	-	-	-
	The following questions are about how you have been during the last four weeks.					
Sleeping problems						
SL1	How often have you slept badly and restlessly?	0.128	0.302	**0.731**	-0.052	0.190
SL2	How often have you found it hard to go to sleep?	0.119	0.227	**0.758**	-0.049	0.164
SL3	How often have you woken up too early and not been able to get back to sleep?	0.153	0.181	**0.822**	-0.069	0.100
SL4	How often have you woken up several times and found it difficult to get back to sleep?	0.125	0.235	**0.843**	-0.056	0.116
Burnout						
BO1	How often have you felt worn out?	0.229	**0.746**	0.292	-0.070	0.230
BO2	How often have you been physically exhausted?	0.214	**0.732**	0.250	-0.074	0.320
BO3	How often have you been emotionally exhausted?	**0.385**	**0.674**	0.333	-0.104	0.119
BO4	How often have you felt tired?	0.245	**0.740**	0.216	-0.076	0.306
Stress						
ST1	How often have you had problems relaxing?	**0.466**	**0.523**	0.265	-0.141	0.230
ST2	How often have you been irritable?	**0.554**	**0.526**	0.168	-0.135	0.103
ST3	How often have you been tense?	0.205	0.334	0.092	-0.129	**0.783**
ST4	How often have you been stressed?	**0.391**	**0.563**	0.188	-0.080	0.342
Depressive symptoms						
DS1	How often have you felt sad?	**0.420**	**0.563**	0.293	-0.164	0.054
DS2	How often have you lacked self-confidence?	**0.671**	0.241	0.070	-0.306	0.165
DS3	How often have you had a bad conscience or felt guilty?	**0.711**	0.054	0.090	-0.046	0.088
DS4	How often have you lacked interest in everyday things?	**0.709**	0.270	0.018	-0.082	0.100
Somatic stress						
SO1	How often have you had stomach ache?	0.299	-0.025	0.268	-0.044	**0.476**
SO2	How often have you had a headache?	0.146	0.267	0.252	-0.046	**0.570**
SO3	How often have you had palpitations?	**0.378**	0.269	0.199	-0.042	**0.414**
SO4	How often have you had tension in various muscles?	0.234	0.293	0.059	-0.092	**0.799**
Cognitive stress	How well do these descriptions fit you as a person?					
CS1	How often have you had problems concentrating?	**0.632**	**0.411**	0.156	-0.076	0.196
CS2	How often have you found it difficult to think clearly?	**0.696**	0.266	0.189	-0.106	0.284
CS3	How often have you had difficulty in taking decisions?	**0.699**	0.172	0.184	-0.246	0.170
CS4	How often have you had difficulty with remembering?	**0.616**	0.186	0.054	-0.081	0.224
Self-efficacy						
SE1	I am always able to solve difficult problems if I try hard enough	-0.082	-0.168	0.005	**0.609**	-0.061
SE2	If people work against me, I find a way of achieving what I want	0.097	-0.146	-0.033	**0.607**	0.093
SE3	It is easy for me to stick to my plans and reach my objectives	-0.018	-0.069	-0.036	**0.664**	0.006
SE4	I feel confident that I can handle unexpected events	-0.231	-0.009	-0.017	**0.739**	-0.075
SE5	When I have a problem, I can usually find several ways of solving it.	-0.215	-0.041	-0.062	**0.683**	-0.160
SE6	Regardless of what happens, I usually manage.	-0.073	0.092	-0.086	**0.631**	-0.107

*Five factors explaining 61% of the total variance; KMO=0.943; Bartlett's Test of Sphericity: p < 0.001. Bold values indicate factor loading of greater than 0.3. Grey shading values indicate the highest loading for each item.

*Five factors explaining 61% of the total variance; KMO = 0.943; Bartlett's Test of Sphericity: *p* < 0.001. Bold values indicate factor loading of greater than 0.3. Grey shading values indicate the highest loading for each item

labour markets and the significant increase in employees' feeling of job insecurity (e.g. fear of being hampered in the performance of their function or in their career development and even of losing their job) and the resulting negative impact on employees' health and well-being. As for the floor and ceiling effect, we observed similar results to the original Danish study. The *Family-work conflict* scale showed a high floor effect (65.4%) and a very low mean value (10.7). In accordance with the original authors, this result also indicates that private life is not interfering with work in general.

As for the missing items, in 39 out of the total of 41 scales, the missing items are less than 1.3%. A higher proportion of missing values observed in two scales (*Quality of leadership* and *Social support from supervisors*) should be interpreted cautiously due to the fact that most cases are "not applicable" questions rather than "no answers" from the participants.

The Portuguese COPSOQ II had a moderate response rate of 60.6% for the baseline test (*n* = 745) and a good follow-up rate of 59.5% for the retest (*N* = 394).

Several strengths of this study need to be mentioned. Firstly, the inclusion of international statistical standards enables reliable and comparable national, European and international statistics. In line with this, validation of the long version of COPSOQ II, maintaining its full content and structure, also enables statistics comparable to those of other countries.

Secondly, the adoption of COSMIN methodology, internationally widely accepted recommendations for the assessment of psychometric characteristics, is aimed at ensuring the quality of results. Thirdly, the inclusion of various sectors of economic activity, taking into consideration workers at different hierarchical levels and in different functions in each company, ensured greater confidence in the results.

There were some limitations to the study. Firstly, the study sample in the *Wholesale and retail trade* and *Manufacturing* sectors of economic activity should be improved. Secondly, the online survey data collection had lower response rates than the paper-based ones.

Table 11 Exploratory factor analysis of items in the *Offensive behaviour* dimension (*n* = 729) of COPSOQ II (long version): loadings for each factor and each item in the scale after a varimax rotation and factor extraction using principal components

Scale	Item	Factors *	
		1	2
Sexual harassment			
SH	Have you been exposed to undesired sexual attention at your workplace during the last 12 months?	0.139	**0.410**
Threats of violence			
TV	Have you been exposed to threats of violence at your workplace during the last 12 months?	0.004	**0.718**
Physical violence			
PV	Have you been exposed to physical violence at your workplace during the last 12 months?	0.116	**0.797**
Bullying	Bullying means that a person is repeatedly exposed to unpleasant or degrading treatment, and that the person finds it difficult to defend himself or herself against it.		
BU	Have you been exposed to bullying at your workplace during the last 12 months?	**0.627**	0.123
Unpleasant teasing			
UT	Have you been exposed to unpleasant teasing at your workplace during the last 12 months?	**0.742**	0.288
Conflicts and quarrels			
CQ	Have you been involved in quarrels or conflicts at your workplace during the last 12 months?	**0.796**	0.043
Gossip and slander			
GS	Have you been exposed to gossip and slander at your workplace during the last 12 months?	**0.725**	0.033

*Two factors explaining 51% of the total variance; KMO=0.680; Bartlett's Test of Sphericity: p < 0.001. Bold values indicate factor loading of greater than 0.3.

*Two factors explaining 51% of the total variance; KMO = 0.680; Bartlett's Test of Sphericity: *p* < 0.001. Bold values indicate factor loading of greater than 0.3

Thirdly, the current economic crisis could have an impact on the answers that people give to some of the questions.

Conclusion

Most scales in the Portuguese long version of the COPSOQ II were found to be valid and reliable for the evaluation and study of the implications of psychosocial work factors for the health and well-being of workers. Three scales need further evaluation since the hypothesized factor structure was not supported (Meaning of work, Stress, and Depressive symptoms) while three other scales should be further evaluated due to low reliability in test-retest analyses (Variation, Commitment to the workplace, and Bullying).

The Framework Directive (89/391/EEC) confers a central place in risk assessment to preventive approaches and highlights the use of valid and reliable methods in order to identify all types of risk factors in organisations, with psychosocial risk management being the employers' responsibility. This line of approach establishes the importance of integrated prevention, taking an increasing number of risk factors into consideration and including all aspects of psychosocial risks (e.g. demands at work, work-individual interface, work organisation and job contents, offensive behaviour, etc.). This tool is intended to be a resource for researchers and professionals in Portuguese organisations for the prevention and promotion of health and well-being in the labour context and also to promote the development of a national culture of prevention, in particular as regards psychosocial risk factors.

In future research, gradual use of the COPSOQ in various economic activities will lead to a broader database, thereby allowing researchers and professionals to adjust validation analyses (in particular the scales that indicated less satisfactory results), establish comparisons between companies and advance in the development of Portuguese standards.

Abbreviations

BGW: Institute for statutory accident insurance and prevention in the health and welfare services; CAE – Rev. 3: Portuguese classification of economic activities – revision 3; CIDES: Department of health information and decision sciences; CINTESIS: Centre for research in health technologies and information systems and information and decision sciences department; COPSOQ II: Copenhagen Psychosocial Questionnaire II; COSMIN: COnsensus-based standards for the selection of health measurement instruments; CUF: Companhia União Fabril; Cvcare: Center of excellence for epidemiology and health service research for healthcare professionals; EUROSTAT: Statistical office of the european communities; FFAW GmbH: Freiburg research centre for occupational sciences; GPR: Principles of prevention and rehabilitation department; ICC: Intraclass correlation coefficient; ISCO: International standard classification of occupations; ISIC – Rev. 4: International standard classification of activities – revision 4; IVDP: Institute for health services research in dermatology and nursing; KMO: Kaiser-Meyer-Olkin; LAETA: Associated laboratory for energy, transport and aeronautics; NACE – Rev. 2: Classification of economic activities in the european union – revision 2; NOPain: National observatory of pain; OECD: Organisation for Economic Co-operation and Development; OSH: Occupational Safety and Health;

PORDATA: The data base of contemporary Portugal; SD: Standard deviation; SPSS: Statistical package for the social sciences

Acknowledgments
We would like to thank all the employees who agreed to participate in the study.

Funding
This study received no specific grant from any funding agency in the public, commercial or not-for-profit sectors.

Authors' contributions
SR, LFA, JAF, AN, MN and JTC have made substantial contributions to this study. All of the authors approved and critically reviewed the final version of the manuscript.

Competing interests
The authors declare that they have no competing interests.

Author details
[1]Doctoral Programme in Occupational Safety and Health, Faculty of Engineering of the University of Porto, Rua Dr. Roberto Frias, s/n 4200-465 Porto, Portugal. [2]CINTESIS – Centre for Research in Health Technologies and Information Systems and Information and Decision Sciences Department, Faculty of Medicine of the University of Porto, Rua Dr. Plácido da Costa, s/n 4200-450 Porto, Portugal. [3]Department of Health Information and Decision Sciences (CIDES), Faculty of Medicine of the University of Porto, Rua Dr. Plácido da Costa, s/n 4200-450 Porto, Portugal. [4]National Observatory of Pain – NOPain, Faculty of Medicine of the University of Porto, Alameda Prof. Hernâni Monteiro, 4200-319 Porto, Portugal. [5]Faculty of Medicine of the University of Porto, Alameda Prof. Hernâni Monteiro, 4200-319 Porto, Portugal. [6]Allergy Unit, CUF Porto Institute & Hospital, Estrada da Circunvalação 14341, 4100-180; Rua Fonte das Sete Bicas 170, 4460-188 Porto, Portugal. [7]Centre of Excellence for Epidemiology and Health Services Research for Healthcare Professionals (CVcare), University Medical Center Hamburg-Eppendorf, Institute for Health Services Research in Dermatology and Nursing (IVDP), Martinistraße 52, 20246 Hamburg, Germany. [8]Principles of Prevention and Rehabilitation Department (GPR), Institute for Statutory Accident Insurance and Prevention in the Health and Welfare Services (BGW), Hamburg, Germany. [9]Freiburg Research Centre for Occupational Sciences (FFAW GmbH), Bertoldstr. 63, 79098 Freiburg, Germany. [10]LAETA – Associated Laboratory for Energy, Transport and Aeronautics, Faculty of Engineering of the University of Porto, Rua Dr. Roberto Frias, s/n 4200-465 Porto, Portugal.

References
1. European Commission. Europe 2020: A European Strategy for Smart, Sustainable and Inclusive Growth. Communication from the Commission COM(2010) 2020 Final. Brussels: European Commission; 2010. doi:10.1016/j.resconrec.2010.03.010.
2. European Commission. Communication from the commission to the European Parliament, the council, the European economic and social committee and the Committee of the Regions on an EU strategic framework on health and safety at work 2014–2020. Brussels: European Commission; 2014.
3. European Foundation for the Improvement of Living and Working Conditions (Eurofound), European Agency for Safety and Health at Work (EU-OSHA). Psychosocial risks in Europe: prevalence and strategies for prevention. Luxembourg: Publications Office of the European Union; 2014.
4. EU-OSHA. Estimating the cost of accidents and ill-health at work – a review of methodologies. Luxembourg: Publications Office of the European Union; 2014.
5. European Commission. Council directive 89/391/EEC - OSH "framework directive.". In: Official journal of the European Communities, L183, 29/06/1989; 1989.
6. European Commission. Interpretative document of the implementation of council directive 89/391/EEC in relation to mental health in the workplace. In: Employment, social affairs and inclusion; 2014.
7. European Commission. Guidance on risk assessment at work. Luxembourg: Publications Office of the European Union; 1996.
8. International Labour Office. ILO guidelines on occupational safety and health management systems. Geneva: International Labour Office; 2001.
9. Stravoula L, Cox T. The European framework for psychosocial risk management: PRIMA-EF. Nottingham: World Health Organization; 2008.
10. Nübling M, Vomstein M, Haugh A, Nübling T, Adiwidjaja A. European-wide survey on teachers work related stress - assessment, comparison and evaluation of the impact of psychosocial hazards on teachers at their workplace. Brussels: European Trade Union Committee for Education; 2011.
11. Rosário S, Fonseca J, Nienhaus A, Torres da Costa J. Standardized assessment of psychosocial factors and their influence on medically confirmed health outcomes in workers: a systematic review. J Occup Med Toxicol. 2016;11:19. doi:10.1186/s12995-016-0106-9.
12. EU-OSHA. The second European survey of enterprises on new and emerging risks (ESENER-2). Luxembourg: Publications Office of the European Union; 2015.
13. International Labour Office. SOLVE integrating health promotion into workplace OSH policies: Trainer's guide. Geneva: International Labour Office; 2012.
14. International Labour Office. Emerging risks and new patterns of prevention in a changing world of work. In: World day for safety and health at work, 28 April 2010. Geneva: International Labour Office; 2010.
15. Kristensen TS, Hannerz H, Høgh A, Borg V. The Copenhagen psychosocial questionnaire—a tool for the assessment and improvement of the psychosocial work environment. Scand J Work Environ Health. 2005;31(6):438–49. doi:10.5271/sjweh.948.
16. Pejtersen JH, Kristensen TS, Borg V, Bjorner JB. The second version of the Copenhagen psychosocial questionnaire. Scand J Public Health. 2010;38(3 Suppl):8–24. doi:10.1177/1403494809349858.
17. Karasek RA. Job demands, job decisions latitude and mental strain: implications for job redisign. Adm Sci Q. 1979;24:285–307.
18. Johnson JV, Hall EM. Job strain, work place social support, and cardiovascular disease: a cross-sectional study of a random sample of the Swedish working population. Am J Public Health. 1988;78(10):1336–42. doi:10.2105/AJPH.78.10.1336.
19. Siegrist J. Adverse health effects of high-effort / low-reward conditions. J Occup Health Psychol. 1996;1(1):27–41. doi:10.1037/1076-8998.1.1.27.
20. Siegrist J, Starke D, Chandola T, et al. The measurement of effort-reward imbalance at work: European comparisons. Soc Sci Med. 2004;58(8):1483–99.
21. Williams S, Cooper CL. Measuring occupational stress: development of the pressure management indicator. J Occup Health Psychol. 1998;3(4):306–21. doi:10.1037/1076-8998.3.4.306.
22. Setterlind S, Larsson G. The stress profile: a psychosocial approach to measuring stress. Stress Med. 1995;11(2):85–92.
23. Cousins R, Mackay C, Clarke S, Kelly C, Kelly P, McCaig R. Management standards and work-related stress in the UK: practical development. Work Stress. 2004;18:113–36.
24. Moos R. The work environment scale manual. 3rd ed. Palo Alto: Consulting Psychologists Press; 1994.
25. Elo A-L, Skogstad A, Dallner M, Gamberale F, Hottinen V, Knardahl S. User's Guide for the QPSNordic: General Nordic Questionnaire for Psychological and Social Factors at Work. (2000:603 T, ed.). Copenhagen: Nordic Council of Ministers; 2000.
26. Sims H, Szilagyi A, Keller R. The measurement of job characteristics. Acad Manag J. 1976;19(2):195–212.
27. Hackman JR, Oldham GR. Development of the job diagnostic survey. J Appl Psychol. 1975;60(2):159–70. doi:10.1037/h0076546.

28. Ivancevich M, Matteson T. Stress and work. Glenview, IL: Scott, Foresman and Company; 1980.

29. International Labour Office. Workplace stress: a collective challenge. In: World day for safety and health at work 28 April 2016. Geneva: International Labour Office; 2016.

30. Kristensen TS. A questionnaire is more than a questionnaire. Scand J Public Health. 2010;38(3 Suppl):149–55. doi:10.1177/1403494809354437.

31. Nübling M, Burr H, Moncada S, Kristensen TS. COPSOQ international network: Co-operation for research and assessment of psychosocial factors at work. Public Health Forum. 2014;22(1). doi:10.1016/j.phf.2013.12.019.

32. Nübling M, Stößel U, Hasselhorn H-M, Michaelis M, Hofmann F. Measuring psychological stress and strain at work - Evaluation of the COPSOQ Questionnaire in Germany. Psychosoc Med. 2006;3:Doc05. http://www.ncbi.nlm.nih.gov/pubmed/19742072%5Cn, http://www.pubmedcentral.nih.gov/articlerender.fcgi?artid=PMC2736502.

33. Nübling M, Stößel U, Hasselhorn H, Michaelis M, Hofmann F. Methoden Zur Erfassung Psychischer Belastungen - Erprobung Eines Messinstrumentes (COPSOQ).; 2005.

34. Moncada S, Utzet M, Molinero E, et al. The copenhagen psychosocial questionnaire II (COPSOQ II) in Spain-a tool for psychosocial risk assessment at the workplace. Am J Ind Med. 2014;57(1):97–107. doi:10.1002/ajim.22238.

35. Shang L, Ping L, Lin-bo F, Hua-kang G, Jian L. Psychometric properties of the Chinese version of Copenhagen psychosocial questionnaire. J Env Occup Med. 2008;25(6):572–6.

36. Dupret E, Bocéréan C, Teherani M, Feltrin M, Pejtersen JH. Psychosocial risk assessment: French validation of the Copenhagen psychosocial questionnaire (COPSOQ). Scand J Public Health. 2012;40(5):482–90. doi:10.1177/1403494812453888.

37. Berthelsen H, Hakanen J, Kristensen TS, Lönnblad A, Westerlund H. A qualitative study on the content validity of the social capital scales in the Copenhagen psychosocial questionnaire (COPSOQ II). Scand J Work Organ Psychol. 2016;1(1 (5)):1–13. doi:10.16993/sjwop.5.

38. Alvarado R, Pérez-Franco J, Saavedra N, et al. Validación de un cuestionario para evaluar riesgos psicosociales en el ambiente laboral en Chile. Rev Med Chil. 2012;140:1154–63.

39. Pournik O, Ghalichi L, TehraniYazdi A, Tabatabaee SM, Ghaffari M, Vingard E. Measuring psychosocial exposures: Validation of the Persian of the copenhagen psychosocial questionnaire (COPSOQ). Med J Islam Repub Iran. 2015;29(1).

40. COPSOQ International Network. COPSOQ International Network for scientific research and risk assessment with the Copenhagen Psychosocial Questionnaire (COPSOQ). http://www.copsoq-network.org/.

41. Rosário S, Fonseca J, Torres Da Costa J. Validação e Adaptação Linguística e Cultural da Versão Longa do Questionário Psicossocial de Copenhaga II (COPSOQ II) em Português. In: SHO2014. Guimarães: Simpósio Internacional de Segurança e Higiene Ocupacional; 2014. p. 350–2.

42. Rosário S, Fonseca J, Torres Da Costa J. Cultural and linguistic adaptation and validation of the long version of Copenhagen psychosocial questionnaire II (COPSOQ II) in portuguese. In: Occupational safety and hygiene II - selected extended and revised contributions from the international symposium occupational safety and hygiene, SHO 2014; 2014. p. 441–5.

43. Mokking L, Terwee C, Patrick D, et al. The COSMIN checklist for assessing the methodological quality of studies on measurement properties of health status measurement instruments: an international Delphi study. Qual Life Res. 2010;19:539–49.

44. Terwee CB, Mokkink LB, Knol DL, Ostelo RWJG, Bouter LM, De Vet HC. Rating the methodological quality in systematic reviews of studies on measurement properties: a scoring system for the COSMIN checklist. Qual Life Res. 2012;21(4):651–7. doi:10.1007/s11136-011-9960-1.

45. Mokkink LB, Terwee CB, Patrick DL, et al. The COSMIN study reached international consensus on taxonomy, terminology, and definitions of measurement properties for health-related patient-reported outcomes. J Clin Epidemiol. 2010;63(7):737–45. doi:10.1016/j.jclinepi.2010.02.006.

46. Mokkink L, Terwee B, Patrick L, et al. Cosmin checklist manual. Amsterdam: Center, VU University Medical Biostatistics, Department of Epidemiology Research, EMGO Institute for Health and Care; 2012.

47. Berthelsen H, Lönnblad A, Hakanen J, et al. Cognitive interviewing used in the development and validation of Copenhagen psychosocial questionnaire in Sweden. In: Isidorsson T, Håkansson K, Oudhuis M, Schiller B, editors. Conference paper presented at the 7th Nordic working life conference,

Göteborg, Sweden - stream 26: methodological challenges for working life and labour market studies. Göteborg: The 7th Nordic Working Life Conference; 2014.

48. Berthelsen H, Hakanen J, Kristensen T, Lönnblad A, Westerlund H. A qualitative study on the content validity of the social scales in the Copenhagen in the Copenhagen psychosocial questionnaire (COPSOQ II). Scand J Work Organ Psychol. 2016;1((1) 5):1–13.

49. Copenhagen Psychosocial Questionnaire in Portugal. Scientific research and risk assessment with the Copenhagen Psychosocial Questionnaire (COPSOQ) in Portugal. www.copsoq.pt.

50. Comrey AL, Lee HB. A First Course in Factor Analysis (2nd Ed.). New York: Lawrence Erlbaum Associates; 1992. doi:10.1037/0011756.

51. MacCallum RC, Widaman KF, Zhang S, Hong S. Sample size in factor analysis. Psychol Methods. 1999;4(1):84–99. doi:10.1037/1082-989X.4.1.84.

52. Decreto-Lei n.o 381/2007, 14 de Novembro, 1a série – N.o 219. Estabelece a Classificação Portuguesa de Atividades Económicas (CAE), Revisão 3 (CAE – Rev. 3). 2007:pp 8440–8464. https://dre.pt/application/file/a/629058.

53. European Commission. Eurostat methodologies and working papers: NACE rev.2 statistical classification of economic activities in the European Community. Luxembourg: Office for Official Publications of the European Communities; 2008.

54. Nations U. International Standard Industrial Classfication of All Economic Activities Rev.4.; 2008. doi:10.1007/s13398-014-0173-7.2.

55. Fundação Francisco Manuel dos Santos. Pordata (Base de Dados Portugal Contemporânea). Empresas: Total E Por Sector de Atividade Económica. Lisboa: Fundação Francisco Manuel dos Santos; 2013. http://www.pordata.pt/.

56. Instituto Nacional de Estatística. Classificação Portuguesa Das Profissões 2010. Lisboa: Instituto Nacional de Estatística I.P; 2011. https://www.ine.pt.

57. United Nations. International Standard Classification of Occupations - ISCO 2008. Vol I. Geneva: United Nations; 2012. http://www.ilo.org/public/english/bureau/stat/isco/.

58. McDowell I. Measuring Health — a Guide To Rating Scales and Questionnaires. 3rd ed. Oxford: Oxford University Press; 2006. doi:10.1179/108331900786166731.

59. Streiner D, Norman G. Health measurement scales – a practical guide to their development and use. 2nd ed. New York: Oxford University Press; 1995.

60. Nunnally J, Bernstein I. Psychometric theory. 3rd ed. New York: McGraw-Hill; 1994. 1994;3:701

61. Fayers P, Machin D. Quality of life: the assessment, analysis and interpretation of patient report outcomes. 2nd ed. Chichester: John Wiley & Sons Ltd; 2007.

62. Roe Y, Haldorsen B, Svege I, Bergland A. Development and reliability of a clinician-rated instrument to evaluate function in individuals with shoulder pain: a preliminary study. Physiother Res Int. 2013;18(4):230–8. doi:10.1002/pri.1555.

63. Terwee C, Mokkink L, Steultjens M, Dekker J. Performance-based methods for measuring the physical function of patients with osteoarthritis of the hip or knee: a systematic review of measurement properties. Rheumatology (Oxford). 2006;45(7):890–902.

64. Cohen J. Statistical power analysis for the Behavioral sciences. 2nd ed. Hillsdale: Lawrence Erlbaum Associates Publishers; 1988.

65. Thompson B. Exploratory and Confirmatory Factor Analysis: Understanding Concepts and Applications. Washington, DC; 2004. doi:10.1037/10694-000.

66. Kang H. The prevention and handling of the missing data. Korean J Anesth. 2013;64(5):402–6. doi:10.4097/kjae.2013.64.5.402.

67. Thorsen S, Bjorner J. Reliability of the Copenhagen Psychosocial Questionnaire. Scand J Public Health. 2010;38(3):25–32.

68. Cortina JM. What is coefficient alpha? An examination of theory and applications. J Appl Psychol. 1993;78(1):98–104. doi:10.1037/0021-9010.78.1.98.

69. Cronbach LJ. Coefficient alpha and the internal structure of tests. Psychometrika. 1951;16(3):297–334. doi:10.1007/BF02310555.

70. Bollen KA. Multiple indicators: Internal consistency or no necessary relationship? Qual Quant. 1984;18(4):377–385. doi:10.1007/BF00227593.

71. Bollen K, Lennox R. Conventional Wisdom on Measurement: Psychol Bull. 1991;110(2):305–14. doi:10.1037/0033-2909.110.2.305.

72. Fayers M, Hand J. Factor analysis, causal indicators and quality of life. Qual Life Res. 1997;6(2):139–50.

73. Fayers M, Hand J. Causal variables, indicator variables and measurement scales:an example from quality of life. J R Stat Soc. 2002;165:233–61.

10

Imbalances in the German public health system - numbers of state-certified occupational physicians and relation to socioeconomic data

Christoph Gyo, Michael Boll, Dörthe Brüggmann, Doris Klingelhöfer[*], David Quarcoo and David A. Groneberg

Abstract

Background: State-certified occupational physicians who work as civil servants in the Federal Republic of Germany are key players in the German Public Health system. They control i.e. the legal compliance in occupational health and participate in the occupational disease procedures. Despite the role model function of the German Public health system for many developing countries, this area of Public health is debated to have been hampered in the past years by a disregard concerning structural developments.

Methods: Different databases were screened for occupational health benchmarks. Obtained data were compared to socioeconomic data and indices were calculated.

Results: The overall numbers of State-certified occupational physicians decreased in Germany between 1992 and 2012 from 136 to 86 (63 %). On the single state level, the ratios of State-certified occupational physicians per 1 Mio. working population ranged from 8 for the state of Saarland to 0.8 for the state of North Rhine Westphalia. A general difference was found for old versus new German states. Also, large differences were present for the ratios of State-certified occupational physicians per 10^6 employees towards public debt per capita (€) and the ratios of State-certified occupational physicians per Gross Domestic Product (GDP) in the 16 German states in 2012.

Conclusions: In striking contrast to the WHO document on the Occupational safety and health (OSH) system that states in its executive summary that the human and institutional capacities of the German occupational health system are very strong in both quantity and quality, we here show extreme imbalances present at the single state levels that developed over the past 20 years. With a regard to the increasing complexity of the economic system a reversal of this trend should be demanded.

Keywords: Public health administration, Occupational health

Background

The German social security system consists of the five pillars of health, pension, accident, long-term care and unemployment insurance. It covers more than 90 % of the German population. Within this system, the occupational health system operates along the conventions of the International Labour Organization (ILO). As in other countries, the system is under current review [1].

A recent WHO document entitled "Country Profile of Occupational Health System in Germany" elegantly summarizes the settings of the German Occupational Health System. It describes that health and safety at work is administered by the Ministries for Labour and Social Affairs at both federal and the level of the 16 German states, thus reflecting the federal structure of Germany [2]. The federal ministry for Labour and Social Affairs (BMAS) has the responsibility within the federal government for health and safety at the federal German level. It is supported by advisory committees on occupational health including i.e. occupational diseases, hazardous chemical substances,

* Correspondence: klingelhoefer@med.uni-frankfurt.de
The Institute of Occupational Medicine, Social Medicine and Environmental Medicine, School of Medicine, Goethe University Frankfurt, Theodor-Stern-Kai 7, 60590 Frankfurt, Germany

biological agents. On the level of the single states, state labour inspection authorities are responsible for implementing Occupational safety and health (OSH) legislation at the state level. There is also an interplay with the statuary accident insurances in this area of supervision and inspection that leads to the term of the "dual OSH system of Germany".

A key player of the state supervision and inspection was established in the State-certified occupational physician (Gewerbearzt) with a long lasting history in Germany. The first state-certified occupational physician dates back to 1905 in Württemberg, Alsace and Lorraine (German territories in 1905) [3], 1906 (Baden) and 1909 (Bavaria, Franz Koelsch). The first Prussian state-certified occupational physician was established in 1921 in Düsseldorf (Ludwig Teleky). In 1939, 40 State-certified occupational physicians were present in Germany. The WHO document on the Occupational safety and health (OSH) system states in its executive summary that the human and institutional capacities of the system are very strong in both quantity and quality [2]. Consequently, this should be reflected by the numbers of State-certified occupational physicians since they play an important role within the system.

We here hypothesize that the development and number of State-certified occupational physicians in the 16 states of Germany and overall in Germany is not reflecting this. In order to address this issue, numbers of State-certified occupational physicians were searched and related to different socio-economic and accidents features.

Methods

Data on state-certified occupational physicians

Data concerning numbers and development of State-certified occupational physicians were retrieved by the use of an internet search. Terms "Gewerbearzt" or "Landesgewerbearzt" were entered in the Google search engine and more than 12000 and 9740 results respectively were obtained. The top 100 entries were screened. Evolution of numbers of State-certified occupational physicians was collected from the platform of the Federal Institute of Occupational Safety and Health at www.baua.de [4].

Socioeconomic data

Socioeconomic data were retrieved from the German Federal Statistical Office. This is a federal institution with about 2,600 employees who gather, collect, process, present and analyse statistical information. The head office consisting of seven departments and the office leadership is located in Wiesbaden and the operating platform to retrieve data is www.destatis.de. Data on the numbers of physicians related to inhabitants were

retrieved from the platform of the Federal chamber of physicians (Bundesärztekammer) [5].

Data on occupational accidents

Data concerning numbers and development of fatal occupational accidents were retrieved by the use of an internet search. The term of fatal occupational accidents ("Tödliche Arbeitsunfälle") was entered to the Google search engine and approx. 228,000 results were found. The top 100 entries were screened and numbers were obtained from two sources [4, 5].

Results

Federal data

The overall number of State-certified occupational physicians gives an important insight in the integrity of the system. Analysing these numbers between 1992 and 2012, it is obvious that there is a strong decrease in workforce (Table 1) despite the increasing complexity of occupations. From a starting point in 1992 with 136 State-certified occupational physicians (100 %), the level raises to a maximum of 160 State-certified occupational physicians in 1995 (118 %). Then, the level decreases to lower than 100 % from 2004 onwards. In 2007, the rates

Table 1 Number of State-certified occupational physicians in Germany between 1992 and 2012 [4]

Year	Number of State-certified occupational physicians	
	Absolute numbers	Numbers in % of 1992
1992	136	100
1993	155	114
1994	157	115
1995	160	118
1996	159	117
1997	158	116
1998	158	116
1999	147	108
2000	148	109
2001	147	108
2002	146	107
2003	147	108
2004	130	96
2005	121	89
2006	110	81
2007	109	80
2008	99	73
2009	95	70
2010	90	66
2011	90	66
2012	86	63

decreases to 80 % in comparison to 1992 and in 2012, the rate is 63 %.

The correlation of the overall numbers of State-certified occupational physicians in Germany between 1992 and 2012 with the Gross domestic product (GDP in bn €) demonstrates that there is a decrease of physician numbers that correlates with an increase in the GDP (Fig. 1a). Similar trends are found when the numbers are correlated with the Gross domestic product per capita, and the Gross domestic product per employee (Fig. 1b and c).

Single state data

When focussing on the single states, it becomes apparent that there are large differences present between the 16 single German states in 2012. In the total number ranking, Bavaria is ranked 1st with a total of 23 physicians, followed by North Rhine-Westphalia with 7 physicians. The last position is held by Mecklenburg West Pomerania and Bremen, Hamburg, and Schleswig-Holstein with 2 physicians (Table 2).

The analysis of socioeconomic data in relation to physician numbers changes the ranking. I.e. the ratio of State-certified occupational physicians per 1 Mio employees is calculated at 8 per 1 Mio employees for Saarland, 5 for Bremen, 4.5 for Brandenburg, 4 for Thuringia, 3.4 for Bavaria, 1.4 for Baden-Württemberg and Lower Saxony and only 0.8 for North Rhine-Westphalia (Fig. 2). The two states of North Rhine-Westphalia and Baden Württemberg with relatively large numbers of employees tend to employ less State-certified occupational physicians per employee than the other states (slope +/− SD 340.2 +/− 99.42, $r^2 = 0.46$, slope significant non-zero ($p = 0.0041$), Fig. 3a). A similar picture is present when the numbers of State-certified occupational physicians are related to the gross domestic product of the single states (slope +/− SD 24.2 +/− 6.9, $r^2 = 0.47$, slope significant non-zero ($p = 0.0035$), Fig. 3b).

When focussing on the relation of State-certified occupational physicians in single states towards the GDP per employee in single states, no significant relations are found and large variations of the relation are present within the cohort of the 16 states (slope +/− SD 425.6 +/− 491.7, $r^2 = 0.05$, slope not significant non-zero ($p = 0.4013$), Fig. 3c).

When the public debt per capita in each state is related to numbers of State-certified occupational physicians per state it is found that states with a rather low public debt tend to have relatively high numbers of physicians, i.e. Bavaria or Baden-Württemberg, but there is no significant relation present (slope +/− SD −560.8 +/− 323.4, $r^2 = 0.18$, slope not significant non-zero ($p = 0.1049$), Fig. 4a).

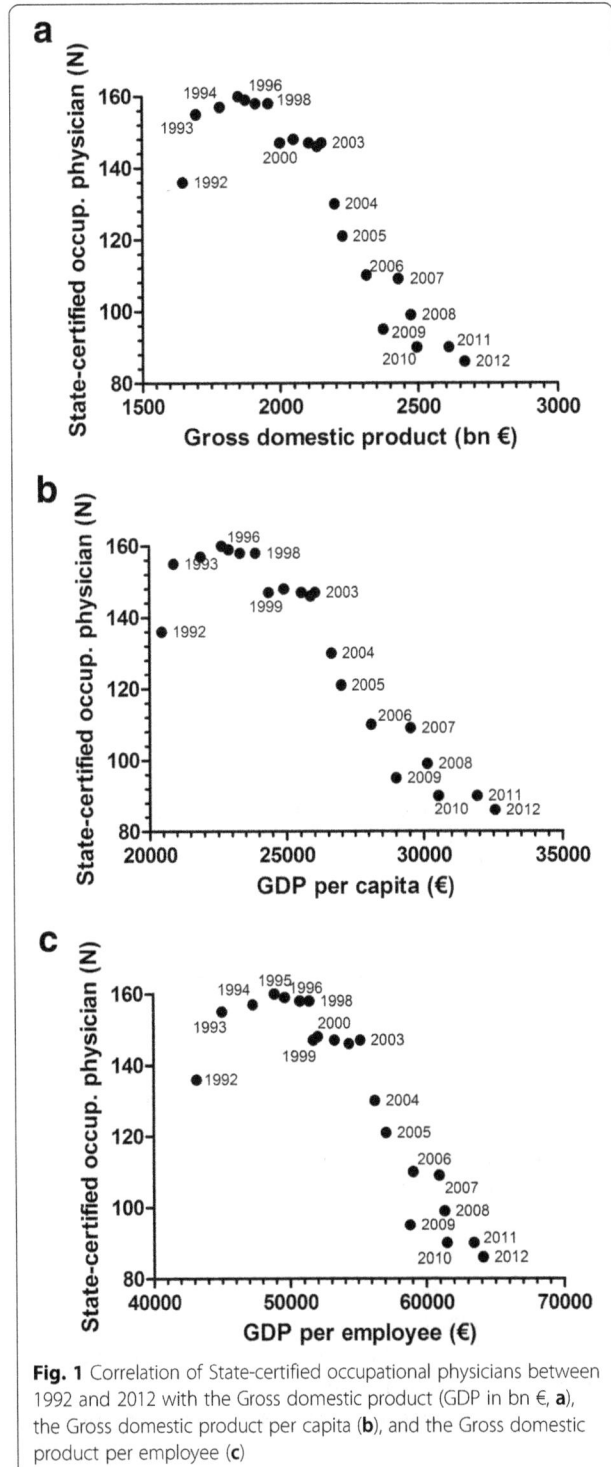

Fig. 1 Correlation of State-certified occupational physicians between 1992 and 2012 with the Gross domestic product (GDP in bn €, **a**), the Gross domestic product per capita (**b**), and the Gross domestic product per employee (**c**)

A comparison of the ratio of State-certified occupational physicians per 10^6 employees with the public debt per capita shows that the state with the highest number of physicians per employees (SL) has a relatively high public depth per capita. Also Bremen fits into this scheme but there is no overall significant relation

Table 2 State-certified occupational physicians in 2012 in the 16 German states.

#	State	State-certified occupational physicians [23]	Working population (Mio.) (https://www.destatis.de/DE/Startseite.html)	State-certified occupational physicians per 1 Mio. Working population
1	Saarland	4	0.5	8.0
2	Bremen	2	0.4	5.0
3	Brandenburg	5	1.1	4.5
4	Thuringia	4	1.0	4.0
5	Bavaria	23	6.7	3.4
6	Saxony-Anhalt	3	1.0	3.0
7	Berlin	5	1.7	2.9
8	Mecklenburg-West Pomerania	2	0.7	2.9
9	Saxony	5	1.9	2.6
10	Rhineland-Palatinate	4	1.9	2.1
11	Hamburg	2	1.1	1.8
12	Hesse	5	3.1	1.6
13	Schleswig-Holstein	2	1.3	1.5
14	Baden-Württemberg	8	5.6	1.4
15	Lower Saxony	5	3.7	1.4
16	North Rhine Westphalia	7	8.7	0.8

State-certified occupational physicians per 1 Mio. Employees

present (slope +/– SD –1281 +/– 927.5, $r^2 = 0.12$, slope not significant non-zero ($p = 0.1887$), Fig. 4b).

Discussion

This study examines the timely evolution of State-certified occupational physicians in Germany between 1992 and 2012. Furthermore, it analyses the data from 2012 on a single state basis. Overall, it can be summarized that the numbers of State-certified occupational physicians continuously decreases. This tendency is opposed by an increase in the wealth of Germany, as measured by different GDP indices. This increase of wealth is contradictory to the decrease of the numbers of State-certified occupational physicians, since an increase of wealth usually goes along with an increase in tax revenues, which should enable the German States to provide for a stable number of State-certified occupational physicians. Thus, it is unlikely that the decrease of the numbers of State-certified occupational physicians has been necessitated by reasons of the public budget. Such decrease rather seems to be caused by focussing public spending on areas more appealing to voters than workplace safety. This development might have been driven also by a shifting of weights from the industrial sector to the service sector, with "typical" work place injuries like fractures, burns, chemical burns, musculoskeletal diseases etc. being on the decline and less obvious work caused diseases like psychological disorders etc. being on the rise.

With regard to the decrease in numbers of deadly working accidents (Fig. 5), one might speculate that this decrease may be reasonable due to a lower workload. However, this assumption is wrong since there is a dramatic increase in the complexity of working processes in the industrialized world. I.e. new technologies including the use of nanoparticles [6, 7] or particles in general [8, 9] and infectious diseases [10, 11] in many working surroundings or musculoskeletal issues [12, 13] enforces federal and state authorities to increase the intellectual capacities in this area of the German occupational health system. Also, psychological and lifestyle issues become more and more important in the field [14–21].

When assessing the structure of the deficit in the State-certified occupational physician workforce in Germany one needs to consult single state data. In this respect, the analysis of the ratio of State-certified occupational physicians per 1 Mio employees in the 16 German states and comparison to the ratio of all physicians to inhabitants per state is interesting, since it demonstrates that the decrease of the ratio of State-certified occupational physicians is not reflected by a comparable development in the ratio of all physicians, even though both are part of the public health system and both are indicators for the quality and quantity of healthcare supply for the population. The first index demonstrates a difference between the old Western German states with the exclusion of Bavaria and Rhineland-Palatinate, and the State of Saarland, which was not a founding state of Western Germany, and the

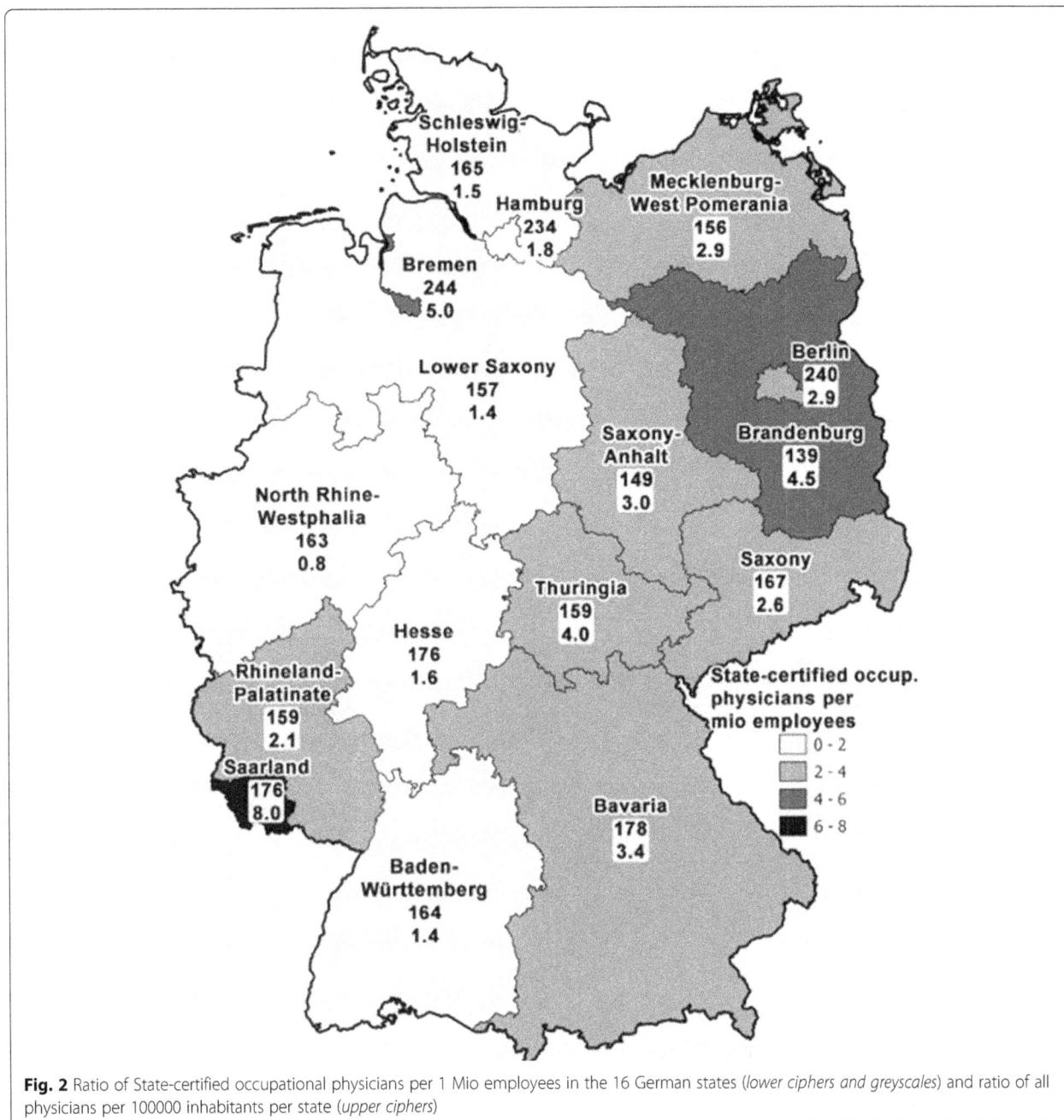

Fig. 2 Ratio of State-certified occupational physicians per 1 Mio employees in the 16 German states (*lower ciphers and greyscales*) and ratio of all physicians per 100000 inhabitants per state (*upper ciphers*)

new, Eastern German states. It shows that these Eastern German States that belonged to the territory of the communistic German Democratic Republic until 1990 have a higher ratio than the Western states. All Eastern states have numbers of 2 or higher State-certified occupational physicians per million inhabitants whereas the Western countries except Rhineland-Palatinate, Bavaria, and the above mentioned Saarland have numbers of less then 2. This might be due to the longstanding tradition of occupational medicine in the former GDR and a transformation process after 1990 that led to efficient state labour authorities in the new German countries.

Interestingly, the only Western German state that has a unique position is the Saarland. This state however does not belong to the founding states of Western Germany after the Second World War. Prior to its creation as the territory of the Saar Basin by the League of Nations after the First World War, the Saarland did not exist as a unified entity. After the Second World War, it was a French-occupied territory from 1947 to 1956. Between 1950 and 1956, Saarland was a member of the council of Europe. In 1955, the inhabitants were offered independence in another plebiscite. However, they decided that their territory should become a state of the Federal Republic of Germany

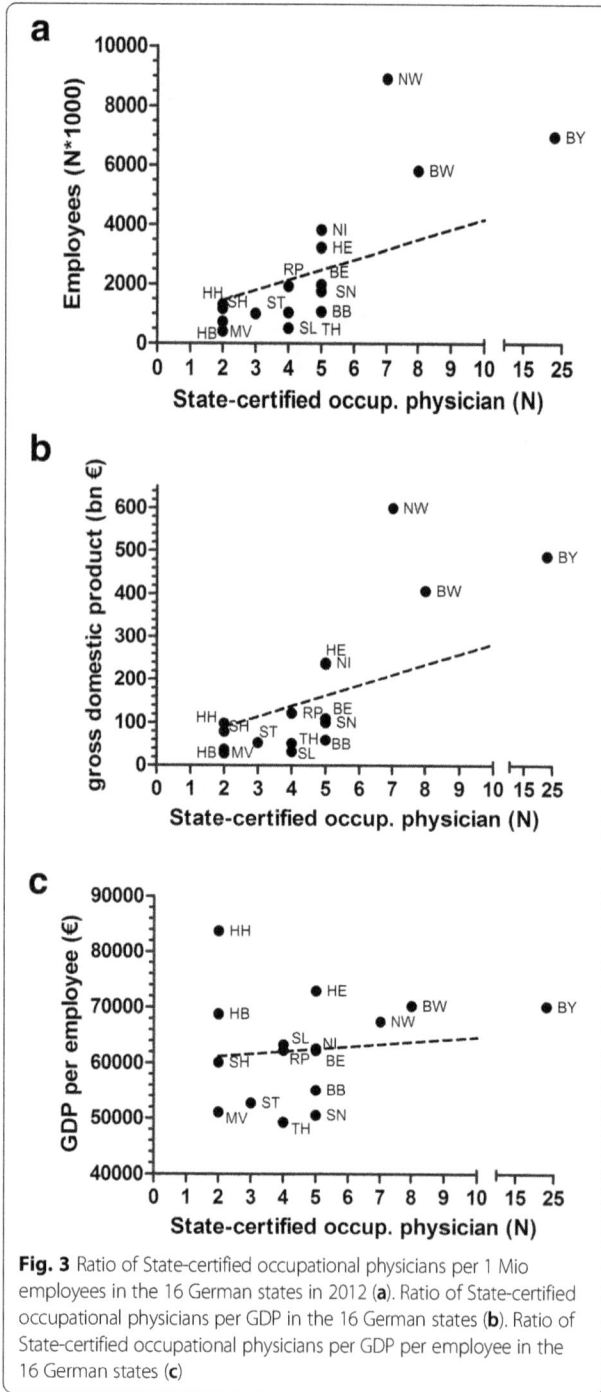

Fig. 3 Ratio of State-certified occupational physicians per 1 Mio employees in the 16 German states in 2012 (**a**). Ratio of State-certified occupational physicians per GDP in the 16 German states (**b**). Ratio of State-certified occupational physicians per GDP per employee in the 16 German states (**c**)

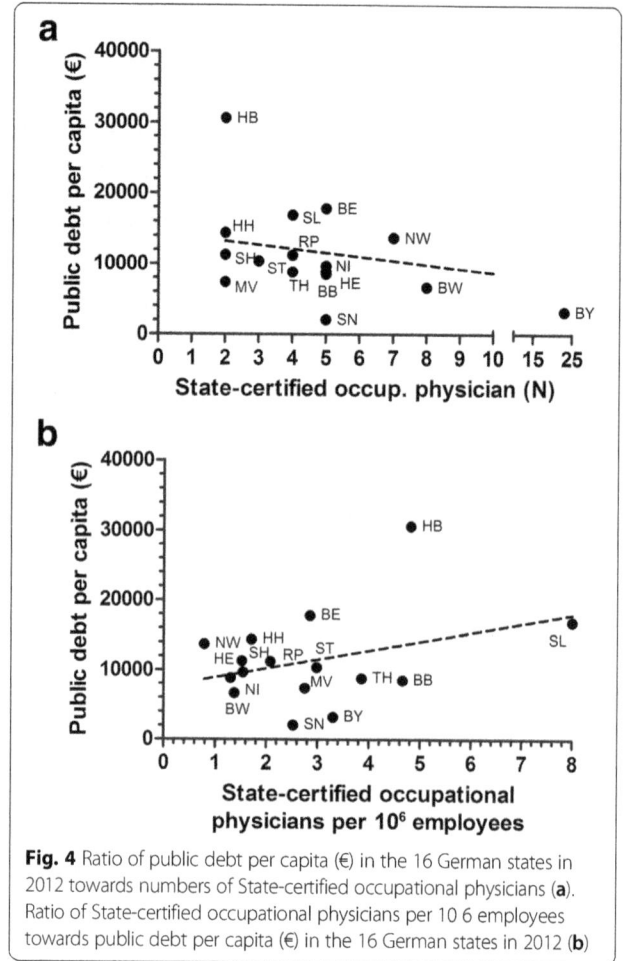

Fig. 4 Ratio of public debt per capita (€) in the 16 German states in 2012 towards numbers of State-certified occupational physicians (**a**). Ratio of State-certified occupational physicians per 10 6 employees towards public debt per capita (€) in the 16 German states in 2012 (**b**)

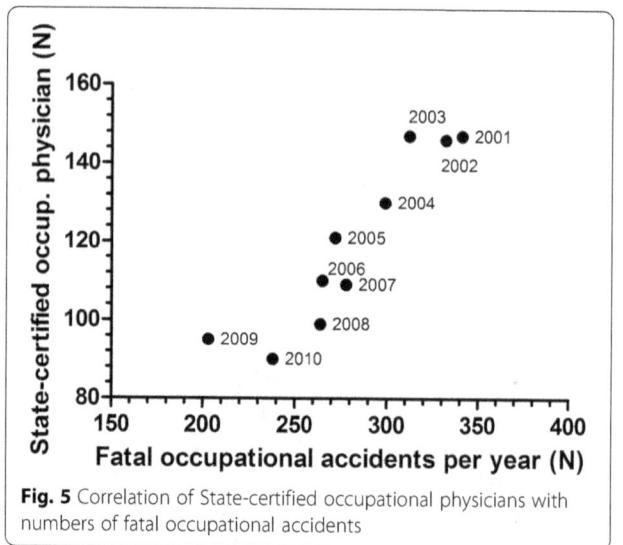

Fig. 5 Correlation of State-certified occupational physicians with numbers of fatal occupational accidents

(Western Germany). Therefore, its current position as the leading German state concerning the ratio of State-certified occupational physician per inhabitant needs to be interpreted on the basis of this history and the wealth of its coal deposits and their large-scale industrial exploitation in the past century. However, the decline of this wealth from the 1980s onwards did not lead to a reduction in the quantity of the occupational health system as measured by the current State-certified occupational physician workforce.

The WHO document on the Occupational safety and health (OSH) system states in its executive summary that the human and institutional capacities of the system are very strong in both quantity and quality [2]. From the present study that revealed extreme imbalances are present in the single state structures of State-certified occupational physicians ranging from about 8 physicians per 1 million employees (Saarland) to 0.8 (North Rhine Westphalia). In an industrialized country such as Germany such inequalities should not be present despite the federal character of the country. Similar trends are also observed for other physicians who serve in the public health area including forensic medicine. Here, since over ten years, a public debate has been started about the shortage of physicians in the area of legal medicine and leading to a reduction of the attractivity to specialize in this area [22].

These inequalities observed here for the Public Health sector are not present in other areas of the German health system. I.e. the juxtaposition of the ratio of State-certified occupational physicians per 1 Mio employees in the 16 German states and the ratio of all physicians to inhabitants per state shows that in the later index which can be regarded as a general index of health system quality, a complete different setting is found (Fig. 2). Here, the federal city-states of Berlin, Hamburg and Bremen have the highest density of physicians with up to 244 physicians per 100,000 inhabitants (Bremen). The territorial states have lower rates but there is not such a gap present as in the ratio of State-certified

occupational physicians per 1 Mio. employees in the 16 German states.

With a regard to the increasing complexity of the German economics it should be unanimously demanded that the overall and single state German State-certified occupational physician workforce should be structured along the Saarland as benchmark with a ratio of about 8 State-certified occupational physicians per 1 million employees. The example of the Saarland demonstrates, that it is both possible and desirable to maintain a high ratio of State-certified occupational physicians per employees even though the industrial landscape and the public budget. This would lead to a structure depicted in Table 3 with an overall number of 325 State-certified occupational physicians who could efficiently counsel German companies, control the legal compliance in occupational health, supervision of around 3.006 occupational medicine physicians dealing with employees directly day per day [5] and participate in the occupational disease procedures.

Conclusions

In summary, the present study identifies inequalities in the occupational health system of the 16 German states of the Federal Republic of Germany by analysing the structure and timely evolution of State-certified occupational physicians. Due to the increase in complexity of the economic system with a multitude of new hazards and technologies, the trend of decreasing numbers of State-certified occupational physicians needs to be

Table 3 Proposed numbers of State-certified occupational physicians in the 16 German states with Saarland as benchmark [23]

#	State	Current number of State-certified occupational physicians [23]	Working population (Mio.) (https://www.destatis.de/DE/Startseite.html)	Proposed State-certified occupational physicians
1	Saarland	4	0.5	4
2	Bremen	3	0.4	3
3	Brandenburg	5	1.1	9
4	Thuringia	4	1.0	8
5	Bavaria	23	6.7	54
6	Saxony-Anhalt	3	1.0	8
7	Berlin	5	1.7	14
8	Mecklenburg-West Pommerania	2	0.7	6
9	Saxony	5	1.9	15
10	Rhineland-Palatinate	4	1.9	15
11	Hamburg	2	1.1	9
12	Hesse	5	3.1	25
13	Schleswig-Holstein	2	1.3	10
14	Baden-Württemberg	8	5.6	45
15	Lower Saxony	5	3.7	30
16	North Rhine Westphalia	7	8.7	70

stopped and reversed in order to prevent serious structural deficiencies in the German health system.

Acknowledgements
We thank Gabriele Volante for editorial help.

Funding
No funding took place.

Authors' contributions
CG, MB, DB, DK, DQ, DAG participated in the construction of the study design, data collection and analysis, manuscript drafting, and critical discussion. All authors read and approved the final manuscript.

Competing interests
The authors declare that they have no competing interests.

References

1. Hakulinen H, Rissanen S, Lammintakanen J. How is the new public management applied in the occupational health care system? - decision-makers' and OH personnel's views in Finland. Health Res Policy Syst. 2011;9:34.
2. WHO Regional Office for Europe: Country Profile of Occupational Health System in Germany (assessed 2015-01-05) [http://www.euro.who.int/__data/assets/pdf_file/0010/178957/OSH-Profile-Germany.pdf].
3. Koelsch F. Beiträge zur Geschichte der Arbeitsmedizin. Bayerische Landesärztekammer. 1967;8.
4. Glynn RW, Scutaru C, Kerin MJ, Sweeney KJ. Breast cancer research output, 1945–2008: a bibliometric and density-equalizing analysis. Breast Cancer Res. 2010;12:R108.
5. Bundesärztekammer: Die ärztliche Versorgung in der Bundesrepublik Deutschland (assessed 2015-01-25) [http://www.bundesaerztekammer.de/page.asp?his=0.3.12002.12003].
6. Ohnishi M, Yajima H, Kasai T, Umeda Y, Yamamoto M, Yamamoto S, Okuda H, Suzuki M, Nishizawa T, Fukushima S. Novel method using hybrid markers: development of an approach for pulmonary measurement of multi-walled carbon nanotubes. J Occup Med Toxicol. 2013;8:30.
7. Gerber A, Bundschuh M, Klingelhofer D, Groneberg DA. Gold nanoparticles: recent aspects for human toxicology. J Occup Med Toxicol. 2013;8(1):32.
8. Fan T, Fang SC, Cavallari JM, Barnett IJ, Wang Z, Su L, Byun HM, Lin X, Baccarelli AA, Christiani DC. Heart rate variability and DNA methylation levels are altered after short-term metal fume exposure among occupational welders: a repeated-measures panel study. BMC Public Health. 2014;14:1279.
9. Song Y, Hou J, Huang X, Zhang X, Tan A, Rong Y, Sun H, Zhou Y, Cui X, Yang Y, et al. The Wuhan-Zhuhai (WHZH) cohort study of environmental air particulate matter and the pathogenesis of cardiopulmonary diseases: study design, methods and baseline characteristics of the cohort. BMC Public Health. 2014;14:994.
10. Tudor C, Van der Walt M, Margot B, Dorman SE, Pan WK, Yenokyan G, Farley JE. Tuberculosis among health care workers in KwaZulu-Natal, South Africa: a retrospective cohort analysis. BMC Public Health. 2014;14:891.
11. Nienhaus A, Costa JT. Screening for tuberculosis and the use of a borderline zone for the interpretation of the interferon-gamma release assay (IGRA) in Portuguese healthcare workers. J Occup Med Toxicol. 2013;8:1.
12. Shuai J, Yue P, Li L, Liu F, Wang S. Assessing the effects of an educational program for the prevention of work-related musculoskeletal disorders among school teachers. BMC Public Health. 2014;14:1211.
13. Lunde LK, Koch M, Knardahl S, Waersted M, Mathiassen SE, Forsman M, Holtermann A, Veiersted KB. Musculoskeletal health and work ability in physically demanding occupations: study protocol for a prospective field study on construction and health care workers. BMC Public Health. 2014;14:1075.
14. Keller M, Bamberg E, Kersten M, Nienhaus A. Instrument for stress-related job analysis for hospital physicians: validation of a short version. J Occup Med Toxicol. 2013;8:10.
15. Munir F, Houdmont J, Clemes S, Wilson K, Kerr R, Addley K. Work engagement and its association with occupational sitting time: results from the Stormont study. BMC Public Health. 2015;15:30.
16. Guglielmi D, Simbula S, Vignoli M, Bruni I, Depolo M, Bonfiglioli R, Tabanelli MC, Violante FS. Solving a methodological challenge in work stress evaluation with the Stress Assessment and Research Toolkit (StART): a study protocol. J Occup Med Toxicol. 2013;8(1):18.
17. Formazin M, Burr H, Aagestad C, Tynes T, Thorsen SV, Perkio-Makela M, Diaz Aramburu CI, Pinilla Garcia FJ, Galiana Blanco L, Vermeylen G, et al. Dimensional comparability of psychosocial working conditions as covered in European monitoring questionnaires. BMC Public Health. 2014;14:1251.
18. Edvardsen HM, Karinen R, Moan IS, Oiestad EL, Christophersen AS, Gjerde H. Use of alcohol and drugs among health professionals in Norway: a study using data from questionnaires and samples of oral fluid. J Occup Med Toxicol. 2014;9:8.
19. Honda T, Chen S, Kishimoto H, Narazaki K, Kumagai S. Identifying associations between sedentary time and cardio-metabolic risk factors in working adults using objective and subjective measures: a cross-sectional analysis. BMC Public Health. 2014;14:1307.
20. Bauer J, Groneberg DA. Perception of stress-related working conditions in hospitals (iCept-study): a comparison between physicians and medical students. J Occup Med Toxicol. 2013;8:3.
21. Aagestad C, Tyssen R, Johannessen HA, Gravseth HM, Tynes T, Sterud T. Psychosocial and organizational risk factors for doctor-certified sick leave: a prospective study of female health and social workers in Norway. BMC Public Health. 2014;14:1016.
22. Gauthier S, Buddeberg-Fischer B, Bucher M, Thali M, Bartsch C. Pilot study on doctors working in departments of forensic medicine in German-speaking areas. J Forensic Leg Med. 2013;20:1069–74.
23. Sicherheit und Gesundheit bei der Arbeit. Bundesministerium für Arbeit und Sozialordnung. 2012. p. 145.

11

An updated re-analysis of the mortality risk from nasopharyngeal cancer in the National Cancer Institute formaldehyde worker cohort study

Gary M. Marsh[1*], Peter Morfeld[2,3], Sarah D. Zimmerman[1], Yimeng Liu[1] and Lauren C. Balmert[1]

Abstract

Background: To determine whether the National Cancer Institute's (NCI) suggestion of a persistent increased mortality risk for nasopharyngeal cancer (NPC) in relation to formaldehyde (FA) exposure is robust with respect to alternative methods of data analysis.

Methods: NCI provided the cohort data updated through 2004. We computed U.S. and local county rate-based standardized mortality ratios (SMRs) and internal cohort rate-based relative risks (RR) in relation to four formaldehyde exposure metrics (highest peak, average intensity, cumulative, and duration of exposure), using both NCI categories and alternative categorizations. We modeled the plant group-related interaction structure using continuous and categorical forms of each FA exposure metric and evaluated the impact of NCI's decision to exclude non-exposed workers from the baseline category.

Results: Overall, our results corroborate the findings of our earlier reanalyses of data from the 1994 NCI cohort update. Six of 11 NPC deaths observed in the NCI study occurred in Plant 1, two (including the only additional NPC death) occurred in Plant 3 among workers in the lowest exposure category of highest peak, average intensity and cumulative FA exposure and in the second exposure category of duration of exposure, and the remaining cases occurred individually in three of eight remaining plants. A large, statistically significant, local rate-based NPC SMR of 7.34 (95 % CI = 2.69–15.97) among FA-exposed workers in Plant 1 contrasted with an 18 % deficit in NPC deaths (SMR = 0.82, 95 % CI = .17–2.41) among exposed workers in Plants 2–10. Overall, the new NCI findings led to: (1) reduced SMRs and RRs in the remaining nine study plants in unaffected exposure categories, (2) attenuated exposure-response relations for FA and NPC for all the FA metrics considered and (3) strengthened and expanded evidence that the earlier NCI internal analyses were non-robust and mis-specified as they did not account for a statistically significant interaction structure between plant group (Plant 1 vs. Plants 2–10) and FA exposure.

Conclusions: Our updated reanalysis provided little or no evidence to support NCI's suggestion of a persistent association between FA exposure and mortality from NPC. NCI's suggestion continues to be driven heavily by anomalous findings in one study plant (Plant 1).

Keywords: Formaldehyde, Nasopharyngeal cancer, Cohort mortality study, Occupational health, National Cancer Institute, Reanalyses

* Correspondence: gmarsh@pitt.edu
[1]Center for Occupational Biostatistics and Epidemiology and Department of Biostatistics, Graduate School of Public Health, University of Pittsburgh, 130 DeSoto Street, Pittsburgh, PA 15261, USA
Full list of author information is available at the end of the article

Background

Formaldehyde (FA) is an important industrial chemical. Production in the U.S. and the European Union exceeds 10 million tons per year [1]. Adhesives and binders are produced from resins based on FA (e.g., for the manufacture of particle board, paper, and vitreous synthetic fibers), to make plastics and coatings, and FA is used in textile finishing [2]. FA is an intermediate in the production of many chemicals, and as formalin it is used as a disinfectant and preservative. In addition, FA is produced in combustion, e.g. in vehicle exhausts and tobacco smoke [2]. Also, FA is formed endogenously in humans [3].

In 2004, the International Agency for Research on Cancer (IARC) reclassified FA from a probable (Group 2A) [4] to a known human carcinogen (Group 1) [1] citing results for nasopharyngeal cancer (NPC) mortality from the follow-up through 1994 of the National Cancer Institute (NCI) formaldehyde cohort study [5]. Based on the same NCI findings, the Group 1 classification was upheld by IARC following the working group meeting for IARC Monograph Volume 100F [2]. Subsequently, the U.S. National Institute of Environmental Health Sciences National Toxicology Program changed the classification of formaldehyde from "anticipated to be carcinogenic in humans" to "known to be a human carcinogen" [6].

In contrast, in 2012, the Committee for Risk Assessment[1] of the European Chemicals Agency[2] disagreed with the proposal to classify FA as a known human carcinogen (Carc. 1A), proposing a lower but still protective category, namely as a substance which is presumed to have carcinogenic potential for humans (Carc. 1B)[3]. Thus, U.S. and European regulatory agencies currently disagree about the potential human carcinogenicity of FA. An overview of open issues and scientific discussions about the health effects of FA exposures is given in Bolt and Morfeld [7].

The National Cancer Institute formaldehyde cohort study

In June 2013, the NCI published the findings of its update through 2004 of mortality from solid tumors among workers in the US industry-wide FA study [8]. This study includes 10 plants and represents the largest cohort study of workers with potential exposure to FA [9]. The purpose of the Beane Freeman et al. update was to extend the mortality follow-up through 2004 and to examine the associations among different exposure characterizations and mortality from several solid tumors. This study also included corrections by Beane Freeman et al. [10] to the earlier update of mortality through 1994 published in 2004 [5]. For an evaluation of the errors that lead to these corrections see Issues 1 and 2 in Marsh et al. [11]. Beane Freeman et al. [8] claim that a persistent increased risk remains for NPC mortality

within the updated cohort associated with peak, average intensity and cumulative FA exposure metrics as reported in Hauptmann et al. [5], although this NPC risk was not reported by Blair et al. [9] in the original FA cohort analysis based on follow-up through 1979. The main conclusion from Beane Freeman et al. [8] is that the update through 2004 suggests a link between FA exposure and NPC mortality that is consistent with some case–control studies [12–17]. Aside from not statistically significantly elevated rate ratios for salivary gland cancer mortality, the authors observed no associations with mortality from other cancer types reported in other studies, including lung, laryngeal, nasal sinus and brain [2, 4].

In 2013, two of us (GM, PM) published a commentary [11] describing why we believe NCI's interpretation regarding the persistent NPC risk is not consistent with available epidemiological evidence including: (1) data from the most recent update of the NCI cohort study [8]; (2) other large and recently updated cohort studies of FA-exposed workers [18–21]; (3) alternative analyses of the 1994 update of the NCI cohort study [22–24] or (4) the independent study of one of the NCI's study plants (Plant 1) [25]. Plant 1, which historically has included the majority of the NPC deaths observed in the NCI cohort [5, 9], was also the focus of our reanalyses of the 1994 update of the NCI cohort [22, 23]. Plant 1, a plastics producing plant operating since 1943 in Wallingford, CT, includes 4261 workers or 17 % of the total NCI cohort of 25,619 workers. Regarding potential for FA exposure, Table 1 shows that workers in the Plant 1 cohort had a median average intensity of exposure (AIE) of 1.023 ppm compared to a range of median AIEs of 0.08 to 2.799 ppm for Plants 2–10.

Siew et al. [26] analyzed a study cohort of all 1.2 million economically active Finnish men born between 1906 and 1945 who participated in the national population census on December 31, 1970. The Finnish job-exposure matrix (FINJEM) was used to calculate occupational FA exposure estimates [27]. The authors analyzed 149 NPC cases and found no association with FA exposure. Although the exposure assessment is limited in this investigation, the large register based study by Sew et al. adds to the cohort studies that showed no elevated NPC risk after FA exposure.

Checkoway et al. [28] performed a re-analysis of the NCI cohort and evaluated associations between cumulative and peak formaldehyde exposure and lympho-hematopoietic malignancies, in particular myeloid leukemia. The authors did not address NPCs. We note that the US National Institute of Environmental Health Sciences National Toxicology Program judged in their decision on FA that "the evidence for nasopharyngeal cancer is somewhat stronger than that for myeloid

Table 1 Selected characteristics and findings for 10 plants in 2004 update of NCI formaldehyde cohort study

UPitt (NCI) plant no.	1 (1)	2 (2)	3 (3)	4 (5)	5 (6)	6 (7)	7 (8)	8 (10)	9 (11)	10 (12)
Entry year	1943	1945	1949	1958	1957	1951	1938	1934	1956	1941
No. Subjects	4261	784	2375	1692	744	5248	4228	1679	1933	2675
Formaldehyde exposure										
% Subjects ever exposed	87.7	99.9	92.7	93.3	64.4	91	81.6	99.3	88.2	95
% Subjects ever in highest peak category	46.1	91.6	0	72.9	20.4	2	.4	1.1	9.3	69.7
Median AIE (ppm) [a]	1.023	2.799	.112	.234	.196	.233	.080	.382	.400	.543
(5–95 %-tile)	.310–1.417	.300–3.927	.010–.222	.100–.596	.029–1.132	.033–.868	.020–.250	.100–2.000	.100–1.615	.216–1.124
Median Cum (ppm-years) [a]	.9	19.0	.1	2.2	1.9	.7	.1	.6	.3	1.3
(5–95 %-tile)	.1–17.2	.4–86.5	.01–2.1	.06–11.9	.08–27.5	.01–16.3	.01–3.5	.03–12.0	.03–5.9	.05–16.4
Median Dur (years) [a]	1.0	11.3	1.1	9.7	16.7	3.6	1.0	1.0	.8	2.3
(5–95 %-tile)	.1–24.4	.3–30.7	.1–20.3	.4–29.5	1.0–34.4	.1–31.3	.1–28.0	.1–25.0	.09–16.5	.1–29.2
Observed and expected deaths and SMRs for NPC										
Obs	6	1	2	0	0	0	1	0	0	1
SMR-US (Exp)	5.44** (1.1)	4.32 (.2)	3.01 (.7)	- (.4)	- (.2)	- (1.1)	.93 (1.1)	- (.4)	- (.3)	1.21 (.8)
(95 % CI)	2–11.85	.11–24.08	.36–10.87	0–9.03	0–18.63	0–3.42	.02–5.18	0–9.39	0–12.79	.03–6.72
SMR-local (Exp)	5.57** (1.1)	4.03 (.2)	7.60 (.3)	- (.5)	- (.2)	- (1.3)	1.24 (.8)	- (0)	- (.4)	1.01 (1.0)
(95 % CI)	2.04–12.12	.10–22.48	.92–27.46	0–7.30	0–21.09	0–2.82	.03–6.89	0–90.04	0–10.14	.03–5.63

[a] Based on exposed jobs only with no lag

** $p < .01$

leukemia" [6]. Thus, it is of specific interest to examine whether the "stronger evidence" for NPC is robust and can be confirmed or refuted in a re-analysis of the updated NCI cohort study [8].

Main methodological issues

Our recent commentary also described several methodological issues in the most recent update of the NCI study that formed the basis for our reanalysis of the updated NCI cohort data on mortality from NPC [11]. In this paper, we addressed three methodological issues: (Issue 1) inappropriateness of excluding unexposed workers from the evaluation of exposure-response relationships; (Issue 2) the trend tests used in the NCI 2004 updates produce misleading results and may be mis-specified and (Issue 3) failure to recognize the important interaction structure between plant group (i.e., Plant 1 vs. Plants 2–10) and FA exposure reported by Marsh et al. [23]. We report here our updated reanalysis of the relationship between FA exposure and mortality from NPC using data from the 2004 update of the NCI FA cohort study.

Methods
Data preparation
We obtained a copy of the updated 2004 NCI formaldehyde cohort study data from NCI. The 2004 NCI cohort file contained the same demographic, work history and formaldehyde exposure data for 25,619 workers first employed at one of 10 industrial plants before January 1, 1966 as the file associated with NCI's 1994 update (1994 NCI cohort file). We were informed by NCI that the only differences between the 1994 and 2004 NCI cohort files were the updated vital status, cause of death, and date of death variables. All event dates (e.g., birth, hire, termination, and death) were limited to month and year to protect subject confidentiality. Further details about the NCI study are provided in Beane Freeman et al. [8] and Blair et al. [9].

Due to the complexity of reformatting the earlier 1994 NCI cohort data file in 2005 to enable analysis with the OCMAP-Plus cohort analysis program [29], and the lack of a common ID (for confidentiality purposes), we matched all deceased employees from the 2004 NCI cohort data file to the 1994 OCMAP cohort data file on all possible variables. We matched 13,883 of 13,951 deaths, or 99.5 %, exactly to the 1994 OCMAP file. For the remaining 68 deaths, we manually selected the closest matches within the 1994 OCMAP file. After the matching was completed, we updated vital status, cause of death, and date of death information for all 13,951 deaths so that the mortality follow-up period was through 2004.

Additionally, we created a new OCMAP file from the 2004 NCI cohort file to ensure that our matched OCMAP file was accurate. This new OCMAP file contained only a portion of the variables as the reformatting was too complex and redundant. We subsequently performed extensive cross-checks and replicated key NCI findings to establish the comparability of the files. Our total person-year count differed by only 11.0 or 0.00001 % of the total person-years reported by NCI [8]. We also matched the plant-specific numbers of subjects, total deaths and deaths from NPC. Compared with Beane Freeman et al. [30], which provided more detailed information, we also matched exactly on median duration of follow-up years (42 years) and median length of employment (2.6 years).

Our general NPC analyses were based on the total of 11 NPC deaths reported in the NCI study. As in our original reanalyses [22, 23], and unlike Hauptmann et al. [5] and Beane Freeman et al. [8], we did not omit from our exposure–response analyses the one NPC death in Plant 11 that had been recoded to oropharyngeal cancer based on findings of a medical record confirmation reported by Lucas [31]. Our concerns about this partial correction of death certificate information are reported elsewhere [32].

Statistical analyses
General methods
In general, our external and internal comparisons of NPC mortality in the NCI 2004 FA cohort were conducted along the lines of our previous reanalysis of NPC [22] and leukemia [33] in the NCI 1994 FA cohort. A main goal was to determine whether our earlier findings were corroborated in this updated reanalysis. Specific goals were to address the three methodological issues noted above, as described below Our results for NCI-replicated analyses differ slightly from those reported by Beane Freeman et al. [8] because the 2004 NCI cohort file did not include the day of events (dates of birth and death and work history dates). We estimated day of event by using the midpoint of the month (15). Also, differences for NCI-replicated exposure-response models occurred because we fit our models with exact conditional logistic regression; whereas, NCI used asymptotic Poisson regression models. Finally, as noted above, our exposure-response models used all 11 NPC deaths; whereas, NCI's were based on 10 deaths. To facilitate comparison, we also present results based on these 10 NPC deaths only.

External mortality comparisons for NPC
For NPC, we computed both U.S. and regional (local county) rate-based SMRs and their 95 % confidence intervals (CI, based on the Poisson distribution) by each of

the 10 plants in the NCI study and by two plant groups (Plant 1 vs. Plants 2–10). SMRs were standardized for race/ethnicity, sex, age group, and time period. Local county area mortality rates for each of the 10 plants in the NCI study were obtained from the Mortality and Population Database System (MPDS) developed at the University of Pittsburgh [34]. For each study plant, the local county area was defined as the county or group of counties surrounding the plant from which most of the work force was drawn (see Marsh and Youk [34] for plant code, plant locations and counties comprising the regional rates). Because MPDS rates are not available before 1950, we applied 1950–1954 rates to previous observation periods for plants that started before 1950. This approximation should have negligible effect on SMRs, as only 3.3 % of the total person-years at risk in the cohort occurred before 1950 [34]. The proportional contribution of expected NPC deaths is likely to be even smaller because these early person-years are associated with relatively young age groups.

We also computed regional rate-based SMRs and 95 % CIs for NPC by each of the four formaldehyde metrics (highest peak, average intensity, cumulative, and duration) used in the NCI study[4]. We used the NCI exposure categories for highest peak exposure (the NCI data were pre-coded into fixed categories) and an alternative categorization for the remaining metrics (approximate tertiles of formaldehyde exposure among all NPC deaths in exposed workers, UPitt categories). Unlike the approximate 60th and 80th percentile cutpoints used by NCI, our categorization produces a more even distribution of NPC deaths among the exposed categories. When evaluating NCI exposure categories we used only 10 NPC deaths as the NCI researchers did in their analyses. We used all 11 NPC deaths in analyses applying UPitt categories.

Internal mortality comparisons

In the NCI study, Poisson regression based on asymptotic estimation was used to examine exposure–response relationships by comparing internal cohort rates for NPC. Alternatively, we used relative risk (RR) regression modeling with both exact and asymptotic estimation to investigate the dependence of the internal cohort rates (modeled as time to death) for NPC on combinations of both categorical and continuous formaldehyde metrics, with adjustment for potential confounding factors through matching or stratification. Study data from the entire 1934–2004 period were modeled. Risk sets were explicitly constructed from the cohort data with age as the primary time dimension, using the RISKSET program module in OCMAP-Plus [29]. To adjust for year of birth ("cohort" or time period) effects, risk sets were caliper-matched, within one year, on date of birth.

Regression models included terms for race/ethnicity (white/black), sex, and payroll category (wage, salary, unknown) to adjust for these potential confounding factors. Trends in RRs relative to the exposure measures considered were based on likelihood ratio tests using either exposed workers or unexposed and exposed workers.

Relative risk regression models were fit using exact and asymptotic conditional logistic regression. The conditional logistic regression likelihood is equivalent to the partial likelihood of Cox regression [35] which can be understood as a refinement of Poisson regression [36]. While the exact models are more appropriate for the small numbers of NPC deaths involved in this analysis, we also ran asymptotic models to enable more direct comparisons with the asymptotic Poisson regression models run by Beane Freeman et al. [8]. Categorical FA exposure models were run in Stata/SE 13.1 [37] and continuous FA exposure models were run in SAS 9.4 [38]. The internal comparisons used the same exposure metric categorization scheme described for the external comparisons. All formaldehyde exposure metrics in the external and internal mortality comparisons incorporated the same 15-year lag period used by NCI. We addressed Methodological Issues 1, 2, and 3 within the internal comparisons.

Methodological issue 1 For Issue 1, we conducted and compared exposure-response analyses using both the lowest FA exposure category (as done by NCI) and the unexposed exposure category as the baseline. We argued (Issue 4 in [23]) that it is inappropriate to exclude unexposed workers from internal analyses as done by Beane Freeman et al. [30]. All workers are from the same factories and, as noted by McLaughlin et al. [39] in a response to a letter by Hauptmann and Ronckers [40], lagging of FA exposure by 15 years results in contributions to the unexposed category from workers who were, in fact, exposed to FA. Indeed, most of the person-time at risk allocated to the unexposed category represents years of follow-up of workers who were eventually exposed to FA. Therefore, it is of major interest to examine whether the statistically significant positive associations between FA exposure and NPC deaths as described by NCI in Bean Freeman et al. [8] can be replicated if unexposed workers are not dropped prior to analyses.

Methodological issue 2 For Issue 2, we avoided the problems associated with using continuous variable trend tests for categorical variables (as done by Beane Freeman et al. [8]; see Issue 5 in Marsh et al. [11] for background and details), by properly matching the trend test with the method of analysis. That is, we modeled the continuous form of the FA metrics (excluding highest peak) to produce a slope estimate that was evaluated for statistical significance (linear trend) via a likelihood ratio test. We used the actual continuous FA exposure in our asymptotic models (referred to in tables as Score 4); whereas, due to the computationally intensive permutation methods inherent in our exact models, we used the median FA exposure value associated with each category of the corresponding pseudo-continuous FA exposure metric (Score 3). As in our earlier reanalysis [23], a pseudo-continuous form of the NCI highest peak exposure variable was defined by scoring each of the categories used by Beane Freeman et al. [8] with the arithmetic mean of the interval, including a reasonable assumption about the score for the last open-ended interval (Scores: unexposed = 0, >0–1.9 = 0.95, 2.0–3.9 = 3.0, 4.0 + = 6.0) (Score 2). Likewise, we also modeled the categorical form of each FA metric and evaluated trend via a likelihood ratio test based on the category-specific score statistics. For all exposure metrics, we used the scores 1, 2, 3, 4 to represent the four categories of FA exposure, respectively (Score 1). In each exposure-response analysis, the main effect of the corresponding exposure metric was assessed with a global test.

Methodological issue 3 The key finding in our previous reanalyses of NPC mortality in the 1994 NCI cohort [22] was that NCI's earlier conclusion of a possible causal association between FA exposure and NPC mortality risk [5] was driven heavily by a large, statistically significant excess in NPC mortality risk for employees from Plant 1. In a later reanalysis using a continuous form of the highest peak FA exposure metric, Marsh et al. [23] showed that the internal analyses of Hauptmann et al. [5] were non-robust and mis-specified as the authors did not account for a statistically significant interaction structure between plant group (Plant 1 vs. Plants 2–10) and highest peak FA exposure. Subsequently, to address plant heterogeneity for NPC mortality risks in the 2004 NCI FA cohort, Beane Freeman et al. [8] refuted the findings of Marsh et al. [23], and through an "influence analysis" concluded that they found "*. . .no evidence of plant heterogeneity for a broad group of metrics, including peak exposure.*" We maintain that Beane Freeman et al. [8] neither correctly interpreted the results of their own influence analysis nor correctly interpreted the results of the interaction evaluation performed by Marsh et al. [23]. For more details see Issue 6 in Marsh et al. [11].

To further address this issue of interaction structure using the 2004 NCI FA cohort data, we extended our earlier models [23], which were based only on the continuous form of the highest peak FA exposure metric, to include continuous forms of the other FA metrics considered (duration of exposure, average intensity of exposure and cumulative exposure). We also considered both exact and asymptotic estimation as described

above. Our continuous form of the highest peak FA exposure metric described above enabled the fitting of an interaction term with the plant group indicator despite analyzing sparse data. We fit different specifications of the interaction model and modeled the continuous form peak exposure metric for Plant 1 and Plants 2–10 separately to gain insights into the meaning of the interaction terms derived from models based on all plants. Finally, we fit interaction models based on the plant group indicator and average FA exposure intensity, cumulative FA exposure or duration of FA exposure. We always evaluated all 11 NPC deaths in these models addressing the interaction issue.

Results
Statistical analyses - external mortality comparisons
Table 1 shows for each of the 10 NCI study plants, selected demographic and FA exposure characteristics and findings from the external mortality comparisons. Because the NCI 2004 update did not include new subjects nor extended work history information, the FA exposure characteristics are identical to those we discussed in our previous reanalysis [22]. We refer to plants by the sequential (UPitt) plant only.

Table 1 shows that the one additional NPC death observed in the 2004 NCI update occurred in Plant 3 resulting in not statistically significant U.S. and local-rate based SMRs of 3.01 and 7.60, respectively, based on two observed deaths. Because of this, U.S. and local rate-based SMRs for NPC in the remaining nine plants decreased from the 1994 update [22]. In particular, six of now 11 NPC deaths occurred in Plant 1 yielding statistically significant ($p < .01$) 5.44-fold and 5.57-fold excesses based on the U.S. and regional comparisons, respectively. In the 1994 update, the corresponding NPC SMRs were 6.62 ($p < .01$) and 7.39 ($p < .01$). The remaining three NPC deaths were scattered individually across three plants (Plants 2, 7, and 10), yielding not statistically significant local rate-based mortality excesses ranging from 1.01-fold (Plant 10) to 4.03–fold (Plant 2). No NPC deaths were observed in Plants 4–6 or 8–9.

Table 2 presents similar data as Table 1 for two plant groups (Plant 1 and Plants 2–10). The now five NPC deaths combined in Plants 2–10 yield a null finding (SMR = 1.06) compared with a statistically significant 5.57-fold excess for Plant 1 based on local NPC rates. An even greater difference in NPC local rate-based SMRs was observed between formaldehyde-exposed workers in Plant 1 (SMR = 7.34, 95 % CI = 2.69–15.97) and Plants 2–10 (SMR = 0.82, 95 % CI = 0.17–2.41), and the NPC SMR among unexposed workers in Plants 2–10 (SMR = 1.88, 95 % CI = 0.23–6.80) was more than twice that among the exposed workers (SMR = 0.82, 95 % CI = 0.17–2.41).

Table 2 Characteristics and findings for Plant 1 (Wallingford) and Plants 2-10 combined in 2004 NCI update

Characteristic/finding	Plant 1 (Wallingford)	Plant 2-10 (all other plants)
Entry year	1940	1934–1958
No. subjects	4261	21358
Formaldehyde exposure		
% Subjects ever exposed	87.7	89.8
% Subjects ever in highest peak category	46.1	20.1
Median AIE (ppm) [a]	1.023	0.366
(5–95 %-tile)	(.310–1.417)	(.052–1.257)
Median Cum (ppm-years) [a]	.9	3.2
(5–95 %-tile)	(.1–17.2)	(.06–23.5)
Median Dur (years) [a]	1.0	13.1
(5–95 %-tile)	(.1–24.4)	(.3–32.1)
Observed deaths and SMRs		
All workers		
Observed deaths	6	5
SMR-US (expected deaths)	5.44** (1.1)	.97 (5.2)
(95 % CI)	(2–11.85)	(.31–2.26)
SMR-local (expected deaths)	5.57** (1.1)	1.06 (4.7)
(95 % CI)	(2.04–12.12)	(.35–2.48)
Exposed workers		
Observed deaths	6	3
SMR-US (expected deaths)	7.23** (.8)	.74 (4.1)
(95 % CI)	(2.65–15.74)	(.15–2.16)
SMR-local (expected deaths)	7.34** (.8)	.82 (3.6)
(95 % CI)	(2.69–15.97)	(.17–2.41)
Unexposed workers		
Observed deaths	0	2
SMR-US (expected deaths)	– (.3)	1.81 (1.1)
(95 % CI)	(0–13.55)	(.22–6.53)
SMR-local (expected deaths)	– (.3)	1.88 (1.1)
(95 % CI)	(0–14.20)	(.23–6.80)

[a]Based on exposed jobs only with no lag
** $p < .01$

Table 3 shows local rate-based NPC SMRs for each of the four FA exposure metrics for all plants combined and by two plant groups (Plant 1 and Plants 2–10). To facilitate comparison, results from the 1994 [22] and 2004 NCI updates are shown side-by-side. In addition to the reasons noted in the Methods section, SMRs differ between the corresponding NCI and UPitt analyses due to the alternative UPitt categorizations used for all but highest peak exposure. Table 3 shows that the one additional NPC death observed in Plant 3 (Table 1) occurred in the lowest FA exposure category (Exp Cat 1) of each of the metrics considered except for duration of exposure (Exp Cat 2). For all plants combined and Plants 2–10, this finding led to an increased SMR for NPC in the corresponding categories. In Plant 1 and for all other categories that did not include the additional death, NPC SMRs decreased between the 1994 and 2004 updates. Similar to our earlier findings [22], SMRs in Table 3 for all plants combined are elevated for nearly all unexposed and exposed categories of each metric considered and are statistically significant for the highest exposure categories of highest peak exposure, average intensity of exposure, and cumulative exposure (UPitt categories only). Many SMRs in the baseline (unexposed) categories exceed those in the corresponding non-baseline categories.

The pattern of NPC SMRs for Plant 1 is similar to those reported in the independent study of Plant 1 [25, 41, 42], namely, very large and often statistically significant excesses in NPC across all non-baseline exposure categories, but little evidence of consistent exposure–response relationships across the formaldehyde exposure metrics considered. All NPC deaths in Plant 1 occurred among exposed workers. For highest peak exposure in Plant 1, all six NPC deaths occurred in the greatest exposure category (4 + ppm) yielding a lower but statistically significant ($p < .01$) SMR of 12.91 (95 % CI = 4.74–28.10). In contrast, for Plants 2–10 combined, two of the five (or two of four for NCI) NPC deaths occurred among workers unexposed to formaldehyde yielding a near 2-fold or greater NPC excess in each of the four baseline categories. For two metrics (highest peak and duration of exposure) the baseline NPC SMR exceeded that observed among the most highly exposed workers.

Statistical analyses - internal mortality comparisons

Additional file 1: Table S1a-d show the results of our internal, exact relative risk (RR) regression analysis for NPC for each of the four FA metrics considered (highest peak, average intensity, cumulative and duration, respectively). Each table shows results for all plants combined, Plant 1 and Plants 2–10, and using both the unexposed category (left portion) and lowest exposure category (right portion) as the baseline category for RR estimates. Also shown are results for each sub-analysis using the NCI categories (based on 10 NPC deaths) [8] and our alternative FA exposure categorization (based on 11 NPC deaths). Each sub-analysis shows slope estimates and corresponding p-values for both categorical and continuous (or pseudo-continuous) forms of the FA metrics considered (Scores 1–4 as noted above), as well as the global test p-value.

Our concern about the inappropriateness of omitting unexposed workers from the baseline category in exposure-response analyses (Issue 1) is evident in the results presented in Additional file 1: Table S1a-d. This

Table 3 NCI FA cohort, NPC SMR results, local comparisons, by FA exposure, update and plant group

Part A — Highest Peak Category[a] and AIE[b]

Metric[c,d]	HPC 2004 NCI Obs	SMR[e]	95% CI	HPC 1994 NCI[f] Obs	SMR[e]	95% CI	AIE 2004 NCI Obs	SMR[e]	95% CI	AIE 1994 NCI[f] Obs	SMR[e]	95% CI
All Plants												
NCI Cats.												
Unexposed	2	1.98	(0.24–7.16)	2	2.22	(0.27–8.00)	2	1.51	(0.18, 5.46)	2	1.62	(0.20–5.84)
Exp Cat 1	1	1.03	(0.03–5.73)	0	0	(0.00–2.46)	1	0.41	(0.01, 2.28)	0	—	(0.00–1.77)
Exp Cat 2	0	—	(0.00, 2.24)	0	0	(0.00–3.47)	1	0.91	(0.02, 5.09)	1	1.17	(0.03–6.50)
Exp Cat 3	7	3.89**	(1.56–8.01)	7	4.84**	(1.94–9.97)	6	6.67**	(2.81, 14.42)	6	8.36**	(3.07–18.21)
UPitt Cats.												
Unexposed	2	1.98	(0.24–7.16)	2	2.22	(0.24–7.16)	2	1.51	(0.18, 5.46)	2	1.62	(0.20–5.84)
Exp Cat 1	1	1.03	(0.03–5.73)	0	—	(0.00–2.46)	4	1.11	(0.30, 2.83)	3	0.99	(0.20–2.90)
Exp Cat 2	0	—	(0.00, 2.24)	0	—	(0.00–3.47)	2	6.33	(0.77, 22.86)	2	7.60	(0.92–27.46)
Exp Cat 3	8	4.50**	(1.94–8.87)	8	5.53**	(2.39–10.90)	3	5.73*	(1.18, 16.75)	3	8.06*	(1.66–23.55)
Plant 1												
UPitt Cats.												
Unexposed	0	—	(0.00, 2.09)	0	0	—	0	—	(0.00, 14.20)	0	—	(0.00–15.97)
Exp Cat 1	0	—	(0.00, 2.90)	0	—	—	2	4.88	(0.59, 17.61)	2	7.46	(0.90–26.94)
Exp Cat 2	0	—	(0.00, 2.90)	0	—	—	2	10.74*	(1.30, 38.79)	2	13.96*	(1.69–50.44)
Exp Cat 3	6	12.91**	(4.74–28.10)	6	17.04**	(6.25–37.08)	2	9.03*	(1.09, 32.64)	2	11.78*	(1.43–42.57)
Plants 2–10												
UPitt Cats.												
Unexposed	2	2.42	(0.29–8.75)	2	2.66	(0.32–9.60)	2	1.88	(0.23, 6.80)	2	1.99	(0.24–7.18)
Exp Cat 1	1	1.04	(0.03–5.77)	0	—	(0.00–2.46)	2	0.62	(0.08, 2.25)	1	0.36	(0.01–2.02)
Exp Cat 2	0	—	(0.00, 2.90)	0	—	(0.00–4.66)	0	—	(0.00, 28.43)	0	—	(0.00–30.78)
Exp Cat 3	2	1.52	(0.18–5.50)	2	1.83	(0.22–6.60)	1	3.31	(0.08, 18.45)	1	4.94	(0.12–27.50)

Part B — Cumulative Exposure (Cum)[b] and Duration of Exposure (Dur)[b]

Metric[c,d]	Cum 2004 NCI Obs	SMR[e]	95% CI	Cum 1994 NCI[f] Obs	SMR[e]	95% CI	Dur 2004 NCI Obs	SMR[e]	95% CI	Dur 1994 NCI[f] Obs	SMR[e]	95% CI
All Plants												
NCI Cats.												
Unexposed	2	1.51	(0.18–5.46)	2	1.62	(0.20–5.84)	2	1.51	(0.18–5.46)	2	1.62	(0.20–5.84)
Exp Cat 1	4	1.50	(0.41–3.83)	3	1.36	(0.28–3.97)	5	1.83	(0.59–4.26)	4	1.80	(0.49–4.62)
Exp Cat 2	1	1.05	(0.03–5.82)	1	1.25	(0.03–6.98)	1	0.98	(0.02–5.45)	1	1.07	(0.03–5.96)
Exp Cat 3	3	3.75	(0.77–10.96)	3	4.57	(0.94–13.37)	2	2.86	(0.35–10.32)	2	3.94	(0.48–14.25)
UPitt Cats.												
Unexposed	2	1.51	(0.18–5.46)	2	1.62	(0.20–5.84)	2	1.51	(0.18–5.46)	2	1.62	(0.20–5.84)
Exp Cat 1	4	1.86	(0.51–4.77)	3	1.69	(0.35–4.94)	3	2.32	(0.48–6.77)	3	2.88	(0.40–8.43)
Exp Cat 2	2	1.08	(0.13–3.89)	2	1.30	(0.16–4.68)	3	1.83	(0.38–5.36)	2	1.49	(0.18–5.38)
Exp Cat 3	3	6.60*	(1.36–19.30)	3	8.80*	(1.82–25.73)	3	1.96	(0.41–5.74)	3	2.35	(0.48–6.86)
Plant 1												
UPitt Cats.												
Unexposed	0	—	(0.00–14.20)	0	—	(0.00–15.97)	0	—	(0.00–14.20)	0	—	(0.00–15.97)
Exp Cat 1	3	8.26*	(1.70–24.14)	3	11.70**	(2.41–34.18)	3	9.14**	(1.89–26.72)	3	12.79**	(2.64–37.37)
Exp Cat 2	2	5.24	(0.63–18.93)	2	7.21	(0.87–26.04)	2	6.30	(0.76–22.75)	2	9.01*	(1.09–32.54)
Exp Cat 3	1	13.66	(0.34–76.10)	1	21.18	(0.53–118.03)	1	5.80	(0.15–32.34)	1	8.03	(0.20–44.75)
Plants 2–10												
UPitt Cats.												
Unexposed	2	1.88	(0.23–6.80)	2	1.99	(0.24–7.19)	2	1.88	(0.23–6.80)	2	1.99	(0.24–7.18)
Exp Cat 1	1	0.56	(0.01–3.12)	1	0.36	(0.00–2.43)	0	—	(0.00–3.82)	0	—	(0.00–4.58)
Exp Cat 2	0	—	(0.00–2.50)	0	—	(0.00–30.78)	1	0.76	(0.02–4.23)	0	—	(0.00–3.29)
Exp Cat 3	2	5.25	(0.64–18.96)	2	6.81	(0.82–24.61)	2	1.48	(0.18–5.33)	2	1.73	(0.21–6.26)

[a] NCI categories based on 60 and 80th percentiles of formaldehyde exposure among cancer deaths who were exposed. Includes only 10/11 deaths

[b] University of Pittsburgh categories based on approx. tertiles of formaldehyde exposure among NPC deaths who were exposed. Include 11 deaths

[c] All exposures lagged 15 years as in NCI study

[d] NCI exposure category cutpoints: highest peak ($>0- < 2.0$, $2.0- < 4.0$, and $4.0+$ ppm); average intensity of exposure ($>0-0.5$, $0.5- < 1.0$, and $1.0+$ ppm); cumulative exposure ($>0-1.5$, $1.5- < 5.5$, and $5.5+$ ppm-years); duration of exposure ($>0- < 5.0$, $5.0- < 15.0$, and $15.0+$ years). UPitt exposure category cutpoints: highest peak (same as NCI) ($>0- < 2.0$, $2.0- < 4.0$, and $4.0+$ ppm); cumulative exposure (<0.734, $0.734-10.150$, and $10.151+$ ppm-years); duration of exposure (<0.617, $0.617-6.263$, and $6.264+$ years); average intensity of exposure (<1.046, $1.046-1.177$, and $1.178+$ ppm)

[e] All SMRs adjusted for sex, race, age group, and time period

[f] From Marsh and Youk (2005)

*$p < 0.05$, **$p < 0.01$

became especially problematic in the 2004 NCI update, as the only additional NPC death observed occurred in the lowest exposure category used by NCI as the baseline for comparison. Specifically, Additional file 1: Table S1a-d show for each of the four FA metrics considered and for all Plants combined and Plants 2–10, a marked difference in results using the lowest exposure category (Exp Cat 1) baseline compared to using the unexposed as baseline, which we believe is more appropriate. Using Exp Cat 1 as baseline, RRs for NPC in the unexposed category (compared with Exp Cat 1) were consistently elevated and for Plants 2–10 often exceeded the RR for the higher two exposure categories (Exp Cats 2–3).

Further, by omitting the unexposed from the assessment of exposure-response, there appears to be some evidence of a trend in RRs with increasing FA exposure based on Exp Cats 1–3 for highest peak (NCI categories: RRs = 4.05, 1.00 (baseline), 1.27, 7.23; Additional file 1: Table S1a) and AIE (NCI categories: RRs = 6.33, 1.00 (baseline), 2.54, 11.29; Additional file 1: Table S1b), as evident by the Scores 1–3 based trend tests[5]. These results lead NCI to conclude that the association between FA and NPC persisted in the 2004 update. We observed similar, yet less pronounced, differences based on our categorization of highest peak and AIE.

Conversely, for each of the four FA metrics, our corresponding analyses using unexposed as baseline yielded lower RRs for Exp Cats 1–3 and little or no evidence of an exposure-response association for highest peak (NCI categories: RRs = 1.00 (baseline), 0.25, 0.28, 1.67; Additional file 1: Table S1a), AIE (NCI categories: RRs = 1.00 (baseline), 0.16, 0.40, 1.69; Additional file 1: Table S1b) or the other FA metrics considered. While our Score 3 based trend test using the NCI categories for AIE was statistically significant (p = .023, Additional file 1: Table S1b), this was based on an unimportant U-shaped distribution of RRs for Exp Cat 1–3. Again, we observed similar, yet less pronounced, differences based on our categorization of highest peak and AIE. Figure 1a, b illustrate using NCI categories the influence of the baseline category on the results for highest peak and AIE, respectively.

Because the one additional NPC death in the NCI 2004 update occurred in Plant 3 (Table 1), the results of our re-analyses of Plant 1 (Additional file 1: Table S1a-d) did not change markedly from those presented earlier [22]. Our results reinforce, however, our earlier findings that the results for all plants combined discussed above, are heavily driven by Plant 1 where 5 of 10 NPC deaths (NCI analysis) or 6 of 11 (our main analysis) occurred [22].

The results of our exposure-response analyses based on asymptotic models (Additional file 2: Table S2a–d) were generally consistent with the corresponding exact models. Most trend test p-values decreased slightly compared to the exact analyses, yet the conclusions are consistent. Only the trend test of pseudo-continuous form of highest peak exposure (Score 2) were statistically significant for all analysis among both exposed and non-exposed workers (UPitt categories: p = .02, Additional file 2: Table S2a) and this was based on an unimportant U-shaped distribution of RRs for the unexposed and Exp Cat 1–3. Moreover, our results based on asymptotic conditional logistic regression are similar to those of Beane Freeman et al. [8], who used asymptotic Poisson regression. For example, in their paper, the overall RR estimate for the unexposed group using low exposure as baseline is 4.39 (95%CI: 0.36–54.05) for highest peak exposure, 6.79 (95%CI: 0.55–83.64) for average intensity of exposure and 1.87 (0.30–11.67) for cumulative exposure. These results are compared to our results in Additional file 2: Table S2 a-c with low exposed group as baseline (4.35 (95%CI: 0.35–54.40), 6.73 (95%CI: 0.53–85.19) and 1.86 (95%CI: 0.29–11.84), respectively.

Statistical analyses - confounding and interaction of NPC risk estimates: the role of plant group

Additional file 3: Table S3a presents the findings of nine different internal modeling approaches of NPC risk in the NCI cohort, evaluating highest peak exposure to FA. All models were adjusted for the standard covariates age, time, sex, race, and payroll category. The regression model findings are described below in terms of the model numbers in the first column of Additional file 3: Table S3a. In Models 1 and 2, the number of observed deaths, the relative risk estimates, the estimated 95 %-confidence intervals (CI) of the relative risks and likelihood ratio trend p-values are shown. Model 2 was adjusted additionally for plant group (Plant 1 vs. Plants 2–10).

The results of Models 1–2 are similar, showing elevated RRs only in the highest exposure category, although far from being statistically significant. After adjustment for plant group, the RR estimate in the highest category was reduced (the estimated relative risk dropped from 1.8 to 1.4 after adjustment). As performed by NCI [8], trend tests (termed Score 1 trend tests here) were based on the full cohort as well as on exposed subjects only. Statistically significant Score 1 trends could only be found if the analysis was restricted to exposed workers. The Score 1 trend p-values were larger than 0.05 when analyzing the full cohort. In Models 3–9, the pseudo-continuous form of the highest peak exposure variable (Score 2) was evaluated in the exact analysis. We report coefficients (βs) of the regression models and the relative risks (RR) linked to coefficients via the formula, exp(β) = RR.

One possible way to identify ill-fitted models is to compare p-values calculated for the same models by different algorithms: the global likelihood ratio p-values

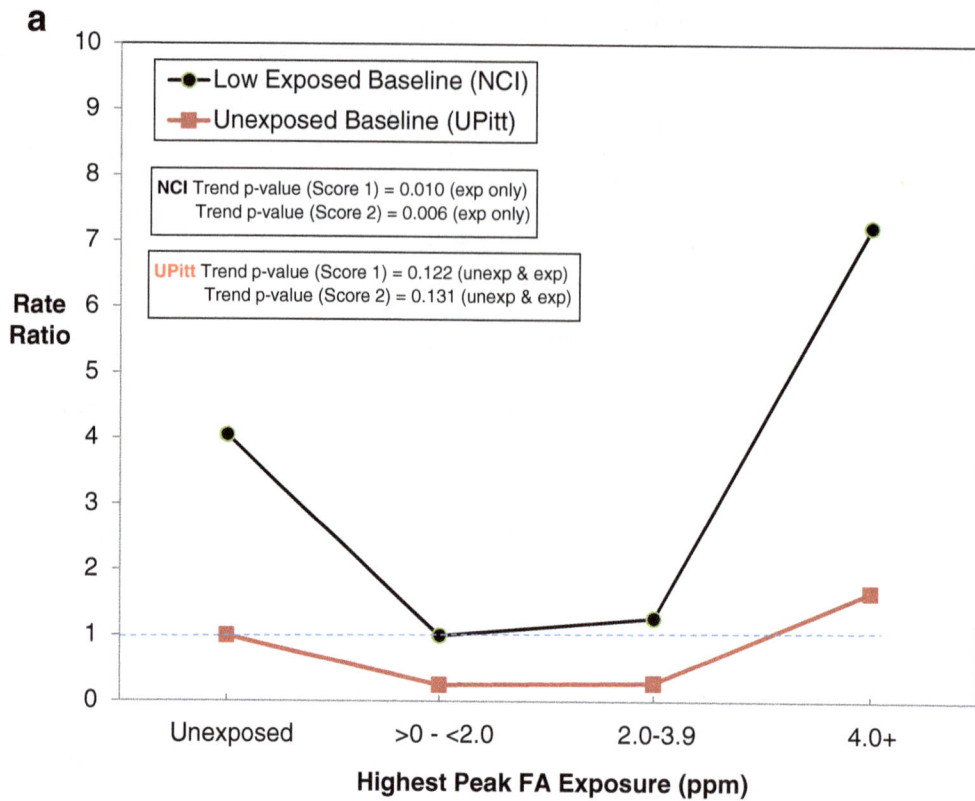

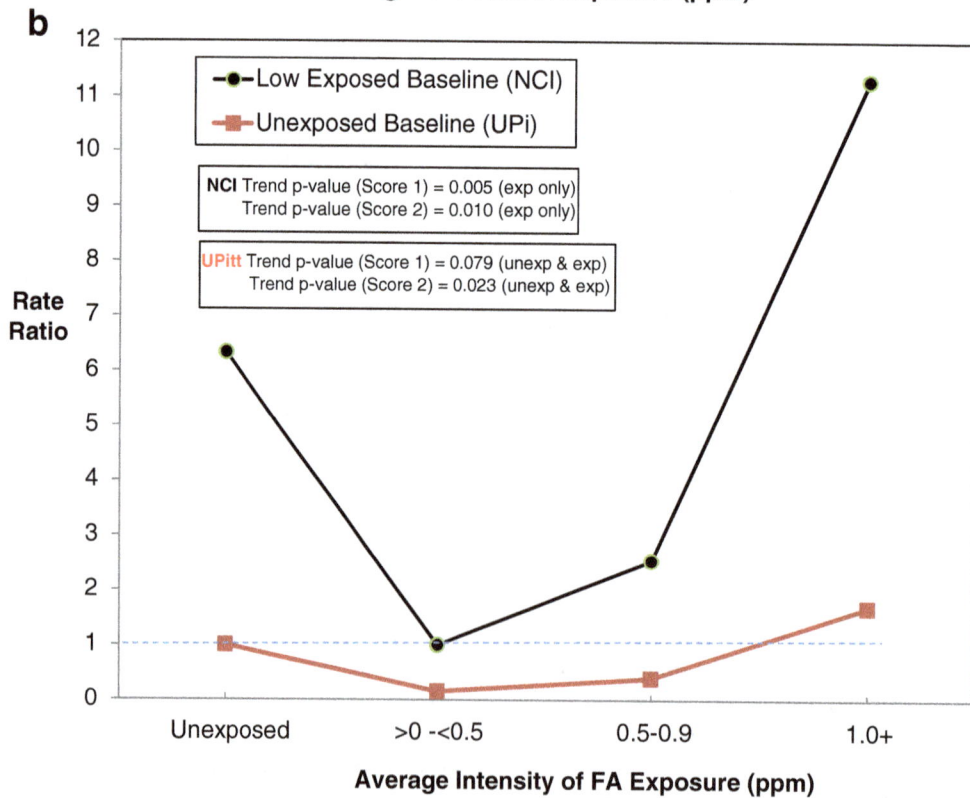

Fig. 1 a RRs and 95 % CIs by Highest Peak Formaldehyde Exposure, Exact Estimation, (from Additional file 1: Table S1a). **b** RRs and 95 % CIs by Average Intensity of Formaldehyde Exposure, Exact Estimation, (from Additional file 1: Table S1b)

shown in the last column of Models 3 to 9 are similar to the Wald p-values (presented together with the 95 %-CIs). Therefore, the model sequence fitted with continuous highest peak FA exposure did not reveal problems when using this p-value criterion.

An analysis similar to categorical Models 1 and 2 is presented in Models 3 and 7 analyzing continuous form highest peak FA exposure (pseudo-continuous highest peak Score 2). In Model 3, only the standard covariates (sex, race & payroll category) were used; Model 7 adjusted additionally for plant group. Again, the effect estimate was somewhat reduced after adjustment, although not remarkably (the coefficient decreased from 0.31 to 0.26 after adjustment, which corresponds to a relative risk reduction from 1.37 to 1.29). The plant group indicator showed a relationship with NPC risk after adjustment for continuous highest peak exposure (global $p = 0.08$, Model 7) and significantly so without adjustment for exposure ($p = 0.015$, Model 6), indicating a higher risk at Plant 1. After Model 6 was extended by an interaction term of continuous highest peak exposure and plant group indicator (shown in Model 9 of Additional file 3: Table S3a), the analysis became much more unstable. The plant group indicator variable and the interaction term were accompanied by confidence interval limits that spread out to infinity on one side each. However, the likelihood ratio test returned a p-value of 0.09 for the interaction term (the Wald test p-value was 0.08). A positive interaction between exposure and plant group is indicated. Analyzing the continuous form highest peak variable separately in both plant groups (Models 4 and 5 of Additional file 3: Table S3a) reproduced this finding from the interaction model: the formaldehyde highest peak exposure effect appears to be restricted to Plant 1 only ($p = 0.05$).

In contrast, for Plants 2–10 the likelihood ratio p-value was 0.67, clearly indicating that the effect was far from being statistically significant in these plants. Accordingly, the coefficient of exposure was estimated to be almost negligible in Plants 2–10 in comparison to Plant 1 (Model 4: 0.0072 vs. Model 5: 0.64). In addition, the confidence interval of the coefficient for Plants 2–10 was situated rather symmetrically around the null. After dropping the main effect of plant group from the full interaction model (full model = Model 9) the estimation process yielded more stable findings (reduced model = Model 8): the interaction between plant group indicator and continuous form highest peak FA exposure was now found to be significant ($p = 0.03$). When fitting asymptotic models (Additional file 4: Table S4a) we obtained similar results for the real continuous highest peak FA exposures with p-values being smaller than in the exact analyses. The global p-values for the interaction terms were 0.011 (Model 8) and 0.015 (Model 9).

Additional file 3: Table S3 b, c, d show results after repeating the exact analyses evaluating average intensity, cumulative exposure or duration of exposure to FA. For all three metrics, we used the continuous-form exposure Score 3 in Model 3–5 and Model 7–9. Model 8 indicate interactions between the plant group variable and the exposure metric in all three analyses: likelihood ratio p-values were 0.06 (average intensity, Additional file 3: Table S3b), 0.004 (cumulative exposure, Additional file 3: Table S3c), and 0.005 (duration of exposure, Additional file 3: Table S3d). We note that findings on cumulative exposure are more unstable because Wald p-values and likelihood ratio p-values differ considerably in many of the returned model findings.

The results of our asymptotic models (Additional file 4: Table S4a b, c, d) were generally consistent with those in the exact analysis. Similar to the asymptotic analysis of highest peak exposure, most of the p-values in the asymptotic analysis of the average intensity, cumulative exposure and duration of exposure to FA decreased compared to the exact analysis. Models 8 indicate interactions between the plant group variable and the corresponding exposure metric in all three asymptotic analyses: likelihood ratio p-values were 0.007 (average intensity, Additional file 4: Table S4-b), 0.015 (cumulative exposure, Additional file 4: Table S4-c), and 0.088 (duration of exposure, Additional file 4: Table S4-d).

Discussion

In this paper, we challenged NCI's claim that an increased mortality risk for nasopharyngeal cancer (NPC) in relation to formaldehyde (FA) exposure persisted in their 2004 update of the FA cohort [8]. As we demonstrated in our re-analyses of the 1994 update of the NCI FA cohort [22, 23], and again here, NCI's claim of a persistent NPC risk stemmed from the use of inappropriate and non-robust statistical analysis methods. The foundation of our current reanalyses was three of the six methodological issues presented earlier: inappropriateness of excluding unexposed workers from exposure-response evaluations; improper trend tests and failure to recognize the important interaction structure between Plant 1 and Plants 2–10 [11].

Our reanalyses included external mortality comparisons via SMRs, in which we compared NPC rates among workers with the corresponding NPC rates of the general populations of both the U.S. and regional CT area. This enabled comparison with NCI's U.S. rate-based only SMRs, and provided new data that accounted for geographic variability in NPC rates. Our reanalyses also included comparisons of NPC mortality among subgroups of workers defined by FA exposure level. In these exposure-response evaluations, we fit relative risk regression models in which subgroups of workers with higher FA exposure were compared to workers with lower or no FA exposure.

We fit many variations of our models to address the three issues noted above. For example, we used both the lowest FA exposure category (as done by NCI) and the unexposed category (our recommended approach) as the baseline category. We also modeled the continuous forms (i.e., not categorized) of the FA exposure metrics and applied corresponding continuous variable trend tests. This enabled a comparison with NCI, where continuous variable trend tests were inappropriately applied to categorical FA exposure variables. Further, to address the dramatic difference in NPC mortality among workers in Plant 1 vs. Plants 2–10, we fit models that included terms to account for this important interaction structure. To date, NCI has not fit models that account explicitly for this interaction. Finally, because NCI relied on Poisson regression based on asymptotic estimation rather than relative risk regression to evaluate exposure-response relationships for FA and NPC, we fit our models using both asymptotic and exact estimation, the latter being better suited for the small number of observed NPC deaths.

Overall, our reanalyses of the 2004 update of the NCI FA cohort do not support an association between FA exposure and NPC as suggested by Hauptmann et al. [5] and Beane Freeman et al. [8]. Our findings and conclusion also corroborate those presented in our earlier re-analysis of the NCI 1994 FA cohort data, and are now even stronger given that the one additional NPC death observed by NCI occurred in Plant 3 among workers in the lowest exposure category of highest peak, average intensity and cumulative FA exposure and in the second exposure category of duration of exposure. This finding led to: (1) reduced SMRs and RRs in the remaining nine study plants in unaffected exposure categories, (2) attenuated exposure-response relations for FA and NPC for all the FA metrics considered and (3) strengthened and expanded evidence that the internal analyses of Hauptmann et al. [5] and Beane Freeman et al. [8] were non-robust and mis-specified as they did not account for an statistically significant interaction structure between plant group (Plant 1 vs. Plants 2–10) and FA exposure (see Models 8 in Additional file 3: Table S3 and Additional file 4: Table S4).

A specific focus of the internal mortality comparisons was to address our concern about the inappropriateness of omitting unexposed workers from the baseline category in exposure-response analyses (Issue 1). We found that analyses using the lowest FA exposure category as the baseline (NCI approach) produced evidence of an exposure-response relationship for FA and NPC for highest peak and average intensity of FA exposure (the basis of NCIs conclusion [8]). In contrast, our corresponding

analyses using unexposed workers as the more appropriate baseline category yielded lower RRs for the exposure categories and little or no evidence of an exposure-response association for any of the FA metrics considered. Again, NCI's finding of only one additional NPC death in the lower FA exposure categories contributed to this null finding.

Our internal analyses also addressed NCI's practice of mixing results of internal mortality comparisons based on categorical analyses with trend tests based on the continuous form of the FA metric considered. More appropriately, our internal analyses matched the results of the analysis (categorical RRs or slope estimates) with the corresponding trend tests based on categorical or continuous (or pseudo-continuous) scores, respectively. While the p-values associated with these two sets of trend tests differed, in most cases these differences were quantitative and the tests consistently rejected or failed to reject the null hypothesis of no association between FA and NPC.

To address Issue 3, we focused on two aspects of risk analysis to explore a possible mis-specification of the models as presented in Beane Freeman et al. [8], confounder adjustment and interaction assessment. Confounding is understood as defined by Greenland and Robins [43] and as explicated graphically in Greenland et al. [44]. We explored confounding in practice by applying the change-in-estimate criterion [45, 46]. Models 1 and 2 of Additional file 3: Table S3 a, b, c, d gave results about the possible confounding effect of the plant group indicator. Although not pronounced, some indication of confounding was indicted in peak exposure and average intensity models because the relative risk in the highest exposure category decreased after taking the plant group indicator into account. Using the continuous peak exposure variable, the same tendency can be seen as a somewhat reduced risk estimate after adjustment for plant group in the peak exposure model but not so in the other analyses. Therefore, the statement of Hauptmann et al. [5] that the risk estimates for FA exposure did not change considerably after adjusting for plants is confirmed again in this re-analysis. We have observed this in our previous analysis too [23].

Beane Freeman et al. [8] did not perform a risk analysis adjusted for plant or plant group. They performed what they called an "influence analysis" by "excluding one plant at a time". Such an analysis cannot contrast the findings of Plant 1 vs Plants 2–10 because it does not cover the important case of studying Plant 1 alone. The authors, however, studied Plants 2–10 as a group: "When Plant 1 was excluded, the number of NPC deaths was two in the highest peak exposure category (RR = 3.36, 95 % CI: 0.3, 37.27), one in the highest average intensity category (RR = 4.09, 95 % CI:

0.25, 66.0), and zero in the highest cumulative exposure category." This can be compared with our findings in Additional file 1: Table S1a-c. The relative estimate is 2.92 (95 % CI: 0.15, 177.22) for the highest peak exposure category, 4.08 (95 % CI: 0.05, 326.39) for the highest average intensity category and 6.74 (95 % CI: 0.32, 428.37) for the highest cumulative exposure category using the low exposure group as the baseline. However, the corresponding relative estimate decreased to 0.43 (95 % CI: 0.02, 7.92) for the highest peak category, 0.42 (95 % CI: 0.01, 9.65) for the highest average intensity category and 0.44 (95 % CI: 0.04, 16.12) for the highest cumulative exposure category with unexposed group as the baseline.

Beane Freeman et al. [8] concluded from their "influence analysis" that they found "... *no evidence of plant heterogeneity for a broad group of metrics, including peak exposure.*" We judge that this statement is wrong. We base our judgement on the findings of our interaction analyses (Issue 3). We begin with stating that the full interaction models (Models 9 in Additional file 3: Table S6 a, b, c, d) showed instabilities: The coefficient for the plant group indicator was always accompanied with a lower 95 % CI limit of −infinity. Accordingly, the likelihood ratio p-values were 100 % for the plant group variable in all analyses with the exception of 42 % when analyzing peak exposures. Thus, it is of interest to reduce the models by dropping the plant variable indicator from the Models 9. This means to force the baseline risk of all plants to be the same and then check for different slopes, although usually recommendations are given not to drop main effects if interactions are explored [45]. These reduced models without the main effect of plant group are presented as Models 8 in Additional file 3: Table S3 a, b, c, d. Because the reduced model uses all cases simultaneously (more power than the separate models) and avoids the problem of relying on the very imprecise baseline risk in Plant 1 (disadvantage of the full interaction model), the estimates are more stable: no median unbiased estimates were necessary and no confidence interval limit approached infinity. The interaction terms were found to be significant at the 5 %-level in all analyses (exception: average exposure analysis returned a likelihood ratio p-value of 0.063).

It has been argued to use the p-value of the interaction term in the decision process when assessing interactions [47]. A conservative approach, however, was recommended, i.e., comparing the p-value of the interaction term with a cut point clearly higher than the usual significance level of 5 %: keep the interaction terms within the models if their p-values are not higher than 25 % [45]. This recommendation is in line with the statement that "in epidemiological settings, the power to detect statistical interactions is typically an order of magnitude less than the power to detect main effects" [48]. Following this advice, our re-analyses found clear evidence of an interaction effect of all three FA exposure metrics and the plant group indicator which cannot be ignored.

We conclude from these analyses that there is no NPC risk identified in Plants 2–10 and all effects of formaldehyde that were described in Beane Freeman et al. [8] stem from Plant 1 only. It is curious that Beane Freeman et al. [8] did not follow the advice given in Marsh et al. [23] to perform a regular interaction analysis, but conducted an "influential analysis" (see above). This type of analysis never analyzed Plant 1 alone and was, therefore, unable to judge the degree of heterogeneity between Plant 1 and Plant 2–10. Marsh et al. [11] explained the misinterpretation by Beane Freeman et al. [8] of the previous interaction analyses performed in Marsh et al. [23] and showed that the results presented by Beane Freeman et al. [8] are entirely consistent with the interaction effect observed in Marsh et al. [23].

We emphasize that the current re-analyses strengthen the argument made in Marsh et al. [23] and Marsh et al. [11], that is, we showed a pronounced positive interaction effect (risk modification) by plant group (Plant 1 vs. Plants 2–10), not only for the continuous peak exposure metric but also for average and cumulative exposure and duration of exposure to FA. It follows that the internal modelling approaches presented by Hauptmann et al. [5] were misspecified and that Beane Freeman et al. [8] did not correct this flaw, but repeated the misleading model set-up.

Conclusions

The results of the analysis of nasopharyngeal cancer risk in the NCI cohort published by Beane Freeman et al. [8] are misleading because they are based on inappropriate regression analyses. The authors repeatedly failed to account for an important interaction structure between the plant group and the exposure variable which prohibits a generalization of formaldehyde effects within the NCI cohort and, in particular, beyond the NCI cohort. Overall, our updated reanalysis provided little or no evidence to support NCI's suggestion of a persistent association between FA exposure and mortality from NPC. NCI's suggestion continues to be driven heavily by anomalous findings in one study plant (Plant 1). Our findings continue to cast considerable additional uncertainty regarding the validity of NCI's suggested persistent association. This may be of particular interest given the conflicting evaluation of FA carcinogenicity by US and EU authorities.

Exemptions

This research was deemed exempt from human subjects review by the University of Pittsburgh Institutional Review Board.

Endnotes

[1]http://echa.europa.eu/web/guest/about-us/who-we-are/committee-for-risk-assessment

[2]ECHA, http://echa.europa.eu

[3]http://echa.europa.eu/web/guest/view-article/-/journal_content/c89bdb13-09e9-497c-8e73-ddae13a842c8

[4]Checkoway et al. [28] redefined the original NCI peak exposure metric in their re-analysis: "at least 1 continuous month of employment in jobs identified in the original exposure characterization as likely having short-term exposure excursions of 2 ppm or more to less than 4 ppm or 4 ppm or more on a weekly or daily basis". This redefinition, however, had no relevant impact on the results: "our re-analysis using redefined 'peak' exposure detected associations similar to those previously reported". Thus, we did not change the NCI definition and used the highest peak exposure metric as originally applied by NCI [8] and in our previous re-analyses [22, 23, 33].

[5]The exact estimation-based RRs based on NCI categories shown in Additional file 1: Table S1a–d differ somewhat from those presented by Beane Freeman et al. [8] who used asymptotic Poisson regression models.

Additional files

Additional file 1: Table S1. a NCI FA cohort, NPC RR results for highest peak FA exposure (ppm) metric, exact estimation. **b** NCI FA cohort, NPC RR results for average intensity of FA exposure (AIE) (ppm) metric, exact estimation. **c** NCI FA cohort, NPC RR results for cumulative FA exposure (Cum) (ppm-years) metric, exact estimation. **d** NCI FA cohort, NPC RR results for duration of FA exposure (Dur) (years) metric, exact estimation. (DOCX 85 kb)

Additional file 2: Table S2. a NCI FA cohort, RR analysis using highest peak FA exposure (ppm), asymptotic estimation. **b** NCI FA cohort, RR analysis using average intensity of FA exposure (ppm), asymptotic estimation. **c** NCI FA cohort, RR analysis using cumulative FA exposure (ppm-years), asymptotic estimation. **d** NCI FA cohort, RR analysis using duration of FA exposure (years), asymptotic estimation. (DOCX 54 kb)

Additional file 3: Table S3. a Observed deaths and interval rate-based RRs or β coefficients by highest peak FA exposure. **b** Observed deaths and interval rate-based RRs or β coefficients by average intensity of FA exposure (ppm). **c** Observed deaths and interval rate-based RRs or β coefficients by cumulative FA exposure (ppm-years). **d** Observed deaths and interval rate-based RRs or β coefficients by duration of FA exposure (years). (DOCX 77 kb)

Additional file 4: Table S4. a Observed deaths and interval RRs or β coefficients by peak FA exposure, asymptotic estimation. **b** Observed deaths and interval RRs or β coefficients by average FA intensity exposure, asymptotic estimation. **c** Observed deaths and RRs or β coefficients by cumulative FA exposure, asymptotic estimation. **d** Observed deaths and RRs or β coefficients by duration of FA exposure, asymptotic estimation. (DOCX 66 kb)

Competing interests

GM's, SZ's, YL's and LB's work on this commentary was performed under a sponsored research contract between the University of Pittsburgh and the Research Foundation Health and Environmental Effects, which is a not-for-profit affiliate of the American Chemistry Council. PM's work was performed under a separate sponsored research agreement between the Institute for Occupational Epidemiology and Risk Assessment of Evonik Industries and RFHEE. Evonik Industries does not produce formaldehyde and has no economical link to production or use of formaldehyde. The funding agencies played no role in the design, writing, interpretation and conclusions. The decision to submit this manuscript for publication is that of the authors.

Authors' contributions

GM and PM were the co-investigators of the reanalyses of the 2004 NCI cohort data and earlier served as co-investigators on reanalyses of the 1994 NCI cohort data. They took lead roles in the drafting of the manuscript. SZ and AL were the primary biostatisticians on the project and contributed to the writing and editing of the manuscript. LB also contributed to the writing and editing of the manuscript. All authors read and approved the final manuscript.

Authors' information

GM is Professor of Biostatistics and Director of the Center for Occupational Biostatistics and Epidemiology at the University of Pittsburgh, Graduate School of Public Health. Since the 1980s, he has been involved epidemiological research on the potential carcinogenicity of formaldehyde, including re- analyses of earlier updates of the NCI formaldehyde cohort and serving as principal investigator of an independent cohort study of workers from one of the NCI study plants.
PM is head of the Institute for Occupational Epidemiology and Risk Assessment of Evonik Industries AG. Evonik Industries and Cologne University have started a public-private partnership to conduct, and participate in investigations, research, and analyses relating to the health, safety, and epidemiological aspects of working conditions. The contract between Evonik Industries and Cologne University guarantees freedom of publication of all research work produced by the Evonik Institute. After his habilitation at Cologne University PM is teaching epidemiology and biostatistics at Cologne University. PM performed re-analyses of NCI's industrial cohort formaldehyde study in cooperation with GM.
SZ is Research Specialist V and Senior Biostatistician in the Center for Occupational Biostatistics and Epidemiology at the University of Pittsburgh, Graduate School of Public Health. YL and LB are PhD students in the Department of Biostatistics at the University of Pittsburgh, Graduate School of Public Health.

Acknowledgments

We obtained the NCI cohort data via a Data Transfer Agreement between the University of Pittsburgh and the National Cancer Institute's (NCI) Technology Transfer Center. We extend special thanks to Dr. Laura Beane Freeman of NCI's Division of Cancer, Epidemiology and Genetics and Dr. Laura Henmueller of the NCI Technology Transfer Center. We also thank Charles Alcorn and Steve Sefcik for computer programming support.

Author details

[1]Center for Occupational Biostatistics and Epidemiology and Department of Biostatistics, Graduate School of Public Health, University of Pittsburgh, 130 DeSoto Street, Pittsburgh, PA 15261, USA. [2]Institute and Policlinic for Occupational Medicine, Environmental Medicine and Preventive Research, University of Cologne, Cologne, Germany. [3]Institute for Occupational Epidemiology and Risk Assessment of Evonik Industries, Essen, Germany.

References

1. Formaldehyde, 2-butoxyethanol and 1-tert-butoxypropan-2-ol. IARC monographs on the evaluation of carcinogenic risks to humans / World Health Organization, International Agency for Research on Cancer. 2006;88:1-478.
2. Chemical agents and related occupations. IARC monographs on the evaluation of carcinogenic risks to humans / World Health Organization, International Agency for Research on Cancer. 2012;100(Formaldehyde):401-35.
3. Swenberg JA, Lu K, Moeller BC, Gao L, Upton PB, Nakamura J, et al. Endogenous versus exogenous DNA adducts: their role in carcinogenesis, epidemiology, and risk assessment. Toxicol Sci. 2011;120 Suppl 1:S130–45. doi:10.1093/toxsci/kfq371.
4. Wood dust. IARC monographs on the evaluation of carcinogenic risks to humans / World Health Organization, International Agency for Research on Cancer. 1995;62:35-215.

5. Hauptmann M, Lubin JH, Stewart PA, Hayes RB, Blair A. Mortality from solid cancers among workers in formaldehyde industries. Am J Epidemiol. 2004; 159(12):1117–30. doi:10.1093/aje/kwh174.

6. NTP. 13th Report on Carcinogens (RoC). 2014. http://ntp.niehs.nih.gov/pubhealth/roc/roc13/index.html. Accessed: June 1, 2015

7. Bolt HM, Morfeld P. New results on formaldehyde: the 2nd International Formaldehyde Science Conference (Madrid, 19-20 April 2012). Arch Toxicol. 2013;87(1):217–22. doi:10.1007/s00204-012-0966-4.

8. Beane Freeman LE, Blair A, Lubin JH, Stewart PA, Hayes RB, Hoover RN, et al. Mortality from solid tumors among workers in formaldehyde industries: an update of the NCI cohort. Am J Ind Med. 2013;56(9):1015–26. doi:10.1002/ajim.22214.

9. Blair A, Stewart P, O'Berg M, Gaffey W, Walrath J, Ward J, et al. Mortality among industrial workers exposed to formaldehyde. J Natl Cancer Inst. 1986;76(6):1071–84.

10. Beane Freeman LE, Blair A, Lubin JH, Stewart PA, Hayes RB, Hoover RN, et al. Supplementary data. Am J Ind Med. 2013;56(9):1015–26.

11. Marsh GM, Morfeld P, Collins JJ, Symons JM. Issues of methods and interpretation in the National Cancer Institute formaldehyde cohort study. Journal of occupational medicine and toxicology (London, England). 2014;9: 22. doi:10.1186/1745-6673-9-22.

12. Vaughan TL, Strader C, Davis S, Daling JR. Formaldehyde and cancers of the pharynx, sinus and nasal cavity: II. Residential exposures. International journal of cancer Journal international du cancer. 1986;38(5):685–8.

13. Vaughan TL, Stewart PA, Teschke K, Lynch CF, Swanson GM, Lyon JL, et al. Occupational exposure to formaldehyde and wood dust and nasopharyngeal carcinoma. Occup Environ Med. 2000;57(6):376–84.

14. Roush GC, Walrath J, Stayner LT, Kaplan SA, Flannery JT, Blair A. Nasopharyngeal cancer, sinonasal cancer, and occupations related to formaldehyde: a case-control study. J Natl Cancer Inst. 1987;79(6):1221–4.

15. Hayes RB, Blair A, Stewart PA, Herrick RF, Mahar H. Mortality of U.S. embalmers and funeral directors. Am J Ind Med. 1990;18(6):641–52.

16. West S, Hildesheim A, Dosemeci M. Non-viral risk factors for nasopharyngeal carcinoma in the Philippines: results from a case-control study. International journal of cancer Journal international du cancer. 1993;55(5):722–7.

17. Hildesheim A, Dosemeci M, Chan CC, Chen CJ, Cheng YJ, Hsu MM, et al. Occupational exposure to wood, formaldehyde, and solvents and risk of nasopharyngeal carcinoma. Cancer Epidemiol Biomark Prev. 2001; 10(11):1145–53.

18. Coggon D, Harris EC, Poole J, Palmer KT. Extended follow-up of a cohort of british chemical workers exposed to formaldehyde. J Natl Cancer Inst. 2003; 95(21):1608–15.

19. Pinkerton LE, Hein MJ, Stayner LT. Mortality among a cohort of garment workers exposed to formaldehyde: an update. Occup Environ Med. 2004; 61(3):193–200.

20. Meyers AR, Pinkerton LE, Hein MJ. Cohort mortality study of garment industry workers exposed to formaldehyde: update and internal comparisons. Am J Ind Med. 2013;56(9):1027–39. doi:10.1002/ajim.22199.

21. Coggon D, Ntani G, Harris EC, Palmer KT. Upper airway cancer, myeloid leukemia, and other cancers in a cohort of British chemical workers exposed to formaldehyde. Am J Epidemiol. 2014;179(11):1301–11. doi:10.1093/aje/kwu049.

22. Marsh GM, Youk AO. Reevaluation of mortality risks from nasopharyngeal cancer in the formaldehyde cohort study of the National Cancer Institute. Regul Toxicol Pharmacol. 2005;42(3):275–83. doi:10.1016/j.yrtph.2005.05.003.

23. Marsh GM, Youk AO, Morfeld P. Mis-specified and non-robust mortality risk models for nasopharyngeal cancer in the National Cancer Institute formaldehyde worker cohort study. Regul Toxicol Pharmacol. 2007;47(1):59–67. doi:10.1016/j.yrtph.2006.07.007.

24. Marsh GM, Youk AO, Morfeld P, Collins JJ, Symons JM. Incomplete follow-up in the National Cancer Institute's formaldehyde worker study and the impact on subsequent reanalyses and causal evaluations. Regul Toxicol Pharmacol. 2010;58(2):233–6. doi:10.1016/j.yrtph.2010.06.001.

25. Marsh GM, Youk AO, Buchanich JM, Erdal S, Esmen NA. Work in the metal industry and nasopharyngeal cancer mortality among formaldehyde-exposed workers. Regul Toxicol Pharmacol. 2007;48(3):308–19. doi:10.1016/j.yrtph.2007.04.006.

26. Siew SS, Kauppinen T, Kyyrönen P, Heikkilä P, Pukkala E. Occupational exposure to wood dust and formaldehyde and risk of nasal, nasopharyngeal, and lung cancer among Finnish men. Cancer Manag Res. 2012;4:223–32. doi:10.2147/cmar.s30684.

27. Kauppinen T, Toikkanen J, Pukkala E. From cross-tabulations to multipurpose exposure information systems: A new job-exposure matrix. Am J Ind Med. 1998;33(4):409–17.

28. Checkoway H, Dell LD, Boffetta P, Gallagher AE, Crawford L, Lees PSJ, et al. Formaldehyde exposure and mortality risks from acute myeloid leukemia and other Lymphohematopoietic Malignancies in the US National Cancer Institute cohort study of workers in Formaldehyde Industries. J Occup Environ Med. 2015;57(7):785–94. doi:10.1097/jom.0000000000000466.

29. Marsh GM, Youk AO, Stone RA, Sefcik S, Alcorn C. OCMAP-PLUS: a program for the comprehensive analysis of occupational cohort data. J Occup Environ Med. 1998;40(4):351–62.

30. Beane Freeman LE, Blair A, Lubin JH, Stewart PA, Hayes RB, Hoover RN, et al. Mortality from lymphohematopoietic malignancies among workers in formaldehyde industries: the National Cancer Institute Cohort. J Natl Cancer Inst. 2009;101(10):751–61. doi:10.1093/jnci/djp096.

31. Lucas LJ. Misclassification of nasopharyngeal cancer. J Natl Cancer Inst. 1994;86(20):1556–8.

32. Marsh GM, Stone RA, Henderson VL. RE: "Misclassification of nasopharyngeal cancer". J Natl Cancer Inst. 1994;86(20):1556–8.

33. Marsh GM, Youk AO. Reevaluation of mortality risks from leukemia in the formaldehyde cohort study of the National Cancer Institute. Regul Toxicol Pharmacol. 2004;40(2):113–24. doi:10.1016/j.yrtph.2004.05.012.

34. Marsh G, Youk A, Sefcik S. Mortality and population data system (MPDS). University of Pittsburgh, Department of Biostatistics Technical Report. Pittsburgh, PA, USA: 2004. p

35. Prentice R, Breslow NE. Retrospective studies and failure time models. Biometrika. 1978;65:153–8.

36. Checkoway H, Pearce N, David K. Research methods in occupational epidemiology. 2nd ed. New York: Oxford University Press; 2004.

37. StataCorp. Stata Statistical Software: Release 12. College Station. TX: StataCorp LP; 2014.

38. SAS Institute Inc. SAS 9.4. Cary: SAS Institute Inc; 2013.

39. McLaughlin JK, Lipworth L, Tarone RE, La Vecchia C, Blot WJ, Boffetta P. Author reply to Hauptmann and Ronckers. Int J Epidemiol. 2010;39:1679–80.

40. Hauptmann M, Ronckers CM. RE: A further plea for adherence to the principles underlying science in general and the epidemiologic enterprise in particular. Int J Epidemiol. 2010;39:1677–9.

41. Marsh GM, Stone RA, Esmen NA, Henderson VL, Lee KY. Mortality among chemical workers in a factory where formaldehyde was used. Occup Environ Med. 1996;53(9):613–27.

42. Marsh GM, Youk AO, Buchanich JM, Cassidy LD, Lucas LJ, Esmen NA, et al. Pharyngeal cancer mortality among chemical plant workers exposed to formaldehyde. Toxicol Ind Health. 2002;18(6):257–68.

43. Greenland S, Robins JM. Identifiability, exchangeability, and epidemiological confounding. Int J Epidemiol. 1986;15(3):413–9.

44. Greenland S, Pearl J, Robins JM. Causal diagrams for epidemiologic research. Epidemiology (Cambridge, Mass). 1999;10(1):37–48.

45. Kleinbaum DG, Kupper LL, Morgenstern H. Epidemiologic research. New York: Van Nostrand Reinhold Company; 1982.

46. Rothman KJ, Greenland S, Lash T. Modern epidemiology. Philadelphia: Lippincott-Raven; 2008.

47. Breslow NE, Day NE. Statistical methods in cancer research. Volume I - The analysis of case-control studies. IARC Sci Publ. 1980;32:5–338.

48. Greenland S. Basic problems in interaction assessment. Environ Health Perspect. 1993;101 Suppl 4:59–66.

12

Risk of lymphoma subtypes by occupational exposure in Southern Italy

Giovanni Maria Ferri[1,6]* (ID), Giorgina Specchia[2], Patrizio Mazza[3], Giuseppe Ingravallo[4†], Graziana Intranuovo[1], Chiara Monica Guastadisegno[1†], Maria Luisa Congedo[1†], Gianfranco Lagioia[1†], Maria Cristina Loparco[1†], Annamaria Giordano[2†], Tommasina Perrone[2†], Francesco Guadio[2†], Caterina Spinosa[3†], Carla Minoia[3†], Lucia D'Onghia[3†], Michela Strusi[3†], Vincenzo Corrado[1†], Domenica Cavone[1†], Luigi Vimercati[1†], Nunzia Schiavulli[1†] and Pierluigi Cocco[5]

Abstract

Background: Occupational exposure is known to play a role in the aetiology of lymphomas. The aim of the present work was to explore the occupational risk of the major B-cell lymphoma subtypes using a case–control study design.

Methods: From 2009 to 2014, we recruited 158 lymphoma cases and 76 controls in the provinces of Bari and Taranto (Apulia, Southern Italy). A retrospective assessment of occupational exposure based on complete work histories and the Carcinogen Exposure (CAREX) job-exposure matrix was performed.

Results: After adjusting for major confounding factors, farmers showed an increased risk of diffuse large B-cell lymphoma (DLBCL) [odds ratio (OR) = 10.9 (2.3–51.6)] and multiple myeloma (MM) [OR = 16.5 (1.4–195.7)]; exposure to the fungicide Captafol was significantly associated with risk of non-Hodgkin lymphoma (NHL) [OR = 2.6 (1.1–8.2)], particularly with the risk of DLBCL [OR = 5.3 (1.6–17.3)].

Conclusions: Agricultural activity seems to be a risk factor for developing lymphoma subtypes, particularly DLBCL, in the provinces of Bari and Taranto (Apulia Region, Southern Italy). Exposure to the pesticides Captafol, Paraquat and Radon might be implicated.

Trial registration: Protocol number UNIBA 2207WEJLZB_004 registered 22/09/2008.

Keywords: Lymphomas, Occupational exposure, CAREX matrix, Pesticides, B-cell lymphoma subtypes, Case–control study

Background

According to 2007–2010 data from the Italian Association of Cancer Registries/Associazione Italiana Registri Tumori (AIRTUM), the estimated standardized incidence rate of haemolymphopoietic cancers was lower in Southern than in Northern Italy; this difference was more significant for non-Hodgkin lymphoma (NHL), multiple myeloma (MM) and chronic lymphocytic leukaemia (CLL) and less significant for Hodgkin lymphomas (HL) [1]. The Apulia areas of reference were the provinces of Bari and Taranto. The estimated standard rates of incidence (× 10,000) of CLL in Taranto Province were 12.8 for males and 12.1 for females. In Bari Province, the rates were 18.1 for males and 11.9 for females. In the Apulia region, they were 14.7 for males and 9.1 for females. The estimated standard rates of incidence of HL were 3.9 for males and 4.1 for females in Taranto Province, 4.5 for males and 5.8 for females in Bari Province and 3.8 for males and 3.7 for females in the Apulia region. The estimated standard rates of incidence of NHL were 14.6 for males and 9.3 females in Taranto Province, 20.7 for males and 15.0 for females in Bari Province, and 14.7 for males and 10.6

* Correspondence: giovannimaria.ferri@uniba.it

Giovanni Maria Ferri, Giorgina Specchia, Patrizio Mazza, Graziana Intranuovo and Pierluigi Cocco jointly supervised this work.

†Equal contributors

[1]Department of Interdisciplinary Medicine (DIM), Section "B. Ramazzini", Regional University Hospital "Policlinico - Giovanni XXIII°", Unit of Occupational Medicine, University of Bari, Piazza G. Cesare, 11, 70124 Bari, Italy

[6]Interdisciplinary Department of Medicine (DIM), University Hospital. Policlinico-Giovanni XXIII, University of Bari, Piazza Giulio Cesare, 11, 70124 Bari, Italy

Full list of author information is available at the end of the article

for females in the Apulia region. The estimated standard rates of incidence of MM were 5.2 for males and 4.1 for females in Taranto Province, 7.4 for males and 6.1 for females in Bari Province and 6.3 for males and 4.8 for females in the Apulia region [2].

The north/south gradients might suggest various causes, including a lesser prevalence of exposure to occupational and environmental carcinogens and to tobacco smoking and a higher prevalence of protective factors such as healthier food habits and a younger age at first pregnancy in Southern Italy. Typical Mediterranean diet items, in particular fruits and vegetables, showed an inverse association with NHL risk [3]. Furthermore, a case–control study of the risk of MM among women in the International Multiple Myeloma Consortium [4] showed a decreased risk of follicular lymphoma (FL) with an increasing number of pregnancies and an association between FL and hormonal contraception [5]. A lower rate of participation in cancer screening programmes in the southern regions of Italy might also reflect a lower detection rate. In terms of mortality, the previously reported North–south gradient has been gradually decreasing in recent years [1]. The observed difference in Taranto and Bari could be explained by different regional industrial activities and other studied factors.

The role of chemical agents (pesticides, solvents), ultraviolet radiation and infectious agents has been extensively studied [6–9].

Male farmers tend to have lower overall cancer incidence and mortality, which might be due to their lower smoking prevalence and increased physical activity [10–13]. However, the risk of certain cancers, including lymphohaematopoietic cancer, has been reported to be increased among farmers [10, 14, 15].

Rieutort et al. found that NHL was associated with various occupational activities and exposures; among them, those involving agricultural or industrial sectors and solvents or pesticides were highlighted, with the highest number of publications and the strongest association with NHL risk [16].

The aim of this case–control study is to assess the association between occupational activities and lymphoma subtypes and to study the occupational risk factors involved in the occurrence of those lymphoma subtypes in the provinces of Taranto and Bari in the Apulia Region (Southern Italy) using the "Carcinogen Exposure" (CAREX) matrix for assessing occupational carcinogen exposure.

Methods

This study reports the activity of a unit of "The Multicentre Italian Study on Gene-Environment Interactions in Lymphoma Etiology" financed by the Italian Projects of National Interest (PRIN) and the Italian Association

for Cancer Research (AIRC) and participated in the InterLymph Consortium initiated by the U.S. National Cancer Institute from 2009 to 2014 and in the Genome-Wide Association Study (GWAS) project. The recruitment of patients was performed in the haematology division of the University Hospital of Bari and in the haematology division of the "Moscati" Hospital of Taranto in the Apulia region (Southern Italy). The study was coordinated by the Occupational Section of the Interdisciplinary Department of Medicine (DIM), University of Bari, Italy.

Study sample

One hundred fifty-eight incident cases of lymphoma first diagnosed during the study period were included: 30 cases of HL and 128 cases of NHL [35 cases of diffuse large B-cell lymphoma (DLBCL), 26 FL, 42 CLL, 3 mantle cell lymphoma, 8 small B-cell lymphoma (SBCL), 11 MM, and 3 mucosa-associated lymphoma tissue (MALT)]. For each case, the diagnosis was reviewed and classified using the 2008 World Health Organization (WHO) classification of lymphoma [17]. During the same period, 76 controls were enrolled and were selected by a matching method (age at first diagnosis, sex and residence); however, due to the small number of controls, no matching analysis was performed. The selection of population controls was performed by accessing the assisted regional register and identifying a list of subjects of the same sex, same age class, and same province of residence (provinces of Bari and Taranto) as the cases. Subsequently, using a simple randomization method, controls were identified and contacted by phone. Outpatient controls were recruited at the ophthalmological and orthopaedic outpatient clinic of Bari Hospital and Taranto Radiology, after the inclusion criteria were verified. In-hospital controls were recruited from the departments of the ophthalmological clinic and the orthopaedic clinic of Bari and Taranto. The inclusion criteria for controls were those without a diagnosis of malignant neoplastic diseases, Acquired Immuno-Deficiency Syndrome (AIDS), eye diseases, thyroid disease, diabetic retinopathy, autoimmune diseases, allergic diseases, viral hepatitis, haematological preneoplastic diseases, such as monoclonal gammopathy of undetermined significance (MGUS), bone marrow aplasia, or myeloproliferative syndromes; similarly, patients undergoing organ transplants were not eligible for inclusion as controls. Cases and controls were recruited from within the same geographic area. The participation rates were 50% for the population controls, 80% for hospitalized controls, and 75% for cases. The population controls, who were selected from among healthy subjects from the regional health service database, were obviously less sensitized. Different methods of control recruitment in the case–control studies were studied, and the method based on the regional health system showed lower compliance (42%) than the method based on the involvement of general practitioners (57%) [18]. All participating cases and controls signed an informed consent form, which described the aims and methods of the study. They all provided a 40 ml blood sample for the biological portion of the study, which was used to study the gene/environment interaction with the assessment of biological exposure parameters (serum polychlorinated biphenyls [PCB], aryl hydrocarbons receptors [AHR], lymphocytic oxidative damage by COMET assay, different genetic polymorphisms, and other biological parameters). This part of the study will produce results only in the coming years.

Questionnaire and exposure assessment by CAREX

All participating subjects were interviewed by a trained interviewer using a semi-structured questionnaire validated in the research project "Epilymph" and provided a complete work history. The questionnaire gathered information on socio-demographics; education; family history of cancer and specifically cancer of the haemolymphatic system; medical history; residential history; tobacco, alcohol and drugs use; work history; diet; physical activity; and reproductive history. We used general questionnaires and specific questionnaires for specific job activity.

The codes used to classify the job titles were allocated on the basis of qualitative crude definitions independent of matrices related to CAREX and contained in the questionnaires completed during the study. In this preliminary analysis, we used the CAREX database to assess occupational exposure to known and suspected carcinogens and pesticides. The same database was used in previous studies in Italy [19], Canada [20], Nicaragua and Panama [21]. The CAREX database sets exposure for occupational sectors. CAREX shows the frequency of reports of exposure to each of the 62 chemical and physical risk factors recognized by the International Agency for Research on Cancer (IARC) (Classes 1 and 2A) [19] for every sector. Every work activity obtained from our semi-structured questionnaires was attributed to an occupational sector that was coded by CAREX. A score was assigned to each risk factor from the report frequencies contained in the CAREX tables for that sector [0 = no exposure (no reports); 1 = low exposure (<75% of report frequency); 2 = medium-high exposure (>75% of frequency of reports)]. For each job activity, the duration (number of years) was recorded. This number was multiplied by the single score. For each subject were evaluated by one to five job activities, and the related products were added. The result of the sum of the products is the CEI. The procedure was based on the following formula:

$$CEI \ (carex) = \Sigma \ (Ordinal \ Score * Years)$$

Categorization of the CEI was as follows: CEI = 0 [no exposure (cumulative indicator = 0)]; CEI = 1 [low exposure (cumulative indicator < = 30)]; CEI = 2 [medium-high exposure (cumulative indicator >30)].

The CEI was not standardized because the statistics used were all non-parametric and therefore normalization was not necessary.

The analysis by job title was conducted only using the most recent job title, while the cumulative exposure was calculated over the entire work history.

Only the pathways of significant chemical substances were considered.

The power of the study was low, and the estimates, with an α type 1 error of 0.05%, were not steady but were equally significant.

Statistical analysis

The statistical analysis was performed using the STATA 12 software, and it was mainly based on the use of non-parametric statistical distributions because of the non-Gaussian distributions of a large number of studied variables.

For the comparison of proportions, the distribution of Z was used as indicated in the "two-sample test of proportions calculator" procedure included in the above-mentioned software.

The univariate analysis was based on the "tab odds" calculations for all the studied variables.

The multivariate analysis was instead based on the use of the "unconditional logistic model", as indicated in the tables, the variables describing sister cancer familiarity, age at diagnosis, province, sex, pack/years (recoded) and level of education. No adjustment was made to the dietary habits because the univariate estimates showed no significant association with lymphoma.

Results

Cases and controls were well distributed in the main categories of age, gender, residence, education level, and job title. However, they were predominantly more than 60 years old (43.7% of cases, 40.8% of controls), male (59.5% of cases, 60.5% of controls), residents of Bari (65.2% of cases, 67% of controls), high school graduates (34.2% of cases, 42.2% of controls), and blue collar workers (31.7% of cases, 31.6% of controls). Specifically, recruited individuals were mostly blue collar workers, clerks and agricultural workers. No significant difference was observed between cases and controls regarding these variables. The two groups were therefore perfectly comparable. The presence of doctors, nurses and researchers, although very low, was only observed among the cases. This finding was also described in the study of t'Mannetje et al. [22] (Table 1).

Univariate analysis

The analysis of lymphoma crude risk (ORs) for all 14 occupational activities was performed (Table 2), and only

Table 1 Distribution of the main variables between cases and controls

Variables	Tot	Cases n	%	Controls n	%	Proportions test z	P
Age							
Less than 20 years	7	6	3.8	1	1.3	0.5	0.3
21–40 years	55	37	23.4	18	23.7	0.0	0.5
41–60 years	72	46	29.1	26	34.2	−0.4	0.7
More than 60 years	100	69	43.7	31	40.8	0.3	0.4
Gender							
Females	94	64	40.5	30	39.5	0.1	0.5
Males	140	94	59.5	46	60.5	0.1	0.5
Province of residence							
Bari	154	103	65.2	51	67.1	−0.3	0.6
Taranto	67	44	27.9	23	30.3	0.2	0.4
Others	13	11	7.0	2	2.6	0.2	0.4
Title of study							
Degree	38	27	17.1	11	14.5	0.2	0.4
High school	86	54	34.2	32	42.1	0.6	0.3
Middle school	64	43	27.2	21	27.6	0.0	0.5
Primary school	46	34	21.5	12	15.8	0.4	0.3
Jobs							
Housewife	16	11	7.0	5	6.6	0.0	0.5
Physician	3	3	1.9	0	0.0	–	–
Blue collar	74	50	31.7	24	31.6	0.0	0.5
Nurse	1	1	0.6	0	0.0	–	–
Teacher	17	9	5.7	8	10.5	−0.4	0.6
Researcher	2	2	1.3	0	0.0	–	–
Craftsman/Merchant	13	11	7.0	2	2.6	0.2	0.4
Agricultural workers	18	14	8.9	4	5.3	0.2	0.4
White collar	43	28	17.7	15	19.7	−0.2	0.6
Military	10	5	3.2	5	6.6	−0.2	0.6
Student/Unemployed/ Retired	3	3	1.9	0	0.0	–	–
Freelancer	8	2	1.3	6	7.9	−0.3	0.6
Technical	5	2	1.3	3	4.0	−0.2	0.6
Missing	21	17	10.8	4	5.3	–	–
Totals	234	158	100	76	100	–	–

Legend

Z = The z-score test for the two proportions is used when you want to know whether two groups differ significantly in some characteristics

the highest estimates (agricultural activity) were used for the multivariate analysis. The same approach was also used to analyse all other studied factors.

Lymphoma risks were analysed for 22 chemical products; none of these was statistically significant. Only higher OR levels were observed for low/medium levels of butadiene [OR = 1.91 (0.68–5.38)]; low/medium levels of acrylonitrile [OR = 1.70 (0.60–4.83)]; low levels of ethylene dibromide [OR = 1.96 (0.59–6.44)]; low levels of ethylene dioxide [OR = 2.58 (0.52–12-64)]; low levels of formaldehyde [OR = 2.31 (0.76–7.02)]; low levels of nitrox dimethylamine [OR = 2.58 (0.52–12.64)]; low levels of toluidine [OR = 1.80 (0.63–5.08)]; medium/high styrene levels [OR = 1.65 (0.67–4.06)]; low levels of tetrachloroethylene [OR = 1.87 (0.83–4.24)]; low levels of trichloroethylene [OR = 1.45 (0.66–3.19)]; low levels of vinyl chloride [OR = 1.71 (0.69–4.21)]; low levels of PAH [OR = 20.31 (2.26–182.23)]; and medium/high PAH levels [OR = 12.50 (1.16–136.4)]. Crude risk associated with low [OR = 20.3 (2.3–182.2)] and medium-high [OR = 12.5 (1.2–134.4)] cumulative exposure to polycyclic aromatic hydrocarbons (PAHs) showed elevated risks, but they were based on very small numbers, and the very unsteady estimates were not used.

Crude risks were also analysed for 10 physical risk factors and none of these was statistically significant. Slightly higher levels of OR were observed only for: low glass wool levels [OR = 2.28 (0.59–8.73)]; low levels of ionizing radiation [OR = 1.78 (0.45–7.03)]; radon medium/high levels [3.28 (0.92–11.71)]; and high levels of solar radiation [OR = 1.76 (0.68–4.59)]. Crude risks were also analysed for seven heavy metals and no significant results were obtained for any of these. There was a higher crude risk only for cobalt [OR = 2.20 (0.62–8.01)]. The crude risks were analysed for nine drugs and no statistical significance was observed. Crude risks for 2 pesticides showed high OR values that were very close to statistical significance: high levels of Captafol [OR = 7.05 (0.90–56.16)]; low levels of dimethilsulfate (Paraquat) [OR = 2.48 (0.96–6.36)]. We also analysed the crude risks for 4 tumour familiarity that did not show any statistical significance; a higher OR was observed only for breast cancer familiarity [OR = 2.15 (0.77–5.99)]. As reported in several experiences [23–26], smoking (pack/years) was not a significant risk factor for lymphomas.

Multivariate analysis

Table 3 shows the multivariate analysis that considered not only subjects with agricultural exposure but also industrial exposure to pesticides. Subjects exposed to Captafol showed a significant increase in risk for all lymphomas [OR = 2.4 (1.1–5.6)], in particular for NHL [OR = 2.6 (1.0–8.2)]. Subjects exposed to low levels of Paraquat also showed an increased risk for all lymphomas [OR = 2.9 (1.0–8.2)], particularly NHL [OR = 2.8 (1.0–8.2)]. Medium high exposure to radon was associated with risk for all lymphomas [OR = 9.5 (1.2–76.8)] and with NHL [OR = 8.8 (1.2–71.4)].

Table 4 presents a significant association between overall exposure to Captafol with NHL [OR = 2.6 (1.1–8.2)] and with DLBCL subtype [OR = 5.3 (1.6–17.3)]. Low exposure to Paraquat was also associated with

Table 2 Distribution of crude risk (ORs) by occupational titles

	DLBCL			FL			CLL			SBCL			MM			NHL			HL			ALL LYMPHOMAS		
	OR	95% LCI	95% UCI	OR	95% LCI	95% UCI	OR	95% LCI	95% UCI	OR	95% LCI	95% UCI	OR	95% LCI	95% UCI	OR	95% LCI	95% UCI	OR	95% LCI	95% UCI	OR	95% LCI	95% UCI
Housewife	0.91	0.15	5.44	0.51	0.04	5.85	0.91	0.11	7.34	0.63	0.03	11.29	4.33	0.29	63.11	1.13	0.29	4.34	–	–	–	1.29	0.36	4.58
Physicians	–	–	–	–	–	–	–	–	–	–	–	–	–	–	–	–	–	–	–	–	–	–	–	–
Blue collars	0.67	0.22	2.07	1.31	0.42	4.12	1.31	0.45	3.75	0.47	0.06	3.29	0.6	0.08	4.1	1.01	0.47	2.13	2.47	0.59	10.39	1.15	0.56	2.36
Nurse	–	–	–	–	–	–	–	–	–	–	–	–	–	–	–	–	–	–	–	–	–	–	–	–
Teacher	0.42	0.07	2.9	1.02	0.15	6.62	1.33	0.28	6.16	–	–	–	1.01	0.06	16.2	0.89	0.28	2.79	–	–	–	0.51	0.17	1.55
Researcher	–	–	–	–	–	–	–	–	–	–	–	–	–	–	–	–	–	–	–	–	–	–	–	–
Craftsman/Merchant	5.74	0.26	124.6	8.39	0.77	9.13	1.99	0.11	34.09	17.87	0.32	380.63	–	–	–	3.91	0.44	34.74	–	–	–	3.6	0.4	32.05
Agricultural workers	9.35	1.99	43.6	–	–	–	2.01	0.36	11.03	–	–	–	8.16	0.7	54.15	2.44	0.64	9.28	–	–	–	2.05	0.54	7.75
Clerk	1.39	0.45	4.27	0.87	0.22	3.38	0.35	0.08	1.5	1.58	0.18	13.93	0.52	0.04	5.59	0.89	0.39	1.94	1.98	0.56	6.96	1.03	0.47	2.23
Military	–	–	–	1.11	0.17	6.9	0.53	0.07	3.69	4.16	0.25	68.81	–	–	–	0.51	0.13	1.94	–	–	–	0.45	0.12	1.72
Student/Unemployed/Retired	–	–	–	–	–	–	–	–	–	–	–	–	–	–	–	–	–	–	–	–	–	–	–	–
Freelancer	–	–	–	–	–	–	–	–	–	–	–	–	–	–	–	–	–	–	–	–	–	–	–	–
Technicians	–	–	–	–	–	–	1.62	0.19	13.84	–	–	–	–	–	–	0.74	0.09	5.85	–	–	–	0.49	0.06	3.85
Food operators	–	–	–	0.73	0.12	4.41	0.92	0.22	3.79	1.22	0.1	14.7	–	–	–	0.6	0.18	1.97	0.23	0.01	3.26	0.58	0.18	1.82

Legend: *HL* Hodgkin Lymphoma, *NHL* Non Hodgkin Lymphoma, *DLBCL* Diffuse Large B-Cell Lymphoma, *FL* Follicular Lymphoma, *CLL* Chronic Lymphocitic Leukemia, *SBCL* Single B Cell Lymphoma, *MM* Multiple Mieloma

Table 3 [a]ORs distribution of main types of lymphomas by different levels of cumulative exposure to selected study factors

Cumulative exposure	Lymphoma types															
	All lymphomas					Hodgkin lymphomas					Non hodgkin lymphomas					
	Cases	Controls	OR[a]	95% LCI	95% UCI	Cases	Controls	OR[a]	95% LCI	95% UCI	Cases	Controls	OR[a]	95% LCI	95% UCI
[b] Captafol																
No	138	70	1	–	–	30	70	1	–	–	108	70	1	–	–
Low	6	5	0.73	0.2	2.69	0	5	–	–	–	6	5	1.03	0.27	3.89
Medium-high	14	1	–	–	–	0	1	–	–	–	14	1	–	–	–
Overall	158	76	*2.4*	*1.11*	*5.63*	*30*	*76*	1	–	–	128	76	*2.59*	*1.04*	*6.42*
Paraquat																
No	123	66	1	–	–	24	66	1	–	–	99	66	1	–	–
Low	28	6	*2.91*	*1.03*	*8.2*	6	6	1.95	0.38	10.04	22	6	*2.83*	*0.96*	*8.37*
Medium-high	7	4	1.1	0.26	4.59	0	4	–	–	–	7	4	1.27	0.3	5.41
Overall	158	76	1.51	0.8	2.87	30	76	1.52	0.35	6.58	128	76	1.52	0.79	2.94
Radon																
No	113	59	1	–	–	28	59	1	–	–	85	59	1	–	–
Low	26	14	0.97	0.44	2.1	2	14	0.12	0.01	1.25	24	14	1.2	0.54	2.65
Medium-high	19	3	*9.5*	*1.18*	*76.82*	*0*	*3*	0.12	0.01	1.25	19	3	*9.37*	*1.16*	*75.85*
Overall	158	76	1.71	0.97	3.02	30	76	0.12	0.01	1.24	128	76	*1.87*	*1.04*	*3.35*

[a] All the estimates were adjusted by sister cancer familiarity, age at diagnosis, province, sex, packyears and level of education
[b] For this cumulative exposure was difficult perform multiple analysis by exposure dummy variables
All the italicized values represent statistical significant estimates

Table 4 [a]ORs distribution of Non Hodgkin lymphoma subtypes by different levels of Cumulative Exposure to selected study factors and agricultural occupation

CUMULATIVE EXPOSURE	NON HODGKIN LYMPHOMA					NON HODGKIN LYMPHOMA SUBTYPES										
	NHL					DLBCL					FL					
	CASES	CONTROLS	OR[a]	95% LCI	95% UCI	CASES	CONTROLS	OR[a]	95% LCI	95% UCI	CASES	CONTROLS	OR[a]	95% LCI	95% UCI
[b] Captafol																
No	102	70	1.0	–	–	25	70	1.0	–	–	22	70	1.0	–	–
Low	6	5	1.0	0.3	3.7	5	5	3.5	0.8	15.2	0	5	1.0	–	–
Medium-high	14	1	–	–	–	5	1	1.0	–	–	4	1	1.0	–	–
Overall	20	6	*2.6*	*1.1*	*8.2*	10	6	*5.3*	*1.6*	*17.3*	4	6	3.0	0.6	14.1
Paraquat																
No	99	66	1.0	–	–	26	66	1.0	–	–	19	66	1.0	–	–
Low	22	6	2.8	0.9	8.2	7	6	*3.8*	*1.0*	*15.3*	6	6	*4.6*	*1.1*	*20.2*
Medium-high	7	4	1.1	0.3	4.8	2	4	1.6	0.2	12.3	1	4	1.1	0.1	13.8
Overall	29	10	2.1	0.9	5.3	9	10	2.7	0.7	9.6	7	10	3.3	0.9	12.3
Radon																
No	85	59	1.0	–	–	22	59	1.0	–	–	17	59	1.0	–	–
Low	24	14	1.2	0.5	2.6	8	14	1.5	0.5	4.4	5	14	1.2	0.3	4.1
Medium-high	19	3	*8.8*	*1.1*	*71.4*	5	3	*13.7*	*1.3*	*143.0*	4	3	*12.7*	*1.2*	*137.2*
Overall	43	17	1.7	0.8	3.6	13	17	2.2	0.8	5.8	9	17	2.0	0.7	5.8
Agricultural occupation																
No	98	68	1.0	–	–	23	68	1.0	–	–	25	68	1.0	–	–
Yes	14	4	2.4	0.6	9.3	8	4	*9.3*	*2.0*	*43.6*	0	4	1.2	0.7	2.0

[b]For this cumulative exposure wasn't possible perform multiple analysis by exposure dummy variablesLegend: *HL* Hodgkin Lymphoma, *NHL* Non Hodgkin Lymphoma, *DLBCL* Diffuse Large B-Cell Lymphoma, *FL* Follicular Lymphoma, *CLL* Chronic Lymphocitic Leukemia, *SBCL* Single B Cell Lymphoma, *MM* Multiple Mieloma

Table 4 [a]ORs distribution of Non Hodgkin lymphoma subtypes by different levels of Cumulative Exposure to selected study factors and agricultural occupation (Continued)

CUMULATIVE EXPOSURE	NON HODGKIN LYMPHOMA SUBTYPES														
	CLL					SBCL					MM				
	CASES	CONTROLS	OR[a]	95% LCI	95% UCI	CASES	CONTROLS	OR[a]	95% LCI	95% UCI	CASES	CONTROLS	OR[a]	95% LCI	95% UCI
[b] Captafol															
No	38	70	1.0	–	–	8	70	1.0	–	–	9	70	1.0	–	–
Low	0	5	1.0	–	–	0	5	1.0	–	–	1	5	3.0	0.1	59.1
Medium-high	4	1	1.0	–	–	0	1	1.0	–	–	1	1	1.0	–	–
Overall	4	6	1.4	0.3	7.0	0	6	1.0	–	–	2	6	10.9	1.0	125.8
Paraquat															
No	33	66	1.0	–	–	7	66	1.0	–	–	9	66	1.0	–	–
Low	7	6	3.5	0.8	16.1	1	6	–	–	–	0	6	1.0	–	–
Medium-high	2	4	0.9	0.1	6.8	0	4	–	–	–	2	4	3.3	0.2	63.8
Overall	9	10	2.9	0.8	10.3	1	10	1.3	0.1	14.7	2	10	2.0	0.1	26.9
Radon															
No	29	59	1.0	–	–	4	59	1.0	–	–	8	59	1.0	–	–
Low	6	14	0.9	0.3	2.9	2	14	2.9	0.3	29.7	2	14	0.6	0.1	5.5
Medium-high	7	3	10.8	0.9	130.1	2	3	*64.4*	*2.1*	*1959.6*	1	3	*106.1*	*1.3*	*8620.0*
Overall	13	14	1.5	0.5	4.0	4	17	6.6	0.9	45.6	3	17	1.4	0.2	9.0
Agricultural occupation															
No	34	68	1.0	–	–	8	68	1.0	–	–	8	68	1.00	–	–
Yes	4	4	2.1	0.4	11.0	0	4	1.0	–	–	2	4	6.16	0.70	54.15

All the italicized values represent statistical significant estimates

DLBCL [OR = 3.8 (1–15.3)] and FL [OR = 4.6 (1.1–20.2)] subtypes. Medium-high levels of exposure to radon were associated with DLBCL [OR = 13.7 (1.3–143.0)] and SBCL [OR = 64.4 (2.1–1959.6)].th=tlb=

Table 5 illustrates the association between agricultural occupations and the risk of different lymphoma subtypes. This occupation category was associated with DLBCL [OR = 10.9 (2.3–51.6)] and MM [OR = 16.5 (1.4–195.7)]. This finding is consistent with the study of Mester et al. [27].

Discussion

The observed association in this study between DLBCL subtype and agricultural occupations [OR = 10.9 (2.3–51.6)] is consistent with the results of a large pooled analysis of international studies [20, 26]. Moreover, general farm workers were at high risk of developing MM [OR = 16.5 (1.4–195.7)], as reported by Morton et al. [28].

A death certificate case–control study suggests that young agricultural worker residents from Southern Brazil were more likely to die from NHL than non-agricultural workers [29]. A meta-analysis suggested that total organo-chlorine pesticides (OCPs) was significantly positively associated with NHL risk [30].

Our study also showed a significant association between the occurrence of lymphoma and exposure to

Table 5 Association estimates (ORs[a]) between occupation as agricultural worker and different lymphoma subtypes

Agricultural worker		Total	No	Yes	OR	95% LCI	95% UCI
ALL LYMPHOMAS	No	72	68	4	1	–	–
	Yes	141	127	14	2.3	0.6	8.5
HL	No	72	68	4	1	–	–
	Yes	24	24	0	–	–	–
NHL	No	72	68	4	1	–	–
	Yes	117	103	14	2.7	0.7	10.1
NHL-DLBCL	No	72	68	4	1	–	–
	Yes	31	23	8	*10.9*	*2.3*	*51.6*
NHL-FL	No	72	68	4	1	–	–
	Yes	25	25	0	–	–	–
NHL-CLL	No	72	68	4	1	–	–
	Yes	37	33	4	2.4	0.5	13.3
NHL-SBCL	No	72	68	4	1	–	–
	Yes	8	8	0	–	–	–
NHL-MM	No	72	68	4	1	–	–
	Yes	10	8	2	*16.5*	*1.4*	*195.7*

[a]All the estimates were adjusted by sister cancer familiarity, age at diagnosis, province, sex, packyears and level of education
Legend: *HL* Hodgkin Lymphoma, *NHL* Non Hodgkin Lymphoma, *DLBCL* Diffuse Large B-Cell Lymphoma, *FL* Follicular Lymphoma, *CLL* Chronic Lymphocitic Leukemia, *SBCL* Single B Cell Lymphoma, *MM* Multiple Mieloma
All the italicized values represent statistical significant estimates

Captafol, which is used as a fungicide in agriculture, according to Mc Duffie et al. 2001 [OR = 2.51 (1.32–4.76)] [31]. In our data, a positive association was also observed with exposure to Paraquat, an herbicide, but there was an inverse trend with exposure level. Uncertainty in the interpretation of our findings might be related to the small study size and the crude definition of exposure. No data are available in the literature regarding the dose–response correlation of pesticides and lymphoma. Recently, however, some studies have reported a relationship between exposure to fungicides, herbicides or insecticides and NHL occurrence [32–35].

Moreover, sales of Captafol and Folpet, both fungicides, which have similar molecular structures, in the Apulia region increased from 80 kg to 741 kg [36] from 2002 to 2012, while sales of Paraquat in 2002 were 662 kg [37]. The extensive use of this pesticide in the Apulia region also explains its popular use for suicidal purposes [38] and horse poisonings [39]; in France, there was no apparent change in the number of suicide attempts involving Paraquat after its ban in July 2007 [40]. Captafol is a human carcinogen, in fact it was classified by the IARC as probably carcinogenic to humans (Group 2A). The Captafol production for use as a fungicide in the United States stopped in 1987. Its continued use from existing stocks was allowed, but in 1999 the Environmental Protection Agency banned its use on all crops except onions, potatoes, and tomatoes. In 2006 even these exceptions were disallowed, so currently its use on all crops is banned in the United States. Several other countries have followed suit since 2000, and as of 2010, no countries are known to allow the use of Captafol on food crops.

The carcinogenic mechanism of Captafol is attributed to its interaction with the thiol groups of glutathione and cysteine, which reduces the defence against oxidative agents, and the N-S bond formation with other biological substrates, both leading to the formation of metabolites such as tetrahydrophthalamide, which is considered a human carcinogen [41].

Paraquat (N,N'-dimethyl-4,4'-bipyridinium dichloride) is an herbicide widely used in agriculture. It is derived from the alkylating agent dimethyl sulphate.

Results from the Agricultural Health Study showed an increased risk of NHL among Paraquat-exposed pesticide applicators [42]. One study suggested that Paraquat increases superoxide dismutase activity and radiation resistance in mouse lymphoma cells [43]. Another study suggested that increased levels of metallothionein, glutathione S-transferase, Cu, Zn-SOD and Mn-SOD might be protective against Paraquat toxicity in acute myelogenous leukaemia (AML) cells [44]. Moreover, the possibility of Paraquat-induced DNA damage has been suggested [45].

Acute exposure to Paraquat accounted for several cases of fatal poisoning, while chronic exposure appears to be associated with respiratory disease and Parkinson's disease [46]. Animal studies have shown DNA alterations in treated animals. In the past, exposure to Paraquat has been associated with melanoma, leukaemia, and cancer of the penis, cervix and lung. More recent studies found a significantly increased risk of developing NHL among subjects exposed to this substance. Therefore, our understanding of Paraquat carcinogenicity is limited, and further studies are warranted [41].

As indicated in Appendix 1 of the work of Mirabelli et al. [19], exposure to Radon, which was higher among agricultural workers, food and beverage production workers, and electricity workers, was also associated with DLBCL [OR = 2.5 (1.2–5.4)] and SBCL [OR = 5.7 (1.3–25.6)]. Radon is a product of the radioactive decay of radium. Radon is easily inhaled. The level of the Radon-gas hazard differs from location to location. Despite its short lifetime, radon gas from natural sources can accumulate in buildings, especially, due to its high density, in low areas such as basements and crawl spaces. Radon can also occur in ground water. Epidemiological studies have shown a clear link between breathing high concentrations of Radon and incidence of lung cancer. Radon is a contaminant that affects indoor air quality worldwide. According to the United States Environmental Protection Agency, Radon is the second most frequent cause of lung cancer, after cigarette smoking, causing 21,000 lung cancer deaths per year in the United States. As Radon itself decays, it produces other radioactive elements called Radon daughters (also known as Radon progeny) or decay products. Unlike the gaseous Radon itself, Radon daughters are solids and stick to surfaces, such as dust particles in the air. The Radon assessment was currently carried out in the studied Apulia areas and only in particular situations the concentration of Radon was above 300 Bq/m^3. But for agricultural workers this exposure was prolonged in time. Moreover, there was suggestive, though statistically non-significant, evidence of a significant increase of DLBCL among children with a high residential indoor exposure to Radon [47] and an increased risk of CLL and HL incidence, and NHL mortality with increasing γ-ray dose among Uranium miners [48].

Conclusions

This is a preliminary report of occupational risk factors for lymphoma in the provinces of Taranto and Bari (Apulia region, Southern Italy). Although limited in size and utilizing a crude method of retrospective exposure assessment, this work revealed that agricultural workers exposed to Captafol, Paraquat and radon could develop lymphoma subtypes, especially DLBCL. These findings confirm existing knowledge and suggest new hypotheses for research about occupational factors suspected to be associated with lymphoma risk.

One of the weaknesses of the study is the instability of the estimates even when they were significant. Such instability prompts us to be cautious about the conclusions even though they are consistent with previous studies.

Abbreviations

AHR: Aryl hydrocarbons receptors; AIDS: Acquired immuno-deficiency syndrome; AIRC: Associazione Italiana per la Ricerca sul Cancro; AIRTUM: Associazione Italiana Registri Tumori; AML: Acute myeloid leukaemia; CAREX: CARcinogen EXposure; CEI: Cumulative exposure index; CLL: Chronic lymphocytic leukaemia; DIM: Interdisciplinary Department of Medicine; DLBCL: Diffuse large B-cell lymphoma; FL: Follicular lymphoma; GWAS: Genome-Wide Association Study; HL: Hodgkin Lymphoma; IARC: International Agency for Research on Cancer; MALT: Mucosa-Associated Lymphoma Tissue; MGUS: Monoclonal Gammopathy of Undetermined Significance; MM: Multiple myeloma; NHL: Non-Hodgkin Lymphoma; OCPs: Organo-Chlorine Pesticides; OR: Odds ratio; PAHs: Polycyclic aromatic hydrocarbons; PCB: Polychlorinated biphenyls; PRIN: Research Project of National Interest; SBCL: Small B-cell lymphoma; WHO: World Health Organization

Acknowledgements

We thank all the workers of the three hospital units involved in this study for their cooperation.

Funding

Research project of national interest (PRIN 2007–2009; AIRC): "The Multicentre Italian Study on gene-environment interactions in Lymphoma etiology".

Authors' contributions

All authors contributed equally in planning, conduction and data analysis of the study. All authors read and approved the final manuscript.

Authors' information

All the authors are interested in the development of the scientific fields related to this work, including cancer epidemiology and haematology.

Competing interests

The authors declare that they have no competing interests.

Author details

[1]Department of Interdisciplinary Medicine (DIM), Section "B. Ramazzini", Regional University Hospital "Policlinico - Giovanni XXIII°", Unit of Occupational Medicine, University of Bari, Piazza G. Cesare, 11, 70124 Bari, Italy. [2]Department of Emergency and Transplantation (DETO), Regional Universitary Hospital "Policlinico - Giovanni XXIII°, Unit of Hematology, University of Bari, Piazza G. Cesare, 11, 70124 Bari, Italy. [3]ASL Taranto, Moscati Hospital, Unity of Haematology, Via Paisiello 1, 74100 Taranto, Italy. [4]Department of Emergency and Transplantation (DETO), Regional University Hospital "Policlinico - Giovanni XXIII° ", Unit of Pathology, University of Bari, Piazza G. Cesare, 11, 70124 Bari, Italy. [5]Department of Public Health, Clinical & Molecular Medicine, Occupational Health Section, University of Cagliari, 09100 Cagliari, Italy. [6]Interdisciplinary Department of Medicine (DIM), University Hospital. Policlinico-Giovanni XXIII, University of Bari, Piazza Giulio Cesare, 11, 70124 Bari, Italy.

References

1. Gruppo di lavoro AIOM-AIRTUM. I numeri del cancro in Italia. Brescia: Intermedia editore; 2014. p. 61–4.
2. Assennato G, Bisceglia L, Bruno D, et al. Incidenza, mortalità e sopravvivenza delle patologie oncologiche in Puglia. Registro tumori Puglia. Rapporto tumori; 2015. p. 259–82.
3. Campagna M, Cocco P, Zucca M, Angelucci E, Gabbas A, Latte GC, et al. Risk of lymphoma subtypes and dietary habits in a Mediterranean area. Cancer Epidemiol. 2015;39:1093–8.
4. Costas L, Lambert BH, Birmann BM, Moysich KB, De Roos AJ, Hofmann JN, et al. A pooled analysis of reproductive factors, exogenous hormone use, and risk of multiple myeloma among women in the international multiple myeloma consortium. Cancer Epidemiol Biomark Prev. 2016;25:217–21.
5. Kane V, Roman E, Becker N, Bernstein L, Boffetta P, Bracci PM, et al. Menstrual and reproductive factors, and hormonal contraception use: associations with non-Hodgkin lymphoma in a pooled analysis of InterLymph case–control studies. Ann Oncol. 2012;23:2362–74.
6. Beane Freeman LE, Deroos AJ, Koutros S, Blair A, Ward MH, Alavanja M, Hoppin JA. Poultry and livestock exposure and cancer risk among farmers in the agricultural health study. Cancer Causes Control. 2012;23:663–70.
7. Becker N, Falster MO, Vajdic CM, de Sanjose S, Martínez-Maza O, Bracci PM, et al. Self-reported history of infections and the risk of non-Hodgkin lymphoma: an InterLymph pooled analysis. Int J Cancer. 2012;131:2342–8.
8. Boffetta P, van der Hel O, Kricker A, Nieters A, de Sanjosé S, Maynadié M, et al. Exposure to ultraviolet radiation and risk of malignant lymphoma and multiple myeloma: a multicentre European case–control study. Int J Epidemiol. 2008;37:1080–94.
9. Cocco P, Brennan P, Ibba A, de Sanjosé LS, Maynadié M, Nieters A, et al. Plasma polychlorobiphenyl and organochlorine pesticide level and risk of major lymphoma subtypes. Occup Environ Med. 2008;65(2):132–40.
10. Blair A, Freeman LB. Epidemiologic studies of cancer in agricultural populations: observations and future directions. J Agromedicine. 2009;14(2): 125–31.
11. Koutros S, Alavanja MCR, Lubin JH, Sandler DP, Hoppin JA, Lynch CF, et al. An update of cancer incidence in the agricultural health study. J Occup Environ Med. 2010;52(11):1098–105.
12. Waggoner JK, Kullman GJ, Henneberger PK, Umbach DM, Blair A, Alavanja MC, et al. Mortality in the agricultural health study, 1993–2007. Am J Epidemiol. 2011;173(1):71–83.
13. Weichenthal S, Moase C, Chan P. A review of pesticide exposure and cancer incidence in the agricultural health study cohort. Environ Health Perspect. 2010;118(8):1117–25.
14. Schenk M, Purdue MP, Colt JS, Hartge P, Blair A, Stewart P, et al. Occupation/industry and risk of non Hodgkin lymphoma in the United States. Occup Environ Med. 2009;66(1):23–31.
15. Hohenadel K, Harris SA, McLaughlin JR, Spinelli JJ, Pahwa P, Dosman JA, et al. Exposure to multiple pesticides and risk of non-Hodgkin lymphoma in men from six Canadian provinces. Int J Environ Res Public Health. 2011;8(6): 2320–30.
16. Rieutort D, Moyne O, Cocco P, de Gaudemaris R, Bicout DJ. Ranking occupational contexts associated with risk of non-Hodgkin lymphoma. Am J Ind Med. 2016;59(7):561-74. doi:10.1002/ajim.22604.
17. Campo E, Swerdlow SH, Harris NL, Pileri S, Stein H, Jaffe ES. The 2008 WHO classification of lymphoid neoplasms and beyond: evolving concepts and practical applications. Blood. 2011;117(19):5019–32.
18. Castaño-Vinyals G, Nieuwenhuijsen MJ, Moreno V, Carrasco E, Guinó E, Kogevinas M, Villanueva CM. Participation rates in the selection of population controls in a case–control study of colorectal cancer using two recruitment methods. Gac Sanit. 2011;25(5):353–6.
19. Mirabelli D, Kauppinen T. Occupational exposures to carcinogens in Italy: an update of CAREX database. Int J Occup Environ Health. 2005;11(1):53–63.
20. Peters CE, Ge CB, Hall AL, Davies HW, Demers PA. CAREX Canada: an enhanced model for assessing occupational carcinogen exposure. Occup Environ Med. 2015;72(1):64–71.
21. Blanco-Romero LE, Vega LE, Lozano-Chavarría LM, Partanen TJ. CAREX Nicaragua and Panama: worker exposures to carcinogenic substances and pesticides. Int J Occup Environ Health. 2011;17(3):251–7.
22. t'Mannetje A, De Roos AJ, Boffetta P, Vermeulen R, Benke G, Fritschi L, et al. Occupation and risk of non-Hodgkin lymphoma and its subtypes: a pooled analysis from the InterLymph consortium. Environ Health Perspect. 2015; 124(4):396–405.
23. Albini A, Rosano C, Angelini C, Amaro A, Esposito AI, Maramotti S, et al.

Exogenous hormonal regulation in breast cancer cells by phythoestrogens and endocrine disruptors. Curr Med Chem. 2014;21(9):1129–45.

24. Engel LS, Hill DA, Hoppin JA, Lubin JH, Lynch CF, Pierce J, et al. Pesticide use and breast cancer risk among farmers' wives in the agricultural health study. Am J Epidemiol. 2005;161:121–35.

25. Hye SK, Soon WL, Yoon JC, Shin SW, Kim YH, Cho MS, et al. Novel germline mutation of BRCA1 gene in a 56-year-old woman with breast cancer, ovarian cancer, and diffuse large B-cell lymphoma. Cancer Res Treat. 2014;47(3):534–8.

26. Tamaoki M, Nio Y, Tsuboi K, Nio M, Tamaoki M, Maruyama R, et al. A rare case of non-invasive ductal carcinoma of the breast coexisting with follicular lymphoma: a case report with a review of the literature. Oncol Lett. 2014;7:1001–6.

27. Mester B, Nieters A, Deeg E, Elsner G, Becker N, Seidler A, et al. Occupation and malignant lymphoma: a population based case control study in Germany. Occup Environ Med. 2006;63(1):17–26.

28. Morton LM, Slager SL, Cerhan JR, Wang SS, Vajdic CM, Skibola CF, et al. Etiologic heterogeneity among non-Hodgkin lymphoma subtypes: the Interlymph non-Hodgkin lymphoma subtypes project. J Nat Cancer Inst Monogr. 2014;48:130–44.

29. Boccolini PM, Boccolini CS, Chrisman JR, Koifman RJ, Meyer A. Non-Hodgkin lymphoma among Brazilian agricultural workers: a death certificate case–control study. Arch Environ Occup Health. 2017;72(3):139–44.

30. Luo D, Zhou T, Tao Y, Feng Y, Shen X, Mei S. Exposure to organochlorine pesticides and non-Hodgkin lymphoma: a meta-analysis of observational studies. Sci Rep. 2016;6:257–68.

31. McDuffie HH, Pahwa P, McLaughlin JR, Spinelli JJ, Fincham S, Dosman JA, et al. Non-Hodgkin's lymphoma and specific pesticide exposures in men: cross-Canada study of pesticides and health. Cancer Epidemiol Biomark Prev. 2001;10(11):1155–63.

32. Alavanja MC, Hofmann JN, Lynch CF, Spinelli JJ, Fincham S, Dosman JA, et al. Non-hodgkin lymphoma risk and insecticide, fungicide and fumigant use in the agricultural health study. PLoS One. 2014;9(10):e109332.

33. Navaranjan G, Hohenadel K, Blair A, Demers PA, Spinelli JJ, Pahwa P, et al. Exposures to multiple pesticides and the risk of Hodgkin lymphoma in Canadian men. Cancer Causes Control. 2013;24(9):1661–73.

34. Schinasi LH, De Roos AJ, Ray RM, Edlefsen KL, Parks CG, Howard BV, et al. Insecticide exposure and farm history in relation to risk of lymphomas and leukemias in theWomen's health initiative observational study cohort. Ann Epidemiol. 2015;25(11):803–10.

35. Schinasi L, Leon ME. Non-Hodgkin lymphoma and occupational exposure to agricultural pesticide chemical groups and active ingredients: a systematic review and meta-analysis. Int J Environ Res Public Health. 2014; 11(4):4449–527.

36. Alessio-Apostoli. Piccin, editor. Manual of occupational medicine and industrial hygiene. For technical prevention. 7thed.; 2009. p. 165.

37. Provincial Agency for Environmental Protection, Trento. Available from: http://www.appa.provincia.tn.it/fitofarmaci/programmazione_dei_controlli_ambientali/Criteri_vendita_prodotti_fitosanitari/pagina122.html. Accessed 20 Nov 2017.

38. Settimi L, Davanzo F, Urbani E, et al. Sistema informativo nazionale per la sorveglianza delle esposizioni pericolose e delle intossicazioni: casi rilevati nel 2009. Quarto rapporto annuale. Istituto Superiore di Sanità. Rapporto Istisan. http://www.iss.it/binary/publ/cont/13_8_web.pdf.

39. Padalino B, Bozzo G, Monaco D, Ceci E. Avvelenamento da Paraquat in cavalli da carne pugliesi. Ippologia; 2012;23(3):15-21.

40. Kervégant M, Merigot L, Glaizal M, Schmitt C, Tichadou L, de Haro L. Paraquat poisonings in France during the European ban: experience of the poison control center in Marseille. J Med Toxicol. 2013;9(2):144–7.

41. National Toxicological Program. Captafol. Rep Carcinog. 2011;12:83–6.

42. Park SK, Kang D, Beane-Freeman L, Blair A, Hoppin JA, Sandler DP, et al. Cancer incidence among Paraquat exposed pesticide applicators in the agricultural health study. Int J Occup Environ Health. 2009;15(3):274–81.

43. Jaworska A, Rosiek O. Paraquat increases superoxide dismutase activity and radiation resistance in two mouse lymphoma L5178Y cell strains of different radiosensitivities. Int J Radiat Biol. 1991;60(6):899–906.

44. Choi CH, Kim HS, Kweon OS, Lee TB, You HJ, Rha HS, et al. Reactive oxygen species-specific mechanisms of drug resistance in Paraquat-resistant acute Myelogenous leukemia sublines. Mol Cells. 2000;10(I):38–46.

45. Ross WE, Block ER, Chang RY. Paraquat-induced DNA damage in mammalian cells. Biochem Biophys Res Commun. 1979;91(4):1302–8.

46. Rudyk C, Litteljohn D, Syed S, Dwyer Z, Hayley S. Paraquat and psychological stressor interactions as pertains to Parkinsonian co-morbidity. Neurobiol Stress. 2015;2:85–93.

47. Peckham EC, Scheurer ME, Danysh HE, Lubega J, Langlois PH, Lupo PJ, et al. Residential radon exposure and incidence of childhood lymphoma in Texas, 1995–2011. Int J Environ Health. 2015;12:12110–26.

48. Zablotska LB, Lane RS, Frost SE, Thompson PA. Leukemia, lymphoma and multiple myeloma mortality (1950–1999) and incidence (1969–1999) in the Eldorado uranium workers cohort. Environ Res. 2014;130:43–50.

13

Work-related injuries among farmers

Devendra Bhattarai[1], Suman Bahadur Singh[2*], Dharanidhar Baral[1], Ram Bilakshan Sah[1], Shyam Sundar Budhathoki[1] and Paras K. Pokharel[1]

Abstract

Background: Agriculture work is one of the most hazardous occupations across countries of all income groups. In Nepal, 74 % of people are working in the agricultural sector. This study aims to identify patterns and factors associated with injuries among farmers of rural Nepal.

Methods: A community-based cross-sectional study was conducted in a rural village in eastern Nepal. House to house visit was done to collect data from the farmers. The study included 500 farmers from Shanishchare village in Morang district of Nepal. A pre-tested semi-structured questionnaire was used to collect data on socioeconomic profile, agriculture work and injury. Prevalence of injuries among farmers in the last 12 months was calculated along with factors associated with the injuries.

Results: The overall prevalence of work- related injuries among farmers was 69 % in the last 12 months. Common injuries among the farmers were cuts (79.7 %), puncture wound (11.3 %) and laceration (7.5 %). Hand tools were responsible for most of the injuries followed by slipping at work, sharp instruments, animals and fall from height. Upper limb injury comprised of 67 % of all injuries and the most involved part was fingers (43 %). The average number of years worked in farming by the respondents was 23.6 ± 13.6 years. Age and working experience of the farmers was found to be significantly associated with the occurrence of injuries among the farmers.

Conclusions: The prevalence of injury among farmers in this study was high. Further research is needed to identify interventions to reduce the agricultural injuries in Nepal.

Keywords: Occupational Health, Farmers, Injuries, Rural Nepal

Background

About 350,000 deaths occur globally due to fatal occupational injuries [1, 2]. The vulnerable population of South East Asian countries comprising of women, the poor, and children, are primarily employed in the informal sectors. They often lack the basic knowledge of hazards and work for long hours in unsafe work conditions without personal protection at work and with little or no health care insurance [3]. The use of machineries and equipment have led to newer occupational injuries among these workers [4, 5].

Agriculture has traditionally been one of the most hazardous occupations for workers [6, 7]. Agricultural

sector provides a strong foundation for rural economic and for the sustainable economic growth [8]. An estimated 1.3 billion workers are engaged in agricultural production worldwide. This represents half of the total world labour force, and almost 60 % of them are in developing countries [9]. Agricultural injuries are reported from all around the globe [10–14].

In Nepal, agriculture contributes to 39 % of the gross domestic product with 13 % of the total foreign trade. Keeping in view of this contribution, priority is given to the development of the agriculture sector in the Eighth Five Year Plan [15]. In Nepal, 73.9 % of people are working in the agricultural sector and 26.1 % in non-agriculture [16]. The intensive use of machinery has raised the risks of injuries [17]. Musculoskeletal injuries are the predominant form of reported non-fatal occupational injuries. Fractures,

* Correspondence: sumanbahadur.singh@bpkihs.edu
[2]Lifeline Institute of Health Sciences, Damak, Nepal
Full list of author information is available at the end of the article

bruises, lacerations, contusions, penetration by foreign bodies and sprains or strains are the most frequent type of occupational injuries [17–19].

Occupational safety and health in Nepal

Approximately 20,000 work related accidents are estimated to occur every year and 200 lives are lost each year in Nepal due to work related injuries and accidents [20]. Occupational safety and health in Nepal is in its primitive stage [21]. Occupational safety and health has received limited attention by the health sector in Nepal [20, 22, 23]. The existing labour law has a small portion where the safety and health is a brief section with vague provisions for overall health and welfare of workers. The act has highlighted only four occupations; tea estate, construction, transportation and hotel & tourism sector separately. The law seems to focus only on increasing productivity rather than health and safety [21, 24]. Limited research is found in occupational safety and health and no research was found focusing on injuries among farmers [23]. Use of personal protective equipment (PPE) among farmers is not known and is reported low in other occupations [22].

Farmers are working under unsafe conditions, particularly in low income countries, leading to injury and death. Farmers are at risk for injury because agricultural work involves multiple tasks and multiple locations. Most of the tasks are carried out in the open air, exposing the workers to adverse working conditions. The majority of farmers are informal sector workers. Farming in villages is a household-based owned occupation and not a company owned business in Nepal. Literature searches in Pubmed, Google scholar and Nepal journal online resulted in the limited literature on injuries among farmers in Nepal. In Nepal there is no systematized recording and reporting of agricultural injuries. Data on injury at national level is also inadequate. This study was conducted to identify patterns of agricultural injuries and assess the factors associated with work-related injuries among agricultural farmer in rural Nepal.

Methods

Morang district is the largest rice producer district of Nepal [25]. Shanishchare village was chosen randomly using the lottery method out of the 65 villages of Morang district. A community based cross-sectional study was carried out among farmers of the Shanishchare village in the eastern region of Nepal. This village is a highly populated village with a population of 29,804 and 5490 households, according to the population census of 2011. Based on the village data, agriculture work is the primary occupation of 19 % of the households in Shanishchare [26].

The sample size was calculated using the prevalence of work-related injuries among farmers, [10] in Hubei, People's Republic of China. Taking prevalence of 33 % from this study and margin of error, as 15 % of prevalence, the sample size was calculated using the formula.

Sample size (n) = Z^2pq/L^2 n= $(1.96^2 *33*67)/4.35^2$ (where L= 15 % of p) {Z=1.96; p=33 %; q= compliment of p} n= 449.

Adding 10 % sample to correct non response, our expected sample size was decided as 494. Thus, we invited 500 farmers from the Shanishchare village to participate in this study.

Our Study period was from September 2012 to December 2013 which included the protocol designing, ethical approval, data collection and report preparation.

Farmers ≥ 20 years of age, having agricultural land ≥ 5 Katthas (1 Kattha = 3645 square feet), who worked in their own farm in Shanishchare village were included in our study. Farmers who are from Shanishchare village and working in fields outside Shanishchare village or farmers from other villages working on farms in Shanishchare village were excluded from our study. The reason for the exclusion of these farmers is that since farmers who work on other people's land are more mobile and seasonal working for wages, or change occupation frequently, it is not feasible to include them in the study as well as disseminate the study findings afterwards. As per the Village Development Committee (VDC) office, there were 2500 farmers having land ≥5 Katthas for cultivation in Shanishchare. After the list of the 2500 farmers was obtained from VDC office, 500 farmers were selected using Systematic Random Sampling selecting every fifth farmer from the list. The first farmer was selected by generating a computer generated random number. However, some information bias cannot be avoided as the farmers were interviewed about injuries in the last 12 months, which is prone to some recall bias. We approached their home to conduct the interviews. If they were not present, we returned after arranging an appointment.

Socio demographic characteristics, work related data and injury characteristics were collected using a semi-structured questionnaire prepared by a team comprising of a Senior Public Health researcher, two Occupational Physicians, an Environmental health expert, a Biostatistician and a Master in Public Health student. The Semi-structured questionnaire was pretested among 50 farmers of Bayarban village, adjacent to Shanishchare village.

Working duration of the farmers was categorised taking 48 h as a cut off for working hours per week; and 20 years as cut off for years of working experience in this study. Both of these are based on the working duration criteria of the Labour Act of Nepal. The act states that the maximum number of working hours in a week should not exceed 48 h in occupation. It has provision of retirement from work after completion of 20 years in any occupation [24].

The collected data were checked thoroughly for completeness and entered in excel sheet after coding the data for analysis. Data Analysis was done using Statistical Package for Social Sciences (SPSS) version 11.5. Frequency and percentages are used to express descriptive statistics. Bivariate analysis of categorical data was done using χ^2 test. Unadjusted Odds Ratio was calculated using Epi info 7. We calculated the 95 % confidence interval and the probability of significance was set at 5 %.

Results

All 500 respondents approached for the study participated in this study giving a response rate of 100 %. The mean age of the respondents was 43.6 ± 13.2 years. There was an equal representation of male and female farmers in this study. All respondents in this study owned their own land for farming. The socio-demographic characteristics of the farmers in this study are shown in Table 1.

The average number of years worked in farming by the respondents was 23.6 ± 3.6 years. More than 3/5th of the respondents, did not use any Personal Protective Equipment (PPE) at work. Among those who use PPE, 97.14 % use ordinary cotton mask, 4 % use boots and 1.7 % use gloves at work (Table 2).

Table 1 Socio-demographic characteristics of farmers in Shanishchare village (n = 500)

Characteristics	Categories	Number	Percentage (%)
Age	<30 years	79	15.8
	30–39 years	121	24.2
	40–49 years	122	24.4
	50–59 years	107	21.4
	≥60 years	71	14.2
Gender	Male	246	49.2
	Female	254	50.8
Marital status	Single	57	11.4
	Married	443	88.6
Religion	Hindu	366	73.2
	Buddhist	25	5.0
	Kirant	97	19.4
	Christian	12	2.4
Literacy	Illiterate	86	17.2
	Literate	414	82.8
Types of family	Nuclear	242	48.4
	Joint	258	51.6
Land holding	≤15 Kattha	287	57.4
	>15 Kattha	213	42.6

Table 2 Working characteristics of the respondents (n = 500)

Characteristics	Categories	Number	Percentage (%)
Working hours	≤48 hours	119	42.2
	>48 hours	324	57.8
Work experience	≤20 years	183	36.6
	>20 years	317	63.4
Personal Protective Equipment (PPE) use	Yes	175	35.0
	No	325	65.0
Types of protective device (n = 175)[a]	Ordinary Mask	170	97.2
	Boot	7	4.0
	Gloves	3	1.7

[a]Multiple responses

A total of 345 respondents (69 %) reported being injured in the past one year. Among these 345 respondents, 9 out of 10 respondents were injured more than once in the past 12 months (Table 3).

Hand tool was a frequent mode of injury among the respondents. Hand tools included sickle, axe, spade, hand saw and hoes. Most frequent types of injury were cut, and the site of injury was fingers (Table 4).

A total of 222 (64.3 %) injured workers took some time off work due to injury. The mean ($\pm$SD) number of days lost due to injuries was 11.4 ± 9.6 days. Out of 345 injured respondents, 245 (71 %) of them used local herbs for first aid treatment. There were 233 (67.5 %) injured farmers who went to the health institution for wound treatment. Apart from herbs, human urine, mud, warm oil and toothpaste were used for first aid treatment of the injury. (Not shown in tables)

The association between socio-demographic characteristics and injuries among farmers is displayed in Table 5.

Table 3 Injury related characteristics reported by respondents (n = 345)

Characteristics	Categories	Number	Percentage (%)
Environment where injured	Working field	314	91.0
	On the way	19	5.5
	House	12	3.5
Frequency of injuries (in past one year)	One time	37	10.7
	Two times	161	46.7
	Three times	121	35.1
	More than three times	26	7.6
Season when injured	Rainy season	221	64.1
	Winter season	124	35.9
Time when injured	Morning	107	31.0
	Day	209	60.6
	Evening	29	8.4

Table 4 Mode of injury, type of injuries and body parts injured (n = 345)

Characteristics	Categories	Frequency	Percentage (%)
Mode of injury	Hands tools	258	74.7
	Slipping	29	8.4
	Animals	27	7.8
	Sharp instruments	23	6.7
	Fall	8	2.3
Types of injuries	Cuts	275	79.7
	Punctures	39	11.3
	Laceration	26	7.5
	Fracture	5	1.4
Body parts injured[a]	Finger	151	43.8
	Leg	105	30.5
	Hand	70	20.3
	Head	23	7.9
	Knee	15	4.2
	Trunk	8	2.3
	Eye	5	1.4

[a]Multiple responses

Discussion

While there are only limited hospital or community based studies on injuries of all kinds in Nepal, no published literature was found regarding injuries among farmers in Nepal [27, 28]. This study could provide some evidences for further studies on agricultural injuries in Nepal. All the farmers owned their own land for farming in this study. However, it is a practice to work for another farm owner during need which is paid back by contributing equal number days in each other's farm. This study showed that the majority of the farmers belonged to age group of 40–49 years, accounting for 24.4 % of all farmers. In this study, the mean age (±SD) was found to be 43.6 ± 13.2 years, which was similar to the findings of other studies [10–12, 29]. A cross-sectional study in India reports mean age (±SD) of farmers as 31.9 ± 6.6 years, which is much younger compared to our study [30]. Higher proportion of the injuries occurred among farmers in the age group 40–49 years. Another cross-sectional study in India shows high injury among farmers in the same age group as our study [31]. However, other studies show injuries among farmers in younger age groups [32]. This is explainable as the farmers in our study are comparatively older compared to the farmers in other studies. The overall prevalence of work- related injuries among farmers injury was 69 % in the last 12 months. Similarly, a cross-sectional study among agricultural workers in Ethiopia showed markedly high rates of injuries [11]. Both Nepal and Ethiopia

Table 5 Distribution of association between Socio- demographic characteristics of farmers by injuries in last one year in Shanishchare village

Characteristics	Accidents in last one year		p-value[a]	Unadjusted Odds Ratio	
	Yes (n = 345)	No (n = 155)		OR	95 % CI
Age in years					
<30	35	44	0.001	1	
30–39	86	35		3.08	1.70–5.58
40–49	86	36		3.00	1.66–5.41
50–59	87	20		5.46	2.83–16.56
≥60	51	20		3.20	1.62–6.33
Gender					
Male	162	84	0.134	1	
Female	183	71		1.33	0.91–1.95
Marital status					
Single	27	30	0.001	1	
Married	318	125		2.82	1.61–4.34
Literacy					
Literate	279	135	0.088	1	
Illiterate	66	20		1.59	0.92–2.74
Type of Family					
Nuclear	163	79	0.441	1	
Joint	182	76		1.16	0.79–1.69
Working hours (per week)					
≤48 hours	127	84	0.001	1	
>48 hours	218	71		2.03	1.38–2.98
Working experience (years)					
≤20 years	159	98	0.001	1	
>20 years	186	57		2.01	1.36–2.96

[a]χ^2 test

are developing countries and are agrarian based and thus similar scenario can be seen. In Ethiopia, agriculture holds 41 % contribution to the gross domestic product, which is similar in Nepal, where agriculture contributes a similar proportion to the gross domestic product [16]. A study from India (30.6 %) shows a lower prevalence of agricultural injury compared to our study [33]. Incidence of injury among the farmers was lower in high income countries [34, 35]. The injuries among farmer are higher in low income countries compared to middle and high income countries. A case series study of surgical trauma and associated head injuries attending to a tertiary hospital in Nepal, reports one fifth of the injured patients were farmers [27]. A study of injury in an urban area of Nepal highlights that farmers suffered more injuries compared to workers in other occupations [28].

Out of 345 injured farmers, a large proportion of respondents (91.0 %) pointed farming fields as a spot for injury occurrence. Our study reported more frequent injuries compared to Ethiopia. Though Ethiopia is a low income country like Nepal, the use of machineries in farming and the techniques of farming may be different, which could explain the difference in findings [11].

One third of the farmers in this study report that they use personal protective equipment (PPE), however, almost all of these farmers only use ordinary masks at work, which they consider as PPE to be used in farming. This is a huge gap identified in our study. Use of PPE seems a neglected issue among farmers. They are not aware of any PPE required for farm work. Further researches may be needed to explore ways to increase access and the use of PPE by farmers.

Hand tools are the most frequent cause of injury in this study. The findings are similar in Indian farmers as well [30]. As a neighbouring country, the contexts of Nepal and India are comparable in population, culture, technology and practices. The findings are similar to the farmers from other countries [10, 11, 27, 36, 37]. Hand equipment like sickles and spades are still used routinely in the farms in Nepal. Cutting of grass, rice, wheat weeding, ridge formation, harvesting and irrigation channel making are done manually. This could explain hand tools as a major mode of injury in this study.

The most common types of injuries among farmers were cuts, puncture and laceration. Similar injuries were reported about Ethiopian farmers [11]. Popularity of traditional mechanical tools and not practicing safety measures could explain the prevalent injuries among the farmers.

Injuries were more common in hands than other parts of the body in this study similar to the study from Ethiopia [11]. Regular involvement of the fingers and hands in activities like cutting of grass and crops during working hours might increase risk of injury among them. Further, lack of safety precaution like use of personal protective equipment could put the farmers at more risk for injury.

There is similar proportion of males (49.2 %) and females (50.8 %) involved in agricultural activities. This highlights that women of Nepal are actively involved in agricultural activities besides regular household chores. National data of Nepal show slightly higher proportion (60 %) of women's involvement in agriculture [20]. However, there is no significant difference in injuries among male and female farmers. Farm related injuries in Ethiopia showed that majority of study participants (77.8 %) were males [11]. Multiple studies report injuries among male farmers are more during farming [4, 38]. This could be explained as males are more involved in farming compared to females.

Comparable to the findings from Ethiopia, illiterate farmers were injured more than the literate farmers in this study [11, 15]. Further exploration may be needed as to why illiterate farmers have more injuries.

Farmers who worked for less or equal to 48 h a week, were less injured compared to those who worked for more than 48 h per week. Possible explanation could be that the farmers who work for more hours they will spend more hours exposed to the risk factors for injuries. The finding is similar in Ethiopian farmers [11].

There was a significant association between injury and the number of years worked as farmers. Similar findings were reported from Ethiopia [11]. This finding suggests that there may be a tendency of farmers to be less careful at work if they have worked for many years. This may also need further exploration.

Traditional practices are being practiced for first aid for injuries. This highlights the deep rooted traditional practice in our society. Local herbs are used for first aid and many do not visit a health institution at all. Injuries at work are perceived minor by these farmers. Traditional practices are also reported from India, where urination on wounds are practiced, as first aid [27]. Application of mud or cow dung on the injury site has been reported [33]. This shows that the farmers seem to lack skills and probably any knowledge about basic first aid.

Limitations

The age and land ownership criteria for inclusion in this study may have left out daily wage seasonal agricultural labourers. The seasonal labourers are more migratory and they change working setup from agriculture to construction or other physical labour demanding works based on the availability of opportunities. Interviewing of only one farmer per land parcel may have left out the injury data on other workers in the family from the same farm. Only persons available at the time of study were included and we could not include the farmers who were not at home. There is possibility of recall bias in history of injury for last 12 months. The study could not identify a causal association for injuries at work among farmers. Other workers on the farm and the non-owners farm workers are not represented by this study. We have further plans to build on the findings of this research to conduct further research to address these farm workers.

Conclusion

The most common types of injury among farmers were cuts, puncture and laceration. Most of the agricultural work is mechanical and farmers are found to be using traditional hand tools in Nepal. Laborious work, maximum use of hand tools, challenging work environment and neglecting safety measures could be responsible for occupational injury. While literatures are scanty in Nepal, this study provides evidence regarding injuries faced by farmers in Nepal, a country whose primary occupation is agriculture. Farming related stakeholders at village level, the agriculture administration at the local and national level, policy makers and researchers could use the findings of this study to design further studies to identify appropriate interventions to decrease injuries among farmers and address the occupational health needs of the farmers in Nepal.

Acknowledgements
We acknowledge the cooperation of all the participants of the study.

Funding
None.

Authors' contributions
DB was involved in conception & designing of the study, data collection, analysis, draft writing & final version preparation for publications. SBS was involved in designing of the research, interpretation of data, drafting of manuscript and preparing the final version for publication. DB was involved in designing of the research, data analysis, manuscript revision and preparing the final version for publication. RBS was involved in conceptualizing the research, manuscript revision and preparing the final version for publication. SSB was involved in conceptualizing the research, interpretation of data, preparing draft and revising it for intellectual content and preparing the final version for publication. PKP was involved in conceptualizing the research, interpretation of data, revising the draft manuscript & approving the final version of the manuscript for publication. All authors read and approved the final manuscript.

Authors' information
DB is a MPH graduate working as a lecturer at the Lifeline Institute of Health Sciences, Nepal.
SBS is a Community Physician working in Occupational Health Unit at School of Public Health & Community Medicine, B P Koirala Institute of Health Sciences, Dharan, Nepal. SBS holds an academic post of Additional Professor.
DB is a Statistician and Research Methodologist at the School of Public Health & Community Medicine, B P Koirala Institute of Health Sciences, Dharan, Nepal. SBS holds an academic post of Assistant Professor.
RBS is Community Physician working in Environmental Health unit at the School of Public Health & Community Medicine, B P Koirala Institute of Health Sciences, Dharan, Nepal. RBS holds an academic post of Associate Professor.
SSB is a Community Physician cum Public Health Professional working in Occupational Health unit at the School of Public Health & Community Medicine, B P Koirala Institute of Health Sciences, Dharan, Nepal. SSB holds an academic post of Assistant Professor.
PKP is a senior Community Physician working as Professor of Public Health at the School of Public Health & Community Medicine, B P Koirala Institute of Health Sciences, Dharan, Nepal.

Competing interests
The authors declare that they have no competing interests.

Author details
[1]School of Public Health and Community Medicine, B P Koirala Institute of Health Sciences, Ghopa 18, Dharan, Nepal. [2]Lifeline Institute of Health Sciences, Damak, Nepal.

References
1. Takala J. Introductory Report: Decent Work—Safe Work. XVIth World Congress on Safety and Health at Work. Vienna: International Labor Organization; 2005. p. 6–10.
2. Hämäläinen P. The effect of globalization on occupational accidents. Saf Sci. 2009;47(6):733–42.
3. World Health Organization. Regional Strategy on Occupational Health and Safety in SEAR counties [Internet]. New Delhi; 2005 [cited 2016 Feb 2]. Available from: http://apps.searo.who.int/PDS_DOCS/B0053.pdf. Accessed 2 Feb 2016.
4. Eijkemans G. Occupational Health & Safety in Africa. African Newsl Occup Heal Saf. 2004;14:28–9.
5. Mohammed G. Ergonomics in small-scale grain mills in Nigeria. African Newsl Occup Heal Saf. 2005;15(1):7–10.
6. Crandall CS, Fullerton L, Olson L, Sklar DP, Zumwalt R. Farm-related injury mortality in New Mexico. Accid Anal Prev. 1997;29(2):257–61.
7. Frank AL, McKnight R, Kirkhorn SR, Gunderson P. Issues of agricultural safety and health. Annu Rev Public Health. 2004;25:225–45.
8. Economic JS, Analysis P. Second. Kathmandu: Taleju Prakashan; 2004.
9. International Labor Organization. Safety and health in agriculture [Internet]. International Labor Organization. Geneva; 2011 [cited 2016 Jan 9]. p. 1–350. Available from: http://www.ilo.org/wcmsp5/groups/public/—ed_dialogue/—sector/documents/normativeinstrument/wcms_161135.pdf. Accessed 9 Jan 2016.
10. Xiang H, Wang Z, Stallones L, Keefe TJ, Huang X, Fu X. Agricultural work-related injuries among farmers in Hubei, People's Republic of China. Am J Public Health. 2000;90(8):1269–76.
11. Yiha O, Kumie A. Assessment of occupational injuries in Tendaho Agricultural Development S.C, Afar Regional State. Ethiop J Heal Dev. 2010; 24(3):167–74.
12. Pickett W, Hartling L, Brison RJ, Guernsey JR. Canadian Agricultural Injury Surveillance Program. Fatal work-related farm injuries in Canada, 1991–1995. Can Med Assoc J. 1999;160(13):1843–8.
13. Myers JR, Layne LA, Marsh SM. Injuries and Fatalities to U.S. Farmers and Farm Workers 55 Years and Older. Am J Ind Med. 2009;52(3):185–94.
14. Lee SJ, Kim I, Ryou H, Lee KS, Kwon YJ. Work-related injuries and fatalities among farmers in South Korea. Am J Ind Med. 2012;55(1):76-83.
15. Ministry of Agriculture Development. Welcome to Ministry of Agricultural Development [Internet]. Ministry of Agriculture Development, Government of Nepal. 2012 [cited 2016 Jan 3]. Available from: http://moad.gov.np/en/content.php?id=319. Accessed 3 Jan 2016.
16. Central Bureau of Statistics. Report on Nepal Labor Force Survey 2008. Kathmandu; 2009 [cited 2016 Jan 3]. Available from: http://cbs.gov.np/image/data/Surveys/2015/NLFS-2008%20Report.pdf. Accessed 3 Jan 2016.
17. Levy BS, Wegman DH, Baron SL, Sokas RK. Occupational and Environmental Health: Recognizing and Preventing Disease and Injury. Sixth. Oxford: Oxford University Press; 2011.
18. Fingerhut M, Driscoll T, Nelson DI, Concha-Barrientos M, Punnet L, Pruss-Ustin A, et al. Contribution of occupational risk factors to the global burden of disease— a summary of findings. Scand J Work Environ Heal Suppl. 2005;1:58–61.
19. Sprince NL, Zwerling C, Lynch CF, Whitten PS, Thu K, Gillette PP, et al. Risk factors for falls among Iowa farmers: a case–control study nested in the Agricultural Health Study. Am J Ind Med. 2003;44(3):265–72.
20. Gautam RP, Prasain JN. Current situation of occupational safety and health in Nepal [Internet]. Kathmandu: General Federation of Nepalese Trade Unions (GEOFONT); 2011. [cited 2016 Jan 22]. p. 1–96. Available from: https://gefont.org/assets/upload/downloads/Study_OSH_Nepal.pdf.
21. Carter WS. Introducing occupational health in an emerging economy: a Nepal experience. Ann Occup Hyg. 2009;54(5):477–85.
22. Budhathoki SS, Singh SB, Sagtani RA, Niraula SR, Pokharel PK. Awareness of occupational hazards and use of safety measures among welders: a cross-sectional study from eastern Nepal. BMJ Open. 2014;4(6):e004646.
23. Joshi SK, Shrestha S, Vaidya S. Occupational safety and health studies in Nepal. Int J Occup Saf Heal. 2011;1:19–26.
24. Government of Nepal. Labour Act,2048 (1992). Nepal: Nepal Law Commission; 1992. p. 1–44.
25. Uprety R. System of Rice Intensification (SRI) Performance in Morang district during 2005 main season [Internet]. Biratnagar; 2005 [cited 2016 Aug 5]. p. 1–10. Available from: sri.ciifad.cornell.edu/countries/nepal/nepuprety1205.pdf. Accessed 5 Aug 2016.

26. Central Bureau of Statistics. VDC Profile of Sanischare VDC, Morang District, Nepal. Kathmandu; 2011.

27. Varghese M, Mohan D. Occupational injuries among agricultural workers in rural Haryana, India. J Occup Accid. 1990;12(1–3):237–44.

28. Ghimire A, Nagesh S, Jha N, Niraula SR, Devkota S. An epidemiological study of injury among urban population. Kathmandu Univ Med J. 2009;7(28):402–7.

29. Singh R, Sharma AK, Jain S, Sharma SC, Magu NK. Wheat thresher agricultural injuries: a by-product of mechanised farming. Asia-Pacific J Public Heal. 2005;17(1):36–9.

30. Das B. Agricultural work related injuries among the farmers of West Bengal, India. Int J Inj Contr Saf Promot. 2014;21(3):205–15.

31. Kumar GVP, Dewangan KN. Agricultural accidents in north eastern region of India. Saf Sci Elsevier Ltd. 2009;47(2):199–205.

32. Ohio Commission on the Prevention of Injury. Agriculture-Related Injuries [Internet]. Report from the Ohio Commission on the Prevention of Injury 2003. 2003 [cited 2016 Jan 23]. p. 1–13. Available from: http://www.publicsafety.ohio.gov/links/agriculture.pdf

33. Kalaiselvana G, Dongre AR, Mahalakshmy T. Epidemiology of injury in rural Pondicherry, India. J Inj Violence Res. 2011;3(2):62–7.

34. Lee K, Lim HS. Work-related injuries and diseases of farmers in Korea. Ind Health. 2008;46:424–34.

35. Maltais V. Risk Factors Associated with Farm Injuries in Canada 1991 to 2001. Ottawa; 2007. Report No.: 21–601. [Cited 2016 Jan 3]. Available from: http://publications.gc.ca/Collection/Statcan/21-601-MIE/21-601-MIE2007084.pdf. Accessed 3 Jan 2016.

36. Kumar A, Singh JK, Mohan D, Varghese M. Farm hand tools injuries: a case study from northern India. Saf Sci. 2008;46(1):54–65.

37. Mohan D, Patel R. Design of safer agricultural equipment: application of ergonomics and epidemiology. Int J Ind Ergon. 1992;10(4):301–9.

38. Bhandari GP, Dhimal M, Ghimire U. Epidemiological Study on Injury and Violence in Nepal [Internet]. Kathmandu; 2009 [cited 2015 Dec 10]. Available from: nhrc.org.np/files/download/0884f4dad42041c

14

Drillers and mill operators in an open-pit gold mine are at risk for impaired lung function

Denis Vinnikov

Abstract

Background: Occupational studies of associations of exposures with impaired lung function in mining settings are built on exposure assessment and far less often on workplace approach, so the aim of this study was to identify vulnerable occupational groups for early lung function reduction in a cohort of healthy young miners.

Methods: Data from annual screening lung function tests in gold mining company in Kyrgyzstan were linked to occupations. We compared per cent predicted forced expiratory volume in one second (FEV_1), forced vital capacity (FVC) and FEV_1/FVC between occupational groups and tested selected occupations in multivariate regression adjusted for smoking and work duration for the following outcomes: $FEV_1 < 80$ %, FEV_1/FVC < 70 % and both.

Results: 1550 tests of permanent workers of 41 occupations (mean age 40.5 ± 9.2 years, 29.8 % never smokers) were included in the analysis. The mean overall VC was 103.0 ± 12.9 %; FVC 109.1 ± 13.0 % and FEV_1 100.2 ± 25.9 %. Drillers and smoking food handlers had the lowest FEV_1%. In non-smokers, the lowest FEV_1 was in drillers (94.9 ± 11.3 % compared to 115.2 ± 17.7 % in engineers). Drillers (adjusted odds ratio (OR) 1.53 (95 % confidence interval (CI) 1.11-2.09)) and mill operators (OR 2.01 (1.13-3.57)) were at greater risk of obstructive ventilation pattern (FEV_1/FVC < 70 %).

Conclusions: Drilling and mill operations are the highest risk jobs in an open-pit mine for reduced lung function. Occupational medical clinic at site should follow-up workers in these occupations with depth and strongly recommend smoking cessation.

Keywords: Occupational, Mining, Spirometry, Screening, Workplace

Background

Occupational exposures are linked to a number of respiratory conditions, such as chronic obstructive pulmonary disease (COPD), and population studies identified those exposures to account for 10-15 % of the burden of COPD [1–3]. In workplaces, exposure to dust, vapors and gases comes into play with smoking, and significant number of smokers in dusty workplaces will eventually develop COPD [4]. Therefore, in hazardous enterprise, primary prevention is directed to minimizing exposure to dust and proper use of personal protective equipment.

Studies of occupational role of dust were mainly based on either self-reported or measured exposure assessment,

and in those analyses, epidemiological studies with proper industrial hygiene data and exposure assessment would have the biggest weight [3]. The alternative to such exposure measurement approach [5] could be particular workplace assessment, where exposures come into complex interaction, and this makes multifactorial cause of occupational COPD plausible. For practical reasons, occupational intervention to detect and combat early lung function impairment may be based on workplace assessment with or without exposure data. Such approach has identified occupations with high risk, and those may be machine operators, construction trades and other related types of work [6]. In mining, which is by itself usually a high-risk enterprise (mining at altitude), knowing which occupations and workplace entail the greatest hazard to a worker's respiratory health is important. Identifying vulnerable groups in a mining setting can then guide proactive monitoring.

Correspondence: denisvinnikov@mail.ru
Department of Internal Medicine, Occupational Diseases and Hematology, Kyrgyz State Medical Academy, Akhunbaev street 92, Bishkek 720020, Kyrgyzstan

Annual screening, where spirometry is mandated, can be one of the tools to detect lung function impairment at very early stages to guide worker placement [2]. Spirometry has been shown to identify early lung function changes in those exposed to mineral dust [7], however identifying vulnerable groups at mining site in the absence of industrial hygiene data is still challenging. Just knowing that dust is associated with COPD is not sufficient for selecting high-risk workers for more thorough monitoring. Thus, the aim of this study was to identify vulnerable groups for early lung function reduction in a cohort of healthy young miners employed for gold mining operation, where industrial hygiene data do not exist.

Methods

Study design and population

This analysis used lung function data of workers at a high-altitude gold mine operating at an altitude of 3800–4500 meters above sea level and situated in the Tyan Shan mountain range in Kyrgyzstan. This was an open pit mine, and gold was extracted on site. Local employees worked two- or three-week 12-h per day shifts at altitude and commuted to their homes for two or three more weeks at low or middle altitude. All high-altitude workers underwent pre-employment and annual screening carried out in a specially designated clinic in Bishkek, including lung function testing. Data collected at this examination included smoking habits, life style attributes, former and current medical history. Such annual screening also comprised physical examination by eight narrow specialists, supplemented by ECG, frontal chest X-ray, blood work, urine test, lipid, liver enzymes and nitrogen metabolism biochemical tests, audiometry, night vision test and other tests upon indications (e.g., cardiac ultrasonography). This study was approved by the Committee on Bioethics of Kyrgyz State Medical Academy.

Dataset analyzed in this study were all spirometric tests done during one calendar year, when ideally all workers should be enrolled, and 2102 tests in total were performed. In general, people working at the mine were healthy and fit, as there was a list of legally mandated contraindications for employment at high altitude covered by the Regulation 225 in 2011 (formerly Order 70 of 2004). Only local subjects working at the mine site and a large marshalling yard located 200 km away from the mine were included (foreign nationals excluded), belonging either to Kyrgyz (93.6 %) or other ethnic groups (6.4 %). Job lists with relevant departments for each subject were obtained from human resources department of the company and were not self-reported, accompanying referral letter for annual screening.

Occupations

The list of employed occupations was mainly dictated by the specific attributes of open-pit mining. Drivers were those operating heavy-duty vehicles, such as mine trucks, graders, shovel machines, loaders, and bulldozers. Mechanics and other maintenance staff were employed in the on-site workshops, repairing machines and assembling new vehicles from parts. Food handlers were involved in various stages of storing, cooking and distributing food to workers at site. Drillers were principal operators and their assistants who control drilling equipment right in the pit. Cleaners worked mainly in the camp doing all types of daily cleaning in dwelling premises and non-residential areas in the camp. Samplers and surveyors were specific mining occupations working in an open pit. Lab technicians were those operating chemical analytical lab inside the mill. Finally, mill operators was a heterogeneous group of workers involved in various stages of gold extraction process within the mill.

Spirometry

Spirometry was performed in the occupational clinic located in Bishkek, always in the midpoint of a two-week off-duty period and typically in the morning. Lung function test was done with MicroMedical MicroLab (UK) equipment. The subject was in a standing position, and asked to refrain from smoking at least for two hours prior to the test, as prompted by spirometry guidelines in Kyrgyzstan [8]. All tests were performed by the same staff, who were regularly trained, equipment was daily calibrated and biological quality control was performed once a month. At least three vital capacity maneuvers and at least three forced vital capacity maneuvers with reproducibility less than 4 % were required. Because no reference spirometry data existed for Kyrgyz population, we used the European Coal and Steel Community (ECSC) reference equations values to calculate percent predicted values for forced expiratory volume in one second (FEV_1) and forced vital capacity (FVC) [9]. We also measured vital capacity (VC), peak expiratory flow (PEF), and flows at 75 %, 50 % and 25 % of the remaining FVC (MEFs). Quality control was performed by either one of two physicians trained in such testing. The best curves were those with maximal ($FEV_1 + FVC$).

Smoking status verification

Workers were defined "never-smokers" if they answered "No" to the question "Have you ever smoked a cigarette?". Should they answer "Yes", but stopped smoking at some point before, they were "Former smokers". Those smoking daily at a time when study was carried out were defined as "Current smokers". Self-reported current smoking status was verified by exhaled carbon monoxide (CO) measurement performed just prior to spirometry. A Smokerlyzer CO (Bedfont, UK) was used for this testing; readings below 10 ppm were interpreted as confirmatory of non-active smoking status. Those having CO level 10 ppm and above from any self-report category were treated as "Current smokers".

Statistical analysis

Exposure metrics were jobs obtained through the list from the HR-department, which were coded into 41 occupations. In a univariate analysis all codes were analyzed separately, however in regression models we grouped relevant occupations in bigger groups, such as all drivers in one category. Outcome measures were selected lung function indices, such as VC, FVC, FEV_1, FEV_1/FVC, PEF and MEF_{25-75}. For this analysis, we calculated per cent predicted values of lung function indices, which were based on age, height, and sex, also corrected for ethnicity. For univariate comparisons, we used Wilcoxon test to determine whether differences in lung function indices between occupations and between smokers and non-smokers were due to chance only. For regression models we created three outcomes measures, which we tested separately in multivariate models: 1) reduction of FEV_1 to less than 80 % (reference – 80 % and more); 2) reduction to FEV_1/FVC to less than 70 % (reference – 70 % or more); and 3) reduction of FEV_1 to less than 80 % and reduction to FEV_1/FVC to less than 70 %. We adjusted our regression models for smoking and work duration, as those were identified as potential confounders on a pathway from an exposure to an outcome. Because %predicted values already account for age and sex, their effect was eliminated and the models were not adjusted for those variables. Smoking variable was coded as never-smokers vs. ever-smokers (reference). We also performed regression analysis in never smokers only, but due to loss of power, we only report them briefly. We used NCSS 9 (Utah, USA) software for all tests. The effect measure in regression models of this cross-sectional study was odds ratio (OR) with relevant 95 % confidence interval (CI).

Results

A total of 2102 spirometry tests were performed during the period of 2010. Of those, 344 were new hires, having spirometry tests at their pre-employment screening. Because their previous employment record and exposure history were not available, they were excluded from the analysis. Of remaining 1758 employees, spirometry test records of 208 employees were incomplete, yielding 1550 tests available for final analysis. The mean age of this predominantly male workforce (87.5 %) was 40.5 ± 9.2 years (Table 1).

Table 1 Study participants' profile

Variable	
N	1550
Age, years	40.5 ± 9.2
Male/female, N	1357/193
BMI, kg/m^2	25.8 ± 3.7
Working at high-altitude site, N (%)	1477 (95.3 %)
Smoking	
Current smokers, N (%)	627 (40.5 %)
Cigarettes a day	9.2 ± 4.8
Duration of smoking, years	13.7 ± 7.8
Ex-smokers, N (%)	460 (29.7 %)
Never smokers, N (%)	463 (29.8 %)
Spirometry	
VC, % pred.	103.0 ± 12.9
FVC, % pred.	109.1 ± 13.0
FEV_1, % pred.	100.2 ± 25.9
FEV_1/FVC, %	76.5 ± 20.3
PEF, % pred.	107.5 ± 16.7
MEF_{50}, % pred.	77.7 ± 24.1
Occupations	
Mechanics, N (%)	242 (15.6)
Mine truck drivers, N (%)	221 (14.3)
Bulldozer, Grader and Loader/shovel operators, N (%)	128 (8.3)
Cleaners, N (%)	99 (6.4)
Security staff, N (%)	96 (6.2)
Drillers, N (%)	88 (5.7)
Office staff, N (%)	82 (5.3)
Other drivers, N (%)	72 (4.6)
Engineers, N (%)	61 (3.9)
Food handlers (kitchen), N (%)	58 (3.7)
Mill operators, N (%)	48 (3.1)
Warehouse staff, N (%)	45 (2.9)
Blasters, N (%)	41 (2.6)
Lab technicians, N (%)	36 (2.3)
Welders, N (%)	34 (2.2)
Samplers, N (%)	23 (1.5)
Geologists, N (%)	18 (1.2)
Grinder operators, N (%)	14 (0.9)
Surveyors, N (%)	11 (0.7)
Other, N (%)	133 (8.6)

'Other drivers' include powertrucks, passenger trucks and conveyance vehicles; 'Office staff' include trainers, accountants, management, administrators and interpreters. Data presented as mean ± standard deviation

More than 90 % of personnel worked at high-altitude site, whereas the rest were employed at a marshalling yard at middle altitude, and the workforce of this yard was mainly made of powertruck drivers, security personnel and warehouse staff. The occupational profile of the main operation site was more diverse. Drivers and vehicle operators were the most prevalent occupations, and when combined with maintenance (mechanics, electricians and related occupations), altogether they made 45 % of staff. Smoking prevalence was high, and never smokers made only 29.8 % of the cohort. Smoking intensity was not high, though, and an average smoker smoked 9.2 cigarettes a day.

In general, this cohort were mainly healthy men with excellent lung function. Both volume and flow parameters were above 100 % predicted, and men did not differ from women in spirometric %predicted values. In total, this cohort comprised workers of 41 occupations, which we grouped into larger groups for further lung function analyses. We selected groups with the cumulative prevalence of three or more percent and their selected spirometry data are presented in Table 2. Cleaners showed significantly greater FEV_1% when compared to any other occupation, and the difference with the poorest lung function group (drillers) reached 7.5 % ($p < 0.001$). Similarly, drillers had still the worst lung function, when only non-smokers of each occupational group were included in the analysis. Finally, FEV_1% difference in non-smoking drillers increased to 10.8 % when compared to non-smoking cleaners ($p < 0.001$).

Of note, we could not detect significant differences when comparing never-smokers with smokers within any occupational group (Table 2), except engineers and food handlers. Only in these two occupational groups ever-smokers had significantly lower FVC% and FEV_1% compared to never-smokers, and non-smoking engineers

showed the highest FVC% and FEV_1%: their FEV_1% was as high as 115 %, and the absolute difference of non-smoking engineers with non-smoking drillers exceeded 20 %.

We wished to further investigate the interplay of occupation with smoking in the association with poor lung function using regression model. When the two confounders were included in the model, most occupations were not significantly associated with selected outcomes, except drilling and mill and grinder operation. Table 3 shows that drillers had statistically significant 53 % higher risk of obstruction (FEV_1/FVC < 70 %), whereas work at the mill and grinding increased the risk two-fold (also for FEV_1/FVC < 70 %). This table only shows models with adjusted regressions. We further selected groups with marginally high or close to significantly high risk to test using cleaners as reference group (as the lowest risk occupation). Because of loss of power, most of these models became unstable, however when drillers were compared to cleaners, the OR of FEV_1 < 80 % was 10.2 (95 % CI 1.05-97.80). Similarly, in mill workers the OR of FEV_1/FVC < 70 % was 3.81 (95 % CI 1.37-10.44). Finally, to demonstrate isolated effect of work duration on obstruction, we tested it as predictor for three metrics of obstruction as in Table 3. In all cases the effect of work duration was very small and even non-significant in two metrics of three (ORs 1.06 (95 % CI 1.02-1.10); 1.06 (95 % CI 0.94-1.19); and 1.03 (95 % CI 0.90-1.19).

Discussion

This was a cross-sectional study of lung function at mandatory annual screening of open-pit gold mine in Kyrgyzstan with the aim to ascertain most vulnerable working groups for early lung function impairment in healthy young workers. In general, workers in various workplaces within the company had excellent spirometry, with all main parameters exceeding 100 % predicted

Table 2 Spirometry data of employees with selected occupations (prevalence 3 % or more)

Occupations	FVC, % pred.			FEV_1, % pred.			FEV_1/FVC, %		
	Overall	NS	S	Overall	NS	S	Overall	NS	S
Heavy-duty vehicles operators	107.8 ± 13.3	106.7 ± 13.8	108.1 ± 13.1	98.0 ± 12.9	98.1 ± 13.5	97.9 ± 12.8	75.1 ± 6.5	76.0 ± 5.4	74.9 ± 6.7
Other drivers	109.1 ± 13.6	109.4 ± 14.8	108.9 ± 13.3	100.3 ± 13.2	101.3 ± 13.3	99.9 ± 13.2	75.2 ± 6.0	75.9 ± 5.3	75.0 ± 6.3
Mechanics	109.1 ± 12.5	110.6 ± 11.2	108.7 ± 12.8	99.3 ± 12.4	101.3 ± 12.1	98.8 ± 12.5	75.9 ± 7.0	77.7 ± 7.0	75.9 ± 6.9
Cleaners	116.8 ± 13.4	116.9 ± 13.5	116.6 ± 13.4	105.3 ± 12.4	105.7 ± 12.6	103.6 ± 11.7	77.5 ± 5.7	77.9 ± 5.8	75.8 ± 5.1
Security staff	109.8 ± 11.2	110.0 ± 10.2	109.7 ± 11.6	99.7 ± 11.2	101.1 ± 11.0	99.1 ± 11.2	75.2 ± 5.0	76.4 ± 6.3	74.7 ± 4.4
Drillers	105.7 ± 12.5	103.5 ± 11.9	106.5 ± 12.6	97.8 ± 13.2	94.9 ± 11.3	98.8 ± 13.7	76.7 ± 7.2	75.8 ± 4.7	77.0 ± 7.9
Office staff	108.5 ± 13.3	108.0 ± 13.5	108.8 ± 13.3	100.4 ± 12.9	101.8 ± 13.9	99.6 ± 12.3	77.7 ± 7.1	79.1 ± 8.5	76.3 ± 5.9
Engineers	108.2 ± 13.2	110.8 ± 17.4	105.3 ± 11.8[a]	101.2 ± 16.0	115.2 ± 17.7	96.6 ± 12.8[a]	77.7 ± 7.2	80.8 ± 3.6	76.7 ± 7.8
Food handlers	113.0 ± 13.1	115.4 ± 12.6	106.6 ± 12.8[a]	99.4 ± 11.8	101.6 ± 12.3	93.9 ± 8.2[a]	75.5 ± 7.1	75.8 ± 7.4	74.8 ± 6.4
Mill operators, including grinder operators and metallurgists	108.5 ± 12.4	109.9 ± 12.1	107.8 ± 12.8	98.7 ± 13.4	100.5 ± 14.7	97.7 ± 12.9	75.0 ± 7.4	75.1 ± 7.0	74.7 ± 7.6

NS never smokers, *S* smokers and ex-smokers. Heavy-duty vehicles operators include mine truck operators, bulldozer, grader and loader/shovel operators; [a] significant difference when compared to never-smokers. Data presented as mean ± standard deviation

Table 3 Regression models of an association between an occupation and selected spirometric outcomes

Exposures (occupations)	$FEV_1 < 80\%$	$FEV_1/FVC < 70\%$	$FEV_1/FVC < 70\%$ and $FEV_1 < 80\%$
Drillers	1.46 (0.69–3.11)	1.53 (1.11–2.09)	1.53 (0.60–3.92)
Drivers	1.24 (0.80–1.91)	1.18 (0.88–1.58)	1.03 (0.58–1.84)
Mechanics	0.63 (0.33–1.19)	0.95 (0.65–1.37)	0.80 (0.37–1.71)
Cleaners	0.14 (0.02–1.05)	0.51 (0.24–1.09)	0.26 (0.03–1.93)
Office staff and engineers	1.30 (0.61–2.75)	0.90 (0.51–1.59)	1.68 (0.71–4.02)
Food handlers	1.18 (0.41–3.40)	1.11 (0.53–2.33)	0.99 (0.23–4.25)
Mill operators including grinders	0.73 (0.22–2.36)	2.01 (1.13–3.57)	1.29 (0.39–4.24)
Security staff	0.60 (0.22–1.68)	0.84 (0.47–1.51)	0.28 (0.03–1.80)

data are presented as adjusted for smoking and work duration odds ratios (OR) with relevant 95 % confidence intervals (CI); group 'Drivers' includes all relevant operators. Reference groups in each model are all other occupations combined

values. Even with fairly high overall smoking prevalence, never smoking workers had similar flows with ever-smokers in almost all occupations, which was due to healthy worker effect, when initially most fit subjects were selected for employment. Using regression analysis, we found drilling and work in the mill were significantly associated with FEV_1/FVC reduction, and working in the mill doubled the risk of obstruction.

Mining is an established setting for occupational respiratory morbidity, and silica exposure in mining venues is associated with silicosis and lung cancer [10, 11]. Mining workplaces also have high dust levels, and exposure to dust in workplace can result in an occupational COPD [12]. Because COPD is a chronic progressive inflammatory condition, the disease develops gradually, and occupational spirometric screening should detect abnormality at earlier stage [13, 14]. When no dust and other exposure measurements are available, screening of high-risk groups may only be feasible based on occupation-specific data to identify most vulnerable workers for more effective follow-up. Since the population attributable fraction of occupational exposures for COPD is around 15 %, early prevention is crucial and should be a cornerstone of an occupational screening clinic routine. Identification of high-risk workplaces could help prevent large number of COPD cases, mostly in never-smokers. A study like this a helpful tool to monitor workers employed in drilling and mill operations as well as to identify workplaces where high-quality dust exposure measurements are needed.

The findings of this study also emphasize the need for better enforcement of workplace control in drilling and in the mill, where exposure to dust, gases and vapors during chemical extraction of gold may be high. Regular dust monitoring program with active dust level reduction are essential to sustain good workforce health in these workplaces. When no full dust elimination is possible, only subjects with excellent baseline lung function should be hired for these positions; however, current legislation in Kyrgyzstan does not prohibit employment of

workers with COPD, except workers with "chronic bronchopulmonary diseases" applying for jobs with documented high exposure to silica dioxide. Existing screening regulation does not list specific workplaces, therefore occupational screening program is challenging for an occupational doctor in mining companies. More intense lung function monitoring with relevant clinical assessment could serve an optional way to slow down lung function decline in drillers and mill operators. One of the ways to do so may be lung function test done twice a year in these groups, supplemented with smoking status verification and documentation, followed by strong cessation advice.

This study has a number of limitations. Such occupations of interest as welding, which are known to have high levels of exposure, were not included in the models because of their small sample size. There were very few surveyors, whose field work in an open pit can also predispose them to higher exposure to dust. Another limitation was a significant shift towards healthy workers with excellent lung function and relatively small number of employees with either initial or advanced stage of respiratory conditions. Such selection is a result of healthy worker effect, a typical selection bias in occupational studies. Nevertheless, most pronounced limitation of our epidemiological study was nonexistence of exposure assessment data to relate them to actual workplace data. Historically, exposure data were inaccessible in this mining enterprise, and their introduction in future would dramatically advance risk mapping and guide occupational doctor at site to enhance prevention activities in vulnerable groups. Directed by preliminary findings from this setting, exposure assessment in drilling workplaces and all over the mill should be given priority and are a matter of research in future.

Good occupational practice assumes maximum elimination of exposure and regular surveillance with the aim to improve knowledge, attitudes and behavior of all workers at risk of developing occupational COPD [2].

Primary occupational doctors at site should further enforce annual lung function decline monitoring programs, because accelerated decline more than 10–15 % from baseline should not stay unattended. High altitude by itself poses stress on lung function in those newly employed with accelerated decline [15], and occupational exposures together with smoking will accelerate this decline further. Based on these observations, the highest risk is attributed to newly employed young smoking men in drilling and the mill. They should not only be closely monitored, but strongly advised to cease smoking with effective pharmacological aid and be thoroughly instructed on proper use of personal protection.

This study is noted for a number of strengths. Exposure ascertainment was quite strong, as data on work history and positions were obtained from HR department. Smoking was also accurately measured, because self-reported exposure was verified using biological markers, which is rare for occupational epidemiologic research. Large cohort size in this study, especially of selected occupations, such as heavy-duty drivers, should also be considered a strength, and resulted in a greater power. And finally, using a workplace approach rather than exposure approach enabled to incorporate all the mix of various exposures in a single workplace. Workplaces are very seldom a single-exposure matrix, so just knowing particular exposure measure, such as particulate matter with aerodynamic diameter 10 μm and less (PM_{10}) is far not sufficient for full assessment.

Conclusions

In conclusion, this cross-sectional study of a large sample of workers in an open-pit gold mine has demonstrated that on overall lung function of mine workers was within normal range, and had clear correlations with the workplace. We have identified two workplaces with the highest risk for FEV_1/FVC reduction, including drillers (operators of drilling machines) and employees in the mill. This should guide regular spirometric surveillance of workers in these occupations and identify subjects at risk at earlier stages of lung function decline.

Acknowledgements
Author would like to acknowledge contribution of all the medical staff of Kumtor Operating Company (Kumtor Gold Company), namely medical advisor Rupert Redding-Jones and Professor Nurlan Brimkulov from Kyrgyz State Medical Academy.

Authors' contributions
The sole author of this paper performed most of lung function tests, did the analysis and interpretation, drafted the manuscript and approved the final version.

Competing interests
The author declares that he has no competing interests.

References
1. Blanc PD, Torén K. Occupation in chronic obstructive pulmonary disease and chronic bronchitis: an update. Int J Tubercul Lung Dis. 2007;11(3):251–7.
2. Fishwick D, Sen D, Barber C, et al. Occupational chronic obstructive pulmonary disease: a standard of care. Occup Med. 2015;65(4):270–82.
3. Omland O, Würtz ET, Aasen TB, et al. Occupational chronic obstructive pulmonary disease: a systematic literature. Scand J Work Environ Health. 2014;40(1):19–35.
4. Blanc PD, Iribarren C, Trupin L, et al. Occupational exposures and the risk of COPD: dusty trades revisited. Thorax. 2009;64(1):6–12.
5. Ehrlich RI, Myers JE, Water Naude JM, et al. Lung function loss in relation to silica dust exposure in South African gold miners. Occup Envir Med. 2011; 68(2):96–101.
6. Bang KM. Chronic obstructive pulmonary disease in nonsmokers by occupation and exposure: a brief review. Cur Opin Pul Med. 2015;21(2):149–54.
7. Hochgatterer K, Moshammer H, Haluza D. Dust is in the air: effects of occupational exposure to mineral dust on lung function in a 9-year study. Lung. 2013;191(3):257–63.
8. Brimkulov N, Vinnikov DV, Davletalieva N, et al. Guidelines on Spirometry for Medicals of Kyrgyzstan (In Russian). Bishkek: Kyrgyz-Finnish Lung Health Programme; 2005.
9. Quanjer PH. Standardized lung function testing. Bull Eur Physiopathol Respir. 1983;19:66–92.
10. Brown T. Silica exposure, smoking, silicosis and lung cancer-complex interactions. Occup Med. 2009;59(2):89–95.
11. Steenland K, Mannetje A, Boffetta P, et al. Pooled exposure–response analyses and risk assessment for lung cancer in 10 cohorts of silica-exposed workers: an IARC multicentre study. Cancer Causes Control. 2001;12(9):773–84.
12. Blanc PD, Menezes AMB, Plana E, et al. Occupational exposures and COPD: an ecological analysis of international data. Eur Respir J. 2009;33(2):298–304.
13. Townsend MC. Occupational and Environmental Lung Disorders Committee. Spirometry in the occupational health setting–2011 update. J Occup Envir Med. 2011;53(5):569.
14. Redlich CA, Tarlo SM, Hankinson JL, et al. Official American Thoracic Society technical standards: spirometry in the occupational setting. Am J Respir Crit Care. 2014;189(8):983–93.
15. Vinnikov D, Blanc PD, Brimkulov N, et al. Five-year lung function observations and associations with a smoking ban among healthy miners at high altitude (4000 m). J Occup Envir Med. 2013;55(12):1421–5.

Work related injury among Saudi Star Agro Industry workers in Gambella region

Daniel Haile Chercos[*] and Demeke Berhanu

Abstract

Background: Work injury is an important cause of morbidity and mortality, much of these work injuries burden can be found in industry required heavy manual work such as, agriculture and fishers. Hence; agriculture is consistently cited as one of the most hazardous industry in the world. The objective of this study isto assess the magnitude and associated factors of work related injury among Saudi Star Agro Industry workers in Gambella region, South West Ethiopia.

Methods: An institutional based cross-sectional study design was conducted on Saudi Star Agro Industry located in Gambella region, from February - June 2014 on 449 randomly selected workers who arestratifiedby working department. Anobservation checklist, factory clinical records and a structured interview questioner were used as a data collection tools.

Result: The prevalence of work related injury was 36.7%. Marital status [AOR;1.69, 95%; CI;(1.1–2.7)], service year [AOR;1.9,95%; CI;(1.17–3.1)], working more than 48 h per week [AOR;9.87, 95%; CI;(5.95–16.28)],safety training [AOR;3.38, 95%;CI;1.14–9.98)], regular health checkup [AOR; 12.29, 95%; CI (9–51.35)] and usage of personal protective equipment [AOR; 2.36, 95%; CI; (1.06–5.25)] were significant factors for the occurrence of work related injury.

Conclusion: The prevalence of work related injury was high. Working hours, safety training and regular health checkup increases the risk of work related injury.

Keywords: Agro industry, Ethiopia, Work related injury, Working environment

Background

Occupational injuries are one of the major public health problems in the world. This is because the total consequence of occupational injury extend well beyond direct physical injury and include a wide array of social and economic burdens [1]. Work related injury is an important cause of morbidity and mortality and much of work related injury burden can be found in industries requiring heavy manual work such as agriculture and fishers [2–4]. However most of work related injuries can be prevented by using appropriate occupational safety and health service as well as by using ongoing injury surveillance [5].

Globally, the burden of occupational injury accounts for 100 million cases per year, in which 360,000 are fatal accidents [6]. Reports showed that Developing countries have the highest injury fatality rate, in which 14 death reported per 100,000 workers due to occupational injuries [6, 7]. This results a loss of about 4% of world Gross National Product and the impact is estimated to be 10–20 times more in developing countries [8].

Agriculture is consistently cited as one of the most hazardous industry in the world. As a result, workers and their families are vulnerable to high injury and fatality rates. In 2008, the farmer and rancher occupation had a fatality rate that was 10 times more when compared with all occupations (40.3 Vs 3.7 per 100,000 workers) [5]. This indicates that workers in the agriculture sector suffer from higher rates of accidents and fatal injuries than workers found in other industries [3, 4].

* Correspondence: daniel.haile7@gmail.com
Department of Environmental and Occupational Health and Safety, Institute of Public Health, University of Gondar, P.O. Box 196, Gondar, Ethiopia

Agriculture, have many organizational and environmental characteristics that can affect the health of workers including; exposure to hazardous conditions in the natural environment, use of dangerous machinery and chemicals and unconventional work arrangement [2–4]. On top of that, the introduction of new technologies and new chemical substances have led to new occupational injuries [8].

Agriculture constitutes the major economical share for most of the Sub-Saharan countries including Ethiopia. In Ethiopia, the number of industries in the agricultural sector is increasing recently and it became the backbone of the Ethiopian economy. In Ethiopia; agricultural industries accounts for almost all of the foreign exchange earnings of the country and it provides almost 50% of the country's Growth Domestic Product (GDP), with nearly 80% of the labor force working in this sector [9]. Although there are few studies done so far that had made considerable progress in protecting workers from occupational injury and illness, there are still vast unreported occupational accidents and diseases exists [10]. In addition, a geographical variation is a big factor for fatality rate of occupational injuries. Therefore it is important to study and take preventive measure related to work related injuries in agricultural sector of a country [11].

Methods
Aim of this study
The aim of this study is to assess the prevalence and associated factors of work related injury among Saudi Star Agro Industry workers, Gambella region, South West Ethiopia.

Study design
An institutional based cross-sectional study design was conducted from February - June 2014.

Study area and period
This study was conducted at Saudi Stare Agro Industry. The study area is located in South West of Ethiopia, Gambella region, Aboboworeda, which is about 813 km from the capital city, Addis Ababa. The company was established in 2007 and has a current production capacity of 12800 t of rice per year. Currently, the industry has employed 1064 workers from which 244 (22.94%) are female workers.

Source population
All workers who were working in agricultural production segment of Saudi Stare Agro Industry.

Inclusion and exclusion criteria
Inclusion criteria
All agricultural workers involved in agricultural production segment.

Exclusion criteria
Administrative staffs, workers on annual leave and workers who were absence during data collection period.

Sample size
The sample size was calculated using a single population proportion formula. It was calculated taking 95% confidence interval, marginal error 4%, and work related injury as 78.3% [12]; yielding a sample size of 449 workers.

Three departments were selected as the major area of the enterprise where workers directly involve in agricultural division. Assuming that work related injury varies with the nature of the work; the calculated sample size was distributed across the selected three departments using stratified sampling technique. Study subjects were allocated proportionally from each department and finally subjects were drawn by simple random sampling technique from each department sampling frame.

Operational definitions

- Work related injury; any physical injury condition sustained on worker in connection with the performance of his/her work but not include work related diseases that need exposure assessment and laboratory tests [13].
- Personal protective equipment (PPE); Utilization of the worker specialized clothing or equipment worn by employees for protection against health and safety hazards at the time of interview [14].
- Manual handling; the movement or support of any load effort, including; lifting put down pushing, puling, carrying and moving.
- Sleeping disorder; the presence of sleeping problems when the workers are at work in the factory [14].
- Safety guarding of machine; the machine is safe if it safe guards workers from contacts with dangerous moving parts [7].
- Agricultural injury; is defined as unintentional physical injury or poisoning which occurred during an agricultural activities and which required medical attention [5].
- Incident; any unplanned event resulting in, or having the potential for injury, illness, in health, damage or other loss [5].
- Excessive heat: heat is recorded as excessive if a worker is found sweating when naked or with light clothing; if the investigator feels a sudden heat wave when entering to the work [7].

Data collection tools and procedures
The data was collected using face to face interview administered from pre – tested structured questionnaire developed from International Labor Organization (ILO),

Occupational Safety and Health (OSH) policy 2012 standards and other studies modified for the purpose of this study. Observations were also made by principal investigator using prepared observational checklist to evaluate work environment. Moreover, record reviews from clinic and safety committee group discussion were also used as assertion to the self-reported information made by study respondents. Seven data collector, one supervisor and one principal investigator were enrolled during data collection.

Data quality control

The questionnaire was developed first in English and translated to Amharic and back to English by language experts for consistency validity. The data collectors were trained for 3 days about data collection tool, questioning technique and ethical issues. A pre-test was also conducted on similar industry to assess the validity and reliability of the questionnaire. The completeness of the questionnaires was checked before data entry.

Data processing and analysis

The data was entered in Statistical Package for Social Sciences (SPSS) 16 for analysis. All assumptions applied to binary regression including fitness of model were checked. The findings were present by using frequencies, tables, and graphs. The presence of interaction between independent factors explored. To identify factors associated with work related injury, Binary Logistic regression model was fitted and variables with a $p < 0.2$ in bivariate analysis included in the multi-variant analysis. Those predictors with p-value < 0.05, in the multi-variant analysis was considered as independent and significant predictors for work related injury and Odds ratio (OR) with 95% confidence interval was reported.

Results

Socio-demographic factors

Majority of a study participants, 265 (59%) were male. The minimum and maximum age was 18 and 41 respectively and 232 (51.6%) of respondent were single.

From a total of 449 respondent 152 (33.9%) were primary school (1–8 grade) and 269 (59.9%) respondents had 3 years and below service year experience. Regarding employment pattern, 413 (92%) were temporarily employed and 382 (85.1%) of the respondent were earned less than 1600 ETB (Table 1).

Work related injury characteristics

Prevalence of work related injuries

Among the study participants, 165 (36.7%) had work related injury in the last 12 months with the overall prevalence rate of 367 per 1000 exposed worker per year. Moreover, 18 (4%) respondent were also injured at job in the last 2 weeks. With respect to the frequency of

Table 1 Distribution of socio-demographic characteristics of respondents in Saudi Star Agro Industry in Gambelia region, Ethiopia, 2014 ($n = 449$)

Variable	Frequency(n)	Percent (%)
Sex		
Male	265	59%
Female	184	41%
Age		
18–29	324	72.2%
> 29	125	27.8%
Educational status		
Illiterate	10	2.2%
Read and write	132	29.4%
Primary school(1–8)	152	33.9%
Secondary school (9–12)	114	25.4%
TVT	37	8.2%
First degree and above	4	0.9%
Marital status		
Married	215	47.9%
Single	232	51.7%
Divorce	2	0.4%
Employment type		
Temporary	413	92%
Permanent	36	8%
Monthly income		
≤ 1600	382	85.1%
> 1600	67	14 .9%
Working experience		
≤ 3	269	59.9%
> 3	180	40.1%

injury occurrence in the last 12 months, 110 (24.5%) respondents were injured once, and 55 (12.2%) injured more than once (Fig. 1).

Cause, type and affected body part

From Injured respondents, predominantly affected parts of the body were; hand 46 (27.9%), leg 34 (20.6%), eye 25 (15.15%) and toe 23 (13.93%) (Table 2). With respect to type of injuries, 61 (37.0%) laceration, 25 (15.15%) eye injury, 24 (14.54%) cut and 23 (13.94%) puncture were the most type of injury reported by respondents (Table 3). Hand tool 63 (38.20%), machine 32 (20%), splinting objects 26 (15.75%) and lifting objects 17 (10.3%) were the top sources of work related injures (Table 4).

With regard to the specific days of injuries, 80 (48.48%) were on Monday, 52 (31.51%) were on Tuesday and most respondent injured in the morning at the time of 6A.M – 6P.M (Fig. 2). When we see Absenteeism due

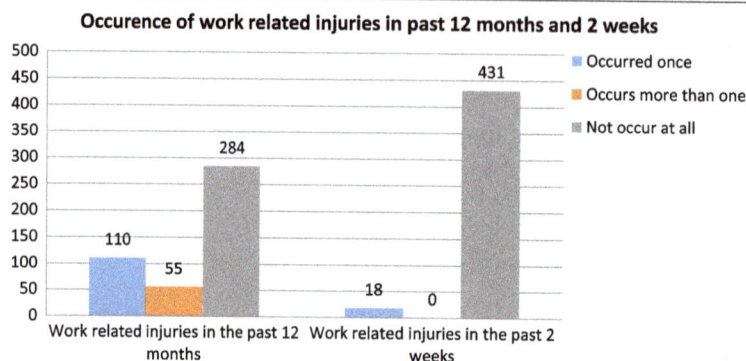

Fig. 1 The prevalence and frequency of work related injuries in the past 12 months and 2 weeks among Saudi Star Agro Industry workers in Gambella region, Ethiopia, 2014

to work related injuries in the industry in the last 12 months, 75 (16.7%) absenteeism occurred for 1 day, 10 (2.2%) for 2 days and 3 (0.2%) for 3 days.

Of those injured respondents 101 (61.2%) workers injured while in production department (cultivating, irrigation, and loading unloading) and 36 (21.8%) were injured in agro mechanization department (mechanic, tractor operator, loader operator and welder). The most frequent reason given by the respondents for the occurrence of injury were working behavior 79 (47.87%).

Severity of work related injury
Out of 165 injured respondents six (1.3%) were hospitalized and 87 working days were lost as the result of work related injury.

Description of work environment
Concerning with working hour, 338 (75.27%) respondents were working for 48 h per week and 111 (24.8%) were working for more than 48 h. From all respondents, 94.2% realized that they have no safety training and 96.88% of

the respondents responded lack of supervision at work place (Fig. 3).

Behavioral characteristics
Among 449 respondents, 59 (13%) were drinking alcohol, 20 (4.5%) were chewing chat, 18 (4%) were smoking cigarette and 42 (4.5%) had sleep disorder. From all respondents 376 (83.75) were not using PPE. Reasons given by respondents for not using PPE are 307 (81.64%) were no PPE, 26 (6.91%) were lack of awareness, 10 (2.65%) don't know how to use the PPE, 15 (3.98%) not comfortable and 18 (4.8%) were due to decrease performance of PPE.

Observation of work environment
During the observation, we have seen that most working section were with excessive heat and dust. In addition, there were no safety division and personnel in the enterprise that help in promoting health and safety condition at work place. Warning sign and health and safety instructions or procedure did not exist in all working section; similarly all working section lacks first aid equipment except they had clinic at central level (Table 5).

Associated factors of work related injury
From the socio-demographic variables, marital status and service years of workers showed significant association

Table 2 Parts of the body injured and types of injury among workers in Saudi Star Agro Industry in Gambelia region, Ethiopia, 2014(n = 165)

Part of the body affected	Frequency	Percent (%)
Hand	46	27.9%
Toe	23	13.9%
Back	17	10.3%
Eye	25	15.2%
Finger	2	1.2%
Leg	34	20.6%
Ear	2	1.2%
Chest	8	4.8%
Upper arm	1	0.6%
Other	7	4.3%

Table 3 Type OF INJURES among injured worker in Saudi Star Agro Industry in Gambelia region, Ethiopia, 2014 (n = 165)

Types of injury	Frequency	Percent (%)
Abrasion/Laceration	61	37.0%
Cut	24	14.5%
Puncture	23	13.9%
Back pain	14	8.5%
Eye injury	25	15.2%
Ear injury	2	1.2%
Others	16	9.7%

Table 4 Source of injury among injured workers in Saudi Star Agro Industry in Gambelia region, Ethiopia, 2014 ($n = 165$)

Source of injury	Frequency	Percent (%)
Machine	33	20%
Falling object	15	9.1%
Splinting object	26	15.8%
Collision	2	1.2%
Acid and acidic substance	8	4.8%
Hand tool	63	38.2%
Lifting object	17	10.3%
Other	1	0.6%

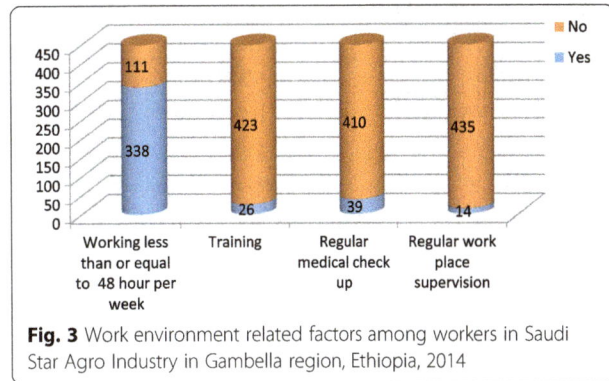

Fig. 3 Work environment related factors among workers in Saudi Star Agro Industry in Gambella region, Ethiopia, 2014

with work related injury. Workers who are single were 1.73 times more likely to report work related injury than workers who are in marriage [AOR; 1.73; 95%; CI (1.09–2.75) and workers whose service year less than or equal to 3 were 1.89 times more likely to report work related injury than whose service year above 3 years [AOR; 1.89; 95%; CI; (1.16–3.08). However sex, age, educational status, income and type of employment have no significance association with work related injury in this study.

Among work environment variables, hours worked per week, safety training and regular health checkup showed significant association with work related injury. Workers who worked more than 48 h per week were 8.33 times more likely to be injured than workers who spend their time in the work place for 48 h and less [AOR; 8.33; 95%; CI (4.87–14.41)]. Similarly, workers without safety and health training were 4.56 times more likely to be injured than who had training [AOR; 4.56; 95%; CI;(1.299–16.1)].In addition, workers who had no regular health checkup were 5.84 times more likely to be injured than who had regular health checkup [AOR; 5.56; 95%; CI (2.04–16.73)]. However, supervision of work place had no significant association with work related injury.

Among behavioral factors, usage of personal protective equipment was significantly associated with work related

injury. Workers who did not used personal protective equipment's were 2.58 times more likely to reported work related injury than workers who did use PPE in the work place [AOR; 2.58, 95%; CI (1.17–5.68). However, smoking cigarettes, drinking alcohol, sleep disorder and chewing chat were not significantly associated with work related injury (Table 6).

Discussion

Magnitude and severity of work related injury

Determining the prevalence of work related injuries and identifying associated factors are essential in the development of injury prevention strategy at the work place. The overall prevalence of work related injury in this study was 36.7% or 367 per 1000 workers per year. This finding is similar with studies done in agricultural workers stating that workers suffer markedly high rate of injuries than any other workers [5, 15]. In addition, most workers in this study are temporary workers (92%) and temporary workers and daily laborers are among the most vulnerable groups in agricultural workplaces [16].

This study indicates high rate of injury compared to a study made on other industries [2, 17, 18]. This could be due to poor promotion and preventive work related to safety and health such as, lack of safety training, lack of regular health checkup, lack of poor usage of personal protective equipment's, and being temporary worker

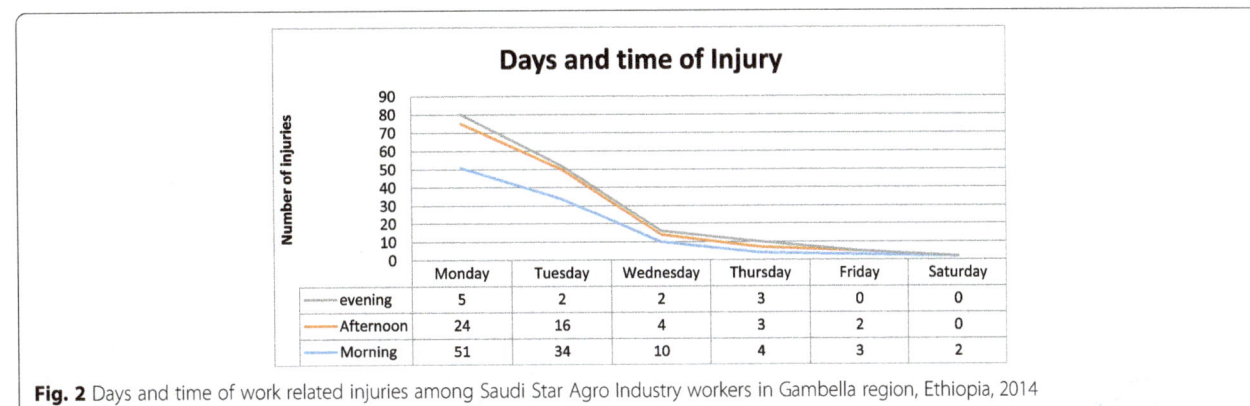

Fig. 2 Days and time of work related injuries among Saudi Star Agro Industry workers in Gambella region, Ethiopia, 2014

Table 5 Occupational health and safety hazards identified in working section, Saudi Star Agro Industry in Gambelia region, Ethiopia, 2014

Type of workplace	Work department	Hazard Identified
Agro mechanization	Farm mechanization	Excessive heat, dust, sharps, gasoline and Sulfuric acid
	Work shop/Garage	Excessive heat, sharps, gasoline and Sulfuric acid
Workshop/Garage	Pest control department	Pesticide and chemicals, and PPE are not Standardized
Others	Seed preparation and rice packing	Noise, Poor ventilation, sharps, dust, and have loaded materials
	Unit farm Irrigation	Excessive heat and dust, Snack bits Dust, and sharps

Table 6 Summery of logistic regression analysis of the relative effect of work related injuries among SAUDI STAR AGRO INDUSTRY IN GAMBELLA REGION, ETHIOPIA, 2014

Characteristics	WRI Yes	WRI No	COR 95% CI	AOR 95% CI
Sex				
Male	86	176	$0.719(0.49-1.06)^x$	$0.63(0.4-1.01)^0$
Female	76	108	1.00	
Age				
≤ 29	126	198	$1.04(0.9-2.18)^0$	$1.28(0.76-2.17)^0$
> 29	39	86	1.00	
Marital status				
Single	107	127	$2.28(1.54-3.39)^{xxx}$	$1.6 (1.01-2.57)^x$
Married	58	157	1.00	1.00
Service				
≤ 3	123	146	$2.77(1.8-4.22)^{xxx}$	$2.05(1.22-3.29)^{xx}$
> 3	42	138	1.00	1.00
Safety				
No	161	262	$3.38(1.14-9.98)^x$	$4.89(1.37-17.4)^x$
Yes	4	22	1.00	1.00
PPE				
No	155	221	$4.42(2.19\_8.89)^{xxx}$	$2.54(1.15-5.64)^x$
Yes	10	63	1.00	1.00
Health checkup				
No	161	248	$5.84(2.04-16.73)^{xx}$	$4.06(1.1-14.99)^x$
Yes	4	36	1.00	1.00
Chewing chat				
No	5	15	$0.55(0.2-1.57)^0$	$0.66(0.14-3.04)^0$
Yes	160	269	1.00	
Working hour				
≤ 48	81	257	1.00	1.00
> 48	84	27	$9.87(5.98-16.28)^{xxx}$	$8.53(4.9-14.73)^{xxx}$

^{0}NB variable whose P-value < 0.3 in bivariate; ^{x}significant at $P < 0.05$; ^{xx}significant at $P < 0.01$; ^{xxx}significant at $P < 0.001$

(temporary workers does not get equal benefits with permanent workers in most industries) may contribute to high rate of injury in this study.

Major work related injury types, part of the body affected, and source of injury

The finding of this study indicates that, abrasion/laceration, eye injury, cut and punctures as the most frequent types of injuries. These findings are consistent with studies conducted in Ethiopia; study conducted in Tendaho agricultural industry and a study done in Gondar on small and medium scale industries [8, 18]. These findings are also consistent with a study done on risk of agricultural injury among African-American farm works from Alabama and Mississippi and a study conducted on eye health and safety among Latino farm workers [19, 20]. In addition literature revealed that the stated findings are common in work related injury [3, 21].

This study also revealed that hand tools, machine and splinting objects are the common source of injury. This finding is consistence with a study done in agricultural injury in rural California [21]. The reason for this may be due to the fact that most of the workers were temporary and daily laborer. These workers are characterized by manual handling and working on environment which is full of pieces of stone and dry soil. The risk of temporary workers and manual worker as the most exposed group in agricultural activities is well documented in study done in Easter U.S [22]. These findings are also in agreement with other studies done in Ethiopia such as Tendho agricultural industry, large scale metal manufacturing industry in Addis Ababa, and on small and medium scale industry in Gondar [7, 8, 18].

In this study we have found that hand, leg, eye and toe were the most common parts of the body injured. This finding is in agreement with the study done in Tendaho agricultural industry in Afar, Ethiopiaand a study done on farm related injury on older Kentucky farmers in U.S. [8, 23].

Determinant of work related injury

The finding of the studies revealed several factors that related to the occurrence, severity and types of injury.

Among the assessed socio-demographic determinant of work related injury marital status and service year were significantly associated with work related injury. This finding is consistent with the study done in Tendho agricultural industry, study done on large scale manufacture industries in Addis Ababa and study done on small and medium scale enterprise in Gondar [7, 8, 17]. In addition, this finding is also consistent with studies done on Kentucky farmers [18].

The finding of this study showed that from all work environmental factors, working hour per week, safety training and regular health checkup were significantly associated with work related injury. These are in agreement with studies done in Tendho manufacturing industry, large manufacturing industries in Addis Ababa, a study done in small and medium enterprise in Gondar, Ethiopia and a study done on occupational injuries in Kombolcha textile factory, Ethiopia [7, 8, 13, 18]. Similarly, the finding of the study is consistent with the studies done on fatal occupational injury among non-governmental employee in Malaysia and injuries and fatalities on older farmers in U.S. [3, 22].

Among the assessed behavioral determinant of work related injury, using of personal protective equipment was significantly associated with injury. This finding is in agreement with studies done in large manufacturing industry in Addis Ababa, study done in Tendho agricultural industry in Afar, study done on small and medium enterprise in Gondar, and study done on occupational injuries among Addis Ababa city municipal solid waste collectors [7, 8, 18, 24]. Similar finding is also observed on studies done on injuries and fatalities in U.S farmers and agricultural injuries on older farmers in Kentucky [22, 23].

Conclusion

The prevalence of work related injury in Saudi Star Agro Industry was high. Marital status, service year, usage of personal protective equipment, safety training regular health checkup and working hours per week were significantly associated with work related injuries.

Acknowledgements

We would further like to thank University of Gondar, College of Medicine and Health Sciences for providing ethical clearance for his study. We also like to express our gratitude to Saudi Star Agro Industry office, State Farm management staffs and study participants.

Funding

This research is funded by University of Gondar, Research and Community Service directorate as an award of winning research projects among academician within the University.

Authors' contributions

DHC participated in proposal research design process, data analysis, and presentation and interpretation process of result, preparation of scientific paper or the manuscript, and corresponding author of the manuscript. DB was responsible for generating the concept of this research paper, literature review and organization, preparation of draft research proposal document, organizing data collection process, and preparation of draft data analysis and interpretation. All authors read and approved the final manuscript.

Competing interests

The authors declare that they have no competing interests.

References

1. Smith TD, DeJoy DM. Occupational injury in America: an analysis of risk factors using data from the General Social Survey (GSS). J Safety Res. 2012;43(1):67–74.
2. Lee SJ, et al. Work-related injuries and fatalities among farmers in South Korea. Am J Ind Med. 2012;55(1):76–83.
3. Abas AB, et al. Fatal occupational injuries among non-governmental employees in Malaysia. Am J Ind Med. 2013;56(1):65–76.
4. Fransen M, et al. Shift work and work injury in the New Zealand Blood Donors' Health Study. Occup Environ Med. 2006;63(5):352–8.
5. Earle-Richardson GB, et al. Improving agricultural injury surveillance: a comparison of incidence and type of injury event among three data sources. Am J Ind Med. 2011;54(8):586–96.
6. Uehli K, et al. Sleep problems and work injuries: a systematic review and meta-analysis. Sleep Med Rev. 2014;18(1):61–73.
7. Habtu Y, Kumie A, Tefera W. Magnitude and factors of occupational injury among workers in large scale metal manufacturing industries in Ethiopia. Open Access Library Journal. 2014;1(08):1.
8. Yiha O, Kumie A. Assessment of occupational injuries in Tendaho Agricultural Development SC, Afar Regional State. Ethiop J Health Dev. 2010;24(3):167–74.
9. Andrews D, et al., The Federal Democratic Republic of Ethiopia: Selected Issues and Statistical Appendix. International Monetary Fund Country Report. 2006(06/122)
10. Kolben K. Labor rights as human rights. Va J Int'l L. 2009;50:449.
11. Karttunen JP, Rautiainen RH. Occupational injury and disease incidence and risk factors in Finnish agriculture based on 5-year insurance records. J Agromedicine. 2013;18(1):50–64.
12. Aderaw Z, Engdaw D, Tadesse T. Determinants of occupational injury: a case control study among textile factory workers in Amhara Regional State, Ethiopia. J Trop Med. 2011;2011:657275.
13. Yessuf Serkalem S, Moges Haimanot G, Ahmed Ansha N. Determinants of occupational injury in Kombolcha textile factory, North-East Ethiopia. Int J Occup Environ Med. 2014;5(2):84–93.
14. Lovelock K, et al. Occupational injury and disease in agriculture in North America, Europe and Australasia: a review of the literature. Dunedin: University of Otago; 2008.
15. ILO. Safety and Health in Agriculture, in SafeWork, h.a.t.e. Programme on safety, Editor. Geneva: International Labour Office; 2000. p. 22.
16. Ezenwa AO. A study of fatal injuries in Nigerian factories. Occup Med (Lond). 2001;51(8):485–9.
17. Tadesse T, Kumie A. Prevalence and factors affecting work-related injury among workers engaged in Small and Medium-scale industries in Gondar wereda, North Gondor zone, Amhara Regional State, Ethiopia. Ethiop J Health Dev. 2007;21(1):25–34.
18. McGwin Jr G, Enochs R, Roseman JM. Increased risk of agricultural injury among African-American farm workers from Alabama and Mississippi. Am J Epidemiol. 2000;152(7):640–50.
19. Verma A, et al. Eye health and safety among Latino farmworkers. J Agromedicine. 2011;16(2):143–52.
20. McCurdy SA, Kwan JA. Agricultural injury risk among rural California public high school students: prospective results. Am J Ind Med. 2012;55(7):631–42.
21. Myers JR, Layne LA, Marsh SM. Injuries and fatalities to U.S. farmers and farm workers 55 years and older. Am J Ind Med. 2009;52(3):185–94.
22. Pfortmueller CA, et al. Injuries in agriculture-injury severity and mortality. Swiss Med Wkly. 2013;143:w13846.

16

"Decision-critical" work: a conceptual framework

Xiangning Fan[1], Charl Els[2], Kenneth J. Corbet[3] and Sebastian Straube[1*]

Abstract

"Safety-sensitive" workers, also termed "safety-critical" workers, have been subject to fitness to work assessments due to concerns that a performance error may result in worker injury, injury to coworkers or the general public, and/or disruption of equipment, production or the environment. However, there exists an additional category of "decision-critical" workers, distinct from "safety-sensitive" workers, in whom impairment may impact workplace performance, relationships, attendance, reliability and quality. Adverse consequences in these latter areas may not be immediately apparent, but a potential "orbit of harm" nevertheless exists. Workplace consequences arising from impairment in "decision-critical" workers differ from those in "safety-sensitive" personnel. Despite their importance in the occupational context, "decision-critical" workers have not previously been differentiated from other workers in the published literature, and we now outline an approach to fitness to work assessment in this group.

Keywords: Decision-critical work, Safety-sensitive work, Fitness to work, Accidents, Occupational safety

Background

A "safety-critical" task has previously been defined to mean "one where certain forms of personal impairment can put other people at risk" [1]. The terms "safety-sensitive" and "safety-critical" have been used in a number of recent occupational health guidance documents [2, 3], outlining the importance of this group of workers. The concept of risk in this operational definition has been further refined in case law to include risks both to the worker as well as to others arising out of performance error due to physical or mental conditions, with consideration of the nature, magnitude and immediacy of the risks. The broader category of "safety-sensitive" work can be thought of as encompassing work in which one or more "safety-critical" tasks are or may be performed, and where possible consequences include death or serious injury of a worker or a member of the general public, or, alternately, damage to or serious disruption of equipment, production or the environment. Of note, opportunities to mitigate harms arising from worker impairment in a "safety-sensitive" role may be limited, as adverse consequences typically occur within a short period of time following a performance error. In this review, we will build on this framework of "safety-sensitive" work, and develop a distinct concept of "decision-critical" work.

Review

The distinction between "safety-sensitive" and "non safety-sensitive" work has been used to justify 1. skills certification requirements for workers on a periodic basis, 2. workplace drug and alcohol policies and testing programs, and 3. more stringent and frequent medical assessments, especially in regulated industries (e.g. transportation). Occupational health professionals evaluating "safety-sensitive" workers are required to document a higher threshold of certainty that no medically-based impairment exists or may be reasonably foreseen to exist. However, there exists considerable ambiguity in the exact meaning of "safety-sensitive" work across industry and occupational categories, as well as among medical practitioners. Outside of administrative definitions in regulated industries, there is no clear consensus on the exact boundary between "safety-sensitive" versus "non safety-sensitive" work. Clarity in this regard would enable a consistent, fair and transparent approach to the assessment of "safety-sensitive" workers, and benefit occupational health professionals, workers, employers and public interest.

* Correspondence: straube@ualberta.ca
[1]Division of Preventive Medicine, Department of Medicine, Faculty of Medicine and Dentistry, University of Alberta, 5-30F University Terrace, 8303-112 Street, Edmonton, AB T6G 2T4, Canada
Full list of author information is available at the end of the article

Despite the importance of the "safety-sensitive" concept, the distinction between "safety sensitive" and "non safety-sensitive" workers is far from the sole delineation of importance when evaluating workers for fitness to work. Given the explicit boundaries of "safety sensitive" work as outlined above, we propose that there exists a second category of "decision-critical" workers, whose continued occupational performance depends on the ability to consistently exercise judgment and insight, but who do not precisely fall under the "safety sensitive" category. Examples of such "decision-critical" workers include corporate executives, schoolteachers, lawyers, information technology workers, and some health professionals, among others. For "decision-critical" workers, adverse workplace consequences may arise from a state of low-grade impairment as well as from a single event or error, with serious consequences that may not be immediately apparent. "Decision-critical" work may affect workers' wellbeing and livelihoods, and impact employer oversight and stewardship of products and services, but without the same direct and near-term adverse effects as "safety-sensitive" work. Despite the less dramatic workplace consequences, impairment in "decision-critical" workers (particularly of the neurocognitive variety) can still pose workplace difficulty with coworkers, supervisors and clients in the domains of attendance, performance, and workplace relationships, and result in financial, legal, reputational or psychological harm, and/or corporate liability. We propose that one definition of "decision-critical" workers is workers whose continued occupational performance depends on the ability to consistently exercise judgment and insight in the workplace, but who would not be considered "safety-sensitive" workers. The case vignettes in the Appendix of this review provide examples of workers who may be considered "decision-critical" and detail how medical conditions in "decision-critical" workers can impact occupational function.

Of note, it is generally accepted that a "safety-sensitive" worker's right to self-determination can be justifiably limited in some circumstances for employers' and the public's interest. However, it is not clear to what extent the same applies to "decision-critical" workers when lesser degrees or different kinds of risk exist, such as when the potential harm is property damage, digital information loss, proprietary breaches, legal liability, delayed completion of time-sensitive job tasks, or economic loss. Indeed, while the language of "safety-sensitive" work is inherently connected to the concept of workplace risk, it is not clear whether the discussion for "decision-critical" workers should always continue to be framed in terms of risk when the potential adverse consequences are less overt and not immediately injurious.

Guidance for occupational health professionals on the topic of fitness to work in both "safety-sensitive" and our proposed "decision-critical" workers has been inconsistent to date. Serra and colleagues [4] have previously reported that, of published guidelines on the assessment of fitness to work, approximately 25 % did not describe the decision-making process by which occupational health professionals should evaluate workers at all, and an additional 25 % indicated that the physician "forms an opinion, or arrives at a clinical judgment," without providing further detail. Of 39 articles on the assessment of fitness to work identified, 34 discussed "health and safety risk," and 31 outlined "determination of capacity." However, of the latter, only 11 addressed the worker's psychological capacity and it is not clear how many guidelines separately considered neurocognitive ability as it applies to decision-making processes.

We propose that the process of assessing fitness to work in "safety-sensitive" and "decision-critical" workers include the explicit identification of important neurocognitive domains from essential job tasks, in the same way that physical demands are separately considered within a physical job demands analysis (e.g. for functional capacity assessment). Indeed, for some "safety-sensitive" and "decision-critical" functions (e.g. driving [5–9]), this has already been attempted in generally applicable medical guidelines. In the workplace, existing cognitive and behavioural job demands analyses (e.g. utilized by the City of Toronto in Toronto, Ontario, Canada [10]) necessitate clear definitions and field-testing to ensure validity [11] but hold promise for standardizing the translation of workplace demands into the health domain (and vice versa). For both "safety sensitive" and "decision-critical" workers, the medical assessment must be relevant, valid, and reliable, comparing the worker's capabilities to the demands of the job. Where neuropsychiatric testing is available, more detailed information on neurocognitive capability can be assessed than by clinical interview alone, although clinical assessment is likely to be the mainstay of assessment for most workers due to practical considerations.

Both episodic and persistent phenomena from medical conditions should be identified in the fitness to work assessment of "safety-sensitive" and "decision-critical" workers. Pertinent conditions may include mental health conditions, personality disorders, and somatic diseases (such as endocrine or cerebrovascular conditions) which may interfere with one or more neurocognitive domains. The worker should be asked about use of medications (e.g. opioids [2]) or illicit substances [12] generally held to preclude "safety-sensitive" work due to impairment of alertness, cognition or judgment. In the context of his/her medical condition, the ability of the worker to function, with or without job accommodation, should then be considered. It has been argued for psychiatric illness [13], and is also true of medical conditions in general, that functional impairment and decision-making capacity should be considered separately from the condition itself. We therefore recommend the following step-wise approach (see Fig. 1):

1. Identify risks in the "orbit of harm" including potentially affected individuals, infrastructure, processes, products, the environment or the public.
2. Identify the "decision-critical" elements of the job and isolate physical and cognitive/behavioural essential job demands.
3. Assess the worker's physical and neurocognitive capacity by clinical examination or appropriate neuropsychological testing. Capacity can be adversely impacted by a medical condition, treatment for a medical condition, medication side

effects, or use of alcohol and/or illicit substances. Include assessment for both persistent/permanent impairment and episodic/fluctuating impairment arising from the above factors.
4. Analyze the degree of match or mismatch between "decision-critical" essential job demands and medical/neurocognitive capacity (impairments). Is job-related critical decision making impaired and, if so, how severely?
5. Negotiate solutions with the employer and worker so that job requirements are met. This may include a formulation of restrictions and limitations [14].

One implication of the distinction between "safety-sensitive" and "decision-critical" workers may be that some

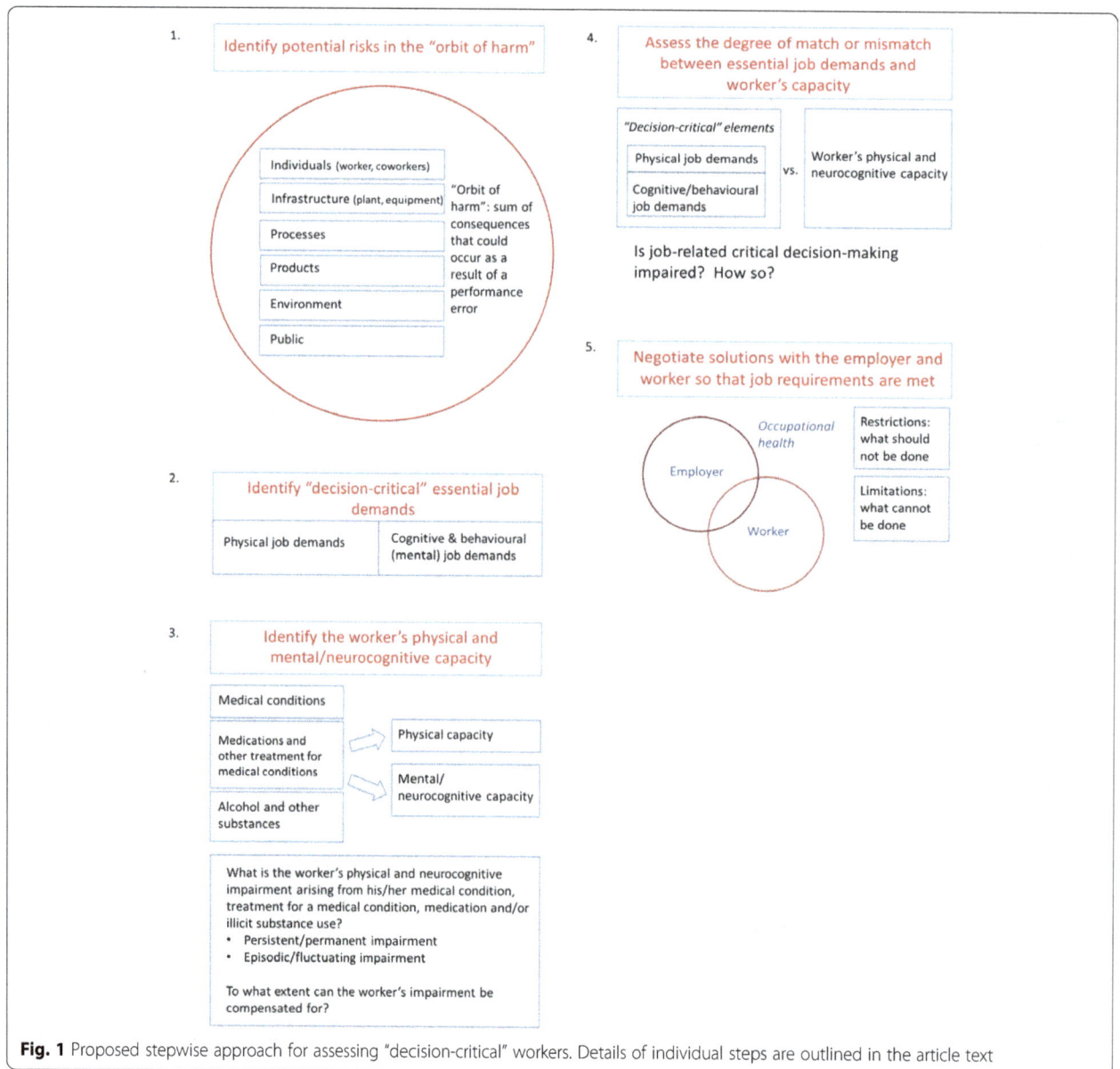

Fig. 1 Proposed stepwise approach for assessing "decision-critical" workers. Details of individual steps are outlined in the article text

workers who are currently classified as "safety-sensitive" should be reclassified as "decision-critical" workers. Another implication of this new categorization of workers is that additional fitness to work evaluation frameworks may be required to assist occupational health professionals in evaluating "decision-critical" workers, as current guidance has been written for "safety-sensitive" or "safety-critical" workers [2, 3], or workers at large. Finally, it is unclear whether certain programs and policies applicable to "safety-sensitive" workers (e.g. workplace drug and alcohol policies and testing programs) can be justified for "decision-critical" workers as well.

Conclusions

To our knowledge, the classification of "decision-critical" workers as a distinct group from "safety-sensitive" workers has not been described previously in the published literature, but this separation provides clarity and utility for occupational health practitioners. Firstly, such a category would allow a narrower and conceptually clearer definition of "safety-sensitive work." Secondly, our description of "decision-critical" work identifies a group of workers whose fitness for work has important occupational and societal implications, and who have not so far been the focus of occupational health professionals. An existing occupational health practice of performing medical assessments of "safety-sensitive" workers can be applied to a broader range of workers in "decision-critical" occupations. We hope the methodology we outline will add validity and reliability to the fitness evaluation of workers in occupations where decision-making is an essential job requirement (e.g. physicians [15]). An advantage of this approach is to convert some questions of putative risk to those of capacity, as these terms are outlined in the popular reference by the American Medical Association [14], and assist treating clinicians in formulating specific, actionable recommendations about fitness to work. The approach we outline is empirical and clinical, as research on developing well-validated measures of cognitive and behavioural job demands, and cognitive ability is ongoing. Judgment and insight are difficult to formally assess by generalist physicians, and poor insight and judgment may exist in the absence of an underlying medical condition. Formal validation of the utility of differentiating between "safety-sensitive" and "decision-critical" workers is required through future research.

Appendix
Case vignettes
Case vignette 1
A Lawyer in a large family legal practice has been observed consuming alcohol over his lunch hour and, at times, in his office throughout the afternoon. On several

occasions he was inaccessible to senior partners, clients, and family members. His appearance in the workplace and regular absences commonly resulted in frequently missed deadlines, miscommunication with clients and partners, and inaccuracies in legal documents. After several meetings with the managing partners regarding his absenteeism and the impact of alcohol use on his work, he was terminated from his position.

Discussion: Professional workers [16] (e.g. lawyers [17, 18] and physicians [19, 20] and workers in higher occupational grades [21], many of whom would be considered "decision-critical" workers, are at risk of substance use disorders, and may encounter special barriers to proper assessment and treatment. An untreated Alcohol Use Disorder may adversely impact an individual's cognitive processes, behaviour, and presentation. This may result in substantial disruption in professional occupational activities, to the detriment of clients, organizations and institutions. Social stigma may deter highly functioning "decision-critical" workers from seeking help for problematic alcohol consumption or substance use, leading to a delay in diagnosis and treatment during which the "decision-critical" worker may continue in a workplace role with substantial responsibilities.

Case vignette 2
A Store Manager working in a community mall presented with a 2-year history of episodes of forgetfulness. She additionally reported sleep disturbance, and decreased energy. Her symptoms made it difficult for her to process orders and inventory, oversee staff, and, on one occasion, secure the store at the time the fire alarm was sounded. Part of her duties included being the person in charge of responses to emergencies in the store. She was diagnosed with Alzheimer's disease after a neurological assessment.

Discussion: Workers with cognitive disorders (e.g. dementia) may present for a fitness to work assessment due to concerns about consistency, judgment, cognitive capacity, and predictability of mental functioning. Some occupational groups (e.g. lawyers, teachers and counsellors) are highly "decision-critical" in having significant cognitive and behavioural job requirements, and workplace performance concerns may be a presenting feature of cognitive disorders in such workers. The physician who is asked to assess a worker who holds a "decision-critical" post should elucidate the specific occupational requirements and attempt to determine whether the worker's functional ability to meet the essential job demands is impaired. Of note, it may be that a "decision-critical" worker is required to exercise insight and judgment only during exceptional workplace events, not on an everyday basis.

Case vignette 3

A Team Leader in a high-profile advertising firm with a history of anxiety reported excessive worries about an upcoming internal company merger. He expressed that his worries about daily activities (i.e., chores, self care, finances) were out of control and were exacerbated by the thought of incorporating additional employees under his oversight. He was often preoccupied with extraneous tasks and thoughts when faced with having to restructure his department. His worries often led to physical symptoms including feelings of panic, upset stomach, shortness of breath, and increased psychomotor agitation.

Discussion: Individuals with Generalized Anxiety Disorder demonstrate impaired judgment, inattention, and fatigue, which may result in substantial impairment in occupational duties. Additionally, somatization may be a component of the presentation, and lead to an extensive work-up for an underlying medical condition (e.g. a work-up for cardiac causes of chest pain), which can raise concerns about fitness to work in both "safety-sensitive" and "decision-critical" roles.

Case vignette 4

A Surgeon was noted to behave erratically in his interactions with patients. Additionally, he had had a number of interactions with coworkers that were perceived as disrespectful, raising concerns as to his ability to continue to function safely in the hospital. A complaint was made to his regulatory college. He was referred for an assessment of his fitness to practice, and diagnosed with a major mood disorder, which had impacted his cognitive capacity. After treatment, he was able to successfully return to the operating theatre, albeit under supervision. The prescribed antidepressants had the potential to result in tremor and sedation, necessitating ongoing assessment of his physical and mental status.

Discussion: Among health care workers, some (e.g. surgeons and anaesthesiologists in the operating theatre) may be considered "safety-sensitive", while others (e.g. with largely administrative or academic roles) may fall into the "decision-critical" category. The distinction can be difficult to make, but in cases where the likelihood of direct patient harm as a result of performance error is high, it may be reasonable to consider such health care workers to be "safety-sensitive" workers. The exact stratification may require a detailed review of job tasks and the working environment.

Competing interests
The authors declare that they have no competing interests.

Authors' contributions
XF and KJC conceived of the idea. XF and SS wrote the draft manuscript. All authors reviewed and revised the manuscript for intellectual content, and read and approved the final manuscript.

Acknowledgements
The authors gratefully acknowledge the assistance of Mr. Mat Milen in contributing to the preparation of illustrative case vignettes for this manuscript.

Funding
Open access publication of this manuscript was facilitated by institutional funding from the Department of Medicine, University of Alberta to SS.

Author details
[1]Division of Preventive Medicine, Department of Medicine, Faculty of Medicine and Dentistry, University of Alberta, 5-30F University Terrace, 8303-112 Street, Edmonton, AB T6G 2T4, Canada. [2]Department of Psychiatry, Faculty of Medicine and Dentistry, University of Alberta, Edmonton, AB, Canada. [3]Department of Community Health Sciences, Cumming School of Medicine, University of Calgary, Calgary, AB, Canada.

References
1. Palmer KT, Brown I, Hobson J, editors. Fitness for work: The medical aspects. 5th ed. Oxford: Oxford University Press; 2013. p. 564.
2. Hegmann KT, Weiss MS, Bowden K, Branco F, DuBrueler K, Els C, et al. ACOEM practice guidelines: opioids and safety-sensitive work. J Occup Environ Med. 2014;56:e46–53.
3. Railway Association of Canada. Canadian railway medical rules handbook, February 2016 edition. Ottawa: Railway Association of Canada; 2016.
4. Serra C, Rodriguez MC, Delclos GL, Plana M, Lopez LIG, Benavides FG. Criteria and methods used for the assessment of fitness for work: a systematic review. Occup Environ Med. 2007;64:304–12.
5. Canadian Medical Association. CMA driver's guide: Determining medical fitness to operate motor vehicles. 8th ed. Canadian Medical Association; 2012.
6. Yale SH, Hansotia P, Knapp D, Ehrfurth J. Neurologic conditions: Assessing medical fitness to drive. Clin Med Res. 2003;1:177–88.
7. The British Psychological Society. Fitness to drive and cognition: A document of the multi-disciplinary working party on acquired neuropsychological deficits and fitness to drive 1999. Leicester: The British Psychological Society; 2001.
8. Hartenbaum N and Janiga D. Medical fitness to drive in the transportation industry and the impact on public safety: Recommended actions [Internet]. American College of Occupational and Environmental Medicine; 2012 May. Available from: http://www.acoem.org/Transportation_PublicSafety.aspx
9. De Valck E, Smeekens L, Vantrappen L. Periodic psychological examination of train drivers' fitness in Belgium. J Occup Environ Med. 2015;57:445–52.
10. Occupational Health, Safety and Workers' Compensation. Job demands analysis procedure manual: behavioural/cognitive job demands analysis. Toronto: City of Toronto; 2003.
11. Lysaght R, Shaw L, Almas A, Jogia A, Larmour-Trode S. Toward improved measurement of cognitive and behavioural work demands. Work. 2008;31:11–20.
12. Phillips JA, Holland MG, Baldwin DD, Meuleveld L, Mueller KL, Perkison B, et al. Marijuana in the workplace: Guidance for occupational health professionals and employers. J Occup Environ Med. 2015;57:459–75.
13. Gold LH, Anfang SA, Drukteinis AM, Metzner JL, Price M, Wall BW, et al. AAPL practice guideline for the forensic evaluation of psychiatric disability. J Am Acad Psychiatry Law. 2008;36(4 Suppl):S3–S50.
14. Talmage JB, Melhorn JM, Hyman MH. AMA guides to the evaluation of work ability and return to work. 2nd ed. USA: American Medical Association; 2011.
15. Anfang SA, Faulkner LR, Fromson JA, Gendel MH. The American Psychiatric Association's resource document on guidelines for psychiatric fitness-for-duty evaluations of physicians. J Am Acad Psychiatry Law. 2005;33:85–8.
16. Coombs. Drug-impaired professionals. Cambridge: Harvard University Press; 2000.

17. Shore ER. The relationship of gender balance at work, family responsibilities and workplace characteristics to drinking among male and female attorneys. J Stud Alcohol. 1997;58:297–302.

18. Association of American Law Schools (AALS). Report of the AALS Special Committee on Problems of Substance Abuse in the Law Schools. Journal of Legal Education. 1994;44:35–80.

19. Weir E. Substance abuse among physicians. Can Med Assoc J. 2000;162:1730.

20. O'Connor PG, Spickard Jr A. Physician impairment by substance abuse. Med Clin North Am. 1997;81:1037–52.

21. Head J, Stansfeld SA, Siegrist J. The psychosocial work environment and alcohol dependence: a prospective study. Occup Environ Med. 2004;61:219–24.

17

Vibration thresholds in carpal tunnel syndrome assessed by multiple frequency vibrometry

Magnus Flondell[1,4], Birgitta Rosén[1,4], Gert Andersson[2,5], Tommy Schyman[3], Lars B. Dahlin[1,4] and Anders Björkman[1,4*] (iD)

Abstract

Background: Carpal tunnel syndrome (CTS) is the most common compression neuropathy, but there is no gold standard for establishing the diagnosis. The ability to feel vibrations in the fingertips is dependent on the function in cutaneous receptors and afferent nerves. Our aim was to investigate vibration perception thresholds (VPTs) in patients with CTS using multi-frequency vibrometry.

Methods: Sixty-six patients (16 men and 50 women) with CTS, diagnosed from clinical signs and by electroneurography, and 66 matched healthy controls were investigated with multi-frequency vibrometry. The VPTs were assessed at seven frequencies (8, 16, 32, 64, 125, 250, and 500 Hz) in the index finger and little finger bilaterally. The severity of the CTS was graded according to Padua and the patient's subjective symptoms were graded according to the Boston carpal tunnel questionnaire. Touch thresholds were assessed using the Semmes-Weinstein monofilaments.

Results: Patients with CTS had significantly higher VPTs at all frequencies in the index finger and in 6 out of 7 frequencies in the little finger compared to the controls. However, the VPT was not worse in patients with more severe CTS. Patients with unilateral CTS showed significantly higher VPTs in the affected hand. There were no correlations between VPTs and electrophysiological parameters, subjective symptoms, or touch threshold.

Conclusions: Patients with CTS had impaired VPTs at all frequencies compared to the controls. Since the VPTs are dependent on function in peripheral receptors and their afferent nerves, multi-frequency vibrometry could possibly lead to diagnosis of CTS.

Keywords: Carpal tunnel syndrome, Vibrometry, Sensibility, Touch thresholds, Vibrotactile sense, Vibration perception threshold

Background

Carpal tunnel syndrome (CTS), where the median nerve is compressed in the carpal tunnel, is the most common compression neuropathy [1] with a prevalence in the general population of 2.7–5.8% [2]. CTS is known to affect both large- and small-diameter myelinated nerve fibers and also unmyelinated nerve fibers [3]. There is no "gold standard" for the diagnosis of CTS, which is generally based on a medical history of sensory disturbances and pain in median nerve-innervated fingers [4] in combination with positive clinical tests. In patients with atypical symptoms and signs, an electroneurography (ENeG) is often used to support the diagnosis. However, there is considerable controversy regarding the need for ENeG in patients with suspected CTS. Some consider ENeG to be mandatory before planning surgery for CTS [5], while others question the need for ENeG [6]. Frequently quoted reasons for not using ENeG in the diagnostic work-up for suspected CTS include treatment delay, inconvenience, patient discomfort, costs, the need for specialist competence to perform and interpret the investigation, and poor correlation between ENeG and clinical symptoms [7, 8].

* Correspondence: anders.bjorkman@med.lu.se
[1]Department of Hand Surgery, Skåne University Hospital, Jan Waldenströms gata 5, 20502 Malmö, SE, Sweden
[4]Department of Translational Medicine – Hand Surgery, Lund University, Malmö, Sweden
Full list of author information is available at the end of the article

The ability to feel vibrations, i.e. vibrotactile sense, is dependent on the function in cutaneous receptors and large-diameter (Aβ) afferent nerves. The vibration perception threshold (VPT), which is the lowest intensity that can be perceived at a particular frequency, is known to be impaired early in different neuropathies [9–11]. Because of this, various methods have been proposed to analyze the VPTs. The VPT can be assessed at a single frequency using a tuning fork (128 Hz) or by vibrometry (100–120 Hz). A technique, multi-frequency vibrometry, whereby the VPT is assessed at seven different frequencies has been shown to increase the sensitivity of detecting neuropathies compared to when a single frequency is used [9, 12, 13].

Altered VPTs at different frequencies may reflect dysfunction of different mechanoreceptors, such as the Pacinian corpuscles (sensitive at a maximum of 250 Hz), the Meissner corpuscles (5–50 Hz), and the Merkel corpuscles (< 15 Hz) and their associated Aβ-sensory fibers [12]. Thus, assessment of VPTs at multiple frequencies has been suggested as a diagnostic tool in diabetic neuropathy and in patients with neuropathy due to long-term exposure to hand-held vibrating tools [14, 15]. Because function in Aβ-sensory fibers is also affected early in compression neuropathies, evaluation of VPTs at different frequencies may be useful in the diagnostic work-up of patients with suspected CTS [14]. Our aim was to investigate VPTs using multi-frequency vibrometry in patients with idiopathic CTS.

Methods

Patients

Over a 6-year period (2009–2015) patients who were referred to the Department of Hand Surgery, Malmö, Sweden with suspected CTS were screened by a hand surgeon for participation in the study.

The inclusion criteria were as follows: subjective symptoms of CTS for more than 3 months, classic or probable CTS according to Katz' hand diagram [4, 16], clinical signs of CTS with a positive Tinels and Phalens test, age between 18 and 70 years, and an ENeG with a fractionated sensory nerve conduction velocity for the median nerve across the wrist of 40 m/s or less. Exclusion criteria were: having been operated for CTS previously, prior wrist or carpal fracture, diabetes, thyroid disease, rheumatoid arthritis, neurological disease, drug abuse, complete conduction block on ENeG or previous regular exposure to hand-held vibrating tools. Participants had to be able to read and understand Swedish in order to be able to fill out the patient-rated outcome measures (PROMs) in the proper way.

For each patient, a similar-aged (within 5 years), gender-matched, and handedness-matched healthy control was identified from a population study cohort collected at our clinic. The same exclusion criteria as used for the study patients were applied. Furthermore, the controls were not to have any sensory deficiencies, pain in the hands, or previous neuropathies.

Assessments

Patients were subjected to a clinical an electrophysiological examination in order to support the diagnosis of CTS. Furthermore, patients and controls were examined with multi-frequency vibrometry.

Clinical assessment

A specialist in hand surgery did all clinical examinations and secured the diagnosis. Subjective symptoms were assesses using Katz' hand diagram [4, 16]. A clinical evaluation was performed where the patients were assessed for weakness in thumb abduction and for signs of atrophy in the thenar muscles. Furthermore Tinels test was performed on the median nerve just proximal to the flexor retinaculum, the test was considered positive if the patient experienced tingling in median nerve innervated fingers during the test [17]. Phalens test for carpal tunnel syndrome was performed as well. The test was considered positive if the patient experienced tingling in median nerve innervated fingers within one minute after commencing the test [17].

Electrophysiology

A standard electrophysiological assessment (ENeG) was performed on both arms. Orthodromic sensory ENeG was performed by stimulating the thumb, the index finger and the long finger for the median nerve and the little finger for assessment of the ulnar nerve. The stimulation ring electrodes were placed at the proximal interphalangeal and distal interphalangeal joints for the index, long, and little finger and just proximal and distal to the interphalangeal joint of the thumb. Recording electrodes were placed over the respective nerves at the proximal wrist crease and three cm more proximal. Fractionated, antidromic sensory neurography was performed on the median nerve with recording ring electrodes placed over the proximal and distal interphalangeal joints of the long finger. The stimulation sites were in the palm, at the proximal wrist crease and proximal to the elbow. The nerve conduction velocity in the segment between the wrist crease and the palm was calculated.

For motor conduction studies, recordings were performed from the abductor pollicis brevis muscle (innervated by the median nerve) and abductor digiti minimi muscle (innervated by the ulnar nerve) with stimulation of the respective nerves 80 mm proximal to the electrode placed over the muscle. The patient's skin temperature was over 30 °C during the ENeG. The ENeG included sensory conduction velocity (SCV), sensory nerve action potential (SNAP), and distal motor latency (DML), and was performed on a Nicolet Viking Select Electromyograph (Nicolet Brand Products, Middleton, WI, USA). All examinations were performed by the same technician and were evaluated independently by the same neurophysiologist.

Based on the results from ENeG, the severity of each patient's CTS was classified according to Padua et al. [18]. However, one inclusion criteria was a fractionated sensory nerve conduction velocity for the median nerve across the wrist of 40 m/s or less. Furthermore, patients with a complete conduction block were excluded. This means that only patients graded as mild and moderate CTS, according to Padua, were eligible for the study.

Multi-frequency vibrometry
Vibration perception thresholds were measured at multiple frequencies using a VibroSense Meter® (Vibrosense Dynamics, Malmö, Sweden) in accordance with previously described technique [19]. Before the examination, the operator explained the examination procedure to the subject. Essentially, the median and ulnar nerves were evaluated by recording bilateral vibration thresholds at the finger pulps of the index finger (innervated by median nerve) and little finger (innervated by the ulnar nerve) bilaterally. The patients wore acoustic ear-muffs to avoid bias from sound emitted by the vibration pin of the measurement unit. Since sensibility varies with temperature [20], the finger temperature was monitored and had to be above 30 °C before assessment. The patient placed the finger to be examined on the vibration pin. When the patient perceived vibration, he or she indicated this by pressing a switch and by holding it depressed until vibrations were no longer felt. The VibroSense Meter® administers vibration at seven different frequencies (8, 16, 32, 64, 125, 250, and 500 Hz), and a median threshold value, expressed in decibel (dB), was recorded for each frequency from the index and little fingers of both hands. The examination, index and little fingers of both hands, took 20 min to complete. The patients and controls were examined in the same way, except that the controls were only assessed in the dominant index finger and little finger. All examinations were performed by one out of two technician who had more than 5-years of experience in doing multifrequency vibrometry.

Assessment of touch threshold
Assessment of cutaneous touch/pressure thresholds was done on the tip of the index and little fingers on both hands in patients with CTS, and on the index finger of the dominant hand in controls, using a set of 20 Semmes-Weinstein monofilaments (SWM) (North Coast Medical Inc., Gilroy, CA, USA). Assessment was started with SWM no. 2.83 (representing a pressure of 70 mg)

and thereafter continued in an ascending or descending order depending on the answer for the first filament. Each filament was applied three times according to a standardized procedure [21]. Results were quantified from 0 to 20, representing the 20 monofilaments, with 20 corresponding to the lowest threshold. To familiarize the test subject with the test procedure and to eliminate the possibility of biased results due to learning effects, testing for touch threshold on the third digit was performed before testing the study fingers.

Patient-rated outcome measures (PROMs)
Symptom severity score (SSS) from the Boston questionnaire [22], which assess subjective severity of symptom in patients with CTS, was recorded at the time of inclusion.

Statistical analysis
IBM SPSS Statistics (Statistical Package for the Social Sciences, version 23 for Mac; IBM Corp., Armonk, NY, USA) was used for the statistical assessment of data. Values are presented as median and interquartile range (IQR).

As this was a matched-control study, there is no need to adjust for confounding variables when comparing cases and controls. Due to this, the Wilcoxon signed-rank test was used to evaluate any statistical difference between patients with CTS and the control group. The same method was used to evaluate whether there was any difference between hands in the same patient. When comparing subgroups according to Padua, the Mann-Whitney U-test was used for continuous and nominal variables. Fisher's exact test was used for categorical variables. Spearman's correlation for non-parametric testing was used for investigation of correlations. Any p-value less than 0.05 were considered significant.

Results
Demographics
Informed consent was obtained from 66 patients (16 men and 50 women, median age 50 years, IQR 13) (Table 1) and 66 age- and gender-matched healthy controls (median age 46.5, IQR 11). Of the 66 patients, 11 were rated as having mild CTS (abnormal SCV and normal DML) and 55 having moderate CTS (abnormal SCV and abnormal DML) according to Padua [18] (Table 1). Thirty-eight patients had unilateral CTS.

There were significantly more women in the group with mild CTS. Age, PROMs and touch thresholds were not significantly different between the Padua groups.

Multi-frequency vibration perception thresholds
The VPTs were significantly higher, indicating poorer capability to detect vibrations, at all frequencies in the index finger in patients with CTS than in the healthy controls (Table 2). In addition, VPTs in the little finger were

Table 1 Characteristics of patients, in total and sub-divided based on severity according to Padua

CTS grade	Mild (n = 11)	Moderate (n = 55)	Total (n = 66)	P-value
Age, years	46[15]	50[13]	50[13]	0.67
Sex, F/M	11/0	39/16	50/16	*0.05*
Bilat./unilat.	2/9	26/29	28/38	0.10
ENeG SCV, m/s	36[7]	30[6]	31[6]	*0.001*
ENeG SNAP, μV	12[9]	5[5]	6[7]	*0.03*
ENeG DML, ms	3.9[0.3]	5.3[1.0]	5.0[1.2]	*< 0.001*
SSS, score	2.72[1.4]	2.45[0.78]	2.55[0.73]	0.34
SWM, no.of filament	18[1]	18[2]	18[2]	0.96

Data are median [IQR]. *P*-values are based on Mann-Whitney U-test for continuous and nominal data and on Fisher's exact test for categorical variables
SCV sensory conduction velocity, *SNAP* sensory nerve action potential, *DML* distal motor latency, *SSS* symptom severity score, *SWM*
Semmes-Weinstein monofilament
Values in italics represent statistically significant differences

significantly higher at all frequencies in patients with CTS than in the controls, except at the highest frequency (500 Hz) (Table 2). When we compared patients who were classified as having mild CTS with their individual controls, the patients had significantly higher VPTs in the index finger at all frequencies except at 500 Hz. Patients with moderate CTS had significantly higher VPTs at all frequencies (Table 3). However, when we compared VPTs in the index finger between patients who were classified as having mild and moderate CTS, there were no significant differences.

When we compared VPTs between the index finger and little finger in the hand with CTS, the VPTs were significantly higher in the index finger at 16, 250, and 500 Hz. However, they were significantly lower in the index finger at 32 and 64 Hz.

Thirty-eight patients had unilateral CTS, as confirmed by symptoms, clinical signs, and ENeG. In these patients, the VPTs in the index finger of the hand with CTS were significantly higher at all frequencies, than in the index finger of the healthy hand.

Correlations

There were no correlations between the VPTs and touch threshold, SSS, or ENeG parameters.

Discussion

This study showed that patients with CTS had significantly higher VPTs in the finger pulps of both the index finger and the little finger than healthy controls, at high as well as low frequencies. Furthermore, patients with unilateral CTS had significantly higher VPTs in the index finger of the hand with CTS than in the index finger of the healthy hand.

Electrodiagnostic studies are often used as reference standard for the diagnosis of CTS. However, these studies have false-positive and false-negative results, and the evidence for the role of electrodiagnostic tests in the diagnostic work-up of patients with suspected CTS is being questioned [17]. ENeG assesses function in the nerves from the basal phalanx of the fingers and proximal up into the forearm, whereas analysis of VPTs at different frequencies assesses function in both the afferent nerves and the peripheral receptors. Thus, compared to ENeG, a multi-frequency vibrometry can provide additional information that may be valuable in some patients.

Based on ENeG, which is thought to reflect the degree of compression of the median nerve, Padua et al. [18] classified CTS into six groups with mild and moderate being the two most common, constituting about 60% of

Table 2 Vibration perception thresholds in patients with carpal tunnel syndrome (CTS) and in healthy controls

Index finger	8 Hz	16 Hz	32 Hz	64 Hz	125 Hz	250 Hz	500 Hz
CTS (n = 66)	108.6[4.9]	115.9[5.1]	117.5[7.8]	109.0[11.7]	110.3[10.3]	120.0[11.3]	133.4[13.1]
Controls (n = 66)	105.0[6.6]	112.5[7.7]	113.1[6.1]	103.1[7.0]	102.0[9.7]	110.1[12.7]	125.9[13.2]
P-value	*< 0.001*	*0.001*	*< 0.001*	*< 0.001*	*< 0.001*	*< 0.001*	*< 0.001*
Little finger	8 Hz	16 Hz	32 Hz	64 Hz	125 Hz	250 Hz	500 Hz
CTS (n = 66)	106.9[7.1]	115.1[7.0]	120.1[7.2]	111.2[10.1]	108.6[9.5]	115.4[14.5]	127.6[14.8]
Controls (n = 66)	105.0[5.1]	111.9[4.7]	115.4[10.1]	107.4[9.8]	104.1[11.2]	111.0[10.0]	125.9[16.2]
P-value	*0.009*	*0.005*	*< 0.001*	*< 0.001*	*0.001*	*0.005*	0.17

Vibration perception thresholds are expressed in dB. Data are median [IQR]. P-values are based on Wilcoxon's signed-rank test
Values in italics represent statistically significant differences

Table 3 Vibration perception thresholds in patients with carpal tunnel syndrome (CTS) sub-divided according to Padua

Index finger	8 Hz	16 Hz	32 Hz	64 Hz	125 Hz	250 Hz	500 Hz
Mild CTS (n = 11)	108.5[4.5]	116.2[10.0]	119.1[9.1]	109.0[11.9]	109.8[8.2]	117.8[10.2]	132.4[9.5]
Controls (n = 11)	99.4[6.3]	108.2[8.5]	107.8[7.3]	101.0[3.9]	97.2[9.6]	108.3[14.3]	125.3[17.1]
P-value	*0.011*	*0.041*	*0.006*	*0.008*	*0.016*	*0.050*	0.062
Moderate CTS (n = 55)	108.9[5.3]	115.6 [4.3]	117.3[7.8]	109.0[11.6]	110.5[10.7]	120.4[12.3]	133.9[15.4]
Controls (n = 55)	105.8[6.0]	113.3 [7.5]	113.6[5.0]	104.9[7.4]	102.8[9.8]	110.2[11.3]	125.9[12.7]
P-values	*0.009*	*0.010*	*0.001*	*0.001*	*< 0.001*	*< 0.001*	*0.003*

Vibration perception thresholds are expressed in dB. Data are median [IQR]. P-values are based on Wilcoxon's signed-rank test
Values in italics represent statistically significant differences

patients. It has been suggested that multi frequency vibrometry can help in staging the degree of nerve compression [14]. However, we could not detect any difference in VPTs between mild and moderate CTS. The differences in ENeG parameters between mild and moderate CTS are subtle. We suggest that studies involving patients from all Padua stages should be done in order to determine whether analysis of VPTs at multiple frequencies can be used to stage the degree of compression of the median nerve in patients with CTS.

The present study corroborates previous results showing pathological nerve conduction [23] and increased VPTs also in the ulnar nerve-innervated little finger in patents with CTS [11]. The carpal tunnel and Guyon's canal - where the ulnar nerve is located - are located next to each other in the wrist, and we speculate that the increased pressure in the carpal tunnel causing the CTS is also transferred to Guyon's canal and the ulnar nerve. Another possibility for the pathological nerve conduction and increased VPTs in both the median and ulnar nerves is a pathological process in the forearm and wrist that results in neuropathy in both the median nerve and the ulnar nerve. CTS is known to result in structural as well as functional changes in the primary somatosensory cortex in the brain [24]. Thus, a third possible explanation, for reduced sensation in the little finger, is that these cerebral changes also effect neurons processing sensory information from the ulnar nerve.

A frequently quoted reason for not using ENeG in the diagnostic work-up for CTS is that there is no absolute correlation of results from nerve conduction studies with clinical symptoms. This was also the case in the present study, where there was no statistically significant correlation between subjective experience of symptoms assessed with the SSS and ENeG or VPTs in patients with mild and moderate CTS according to Padua. However, a correlation between neurophysiological severity, expressed on the seven point Canterbury scale, and surgical prognosis have been described [25]. Furthermore, costs, patient discomfort, and the need for specialized staff have all been advocated as reasons for not doing

ENeG in patients who are suspected of having CTS. However, multi-frequency vibrometry also needs specialized staff and carries a cost, but there is no discomfort. An important difference between the two examinations is that multi-frequency vibrometry requires patient cooperation. In an ENeG examination, the patient has to endure the discomfort from the stimulation current, but patient cooperation is not needed for doing the examination. On the other hand, multi-frequency vibrometry is completely dependent on a cooperating patient who understands the examination, and who can remain focused during the procedure; thus, an unfocused patient and not a disorder in peripheral receptors or the peripheral nerve might cause a pathological VPT.

An alternative diagnostic tool for assessing patients with suspected CTS is neuromuscular ultrasound. Ultrasound of the median nerve has shown strong evidence for accuracy in diagnosing CTS [26] and it is completely painless, specific and sensitive and does not require patient cooperation however, it needs specialized staff.

Further studies are needed to determine the benefit of multi-frequency vibrometry, ENeG and ultrasound, both when they are used as sole diagnostic instrument but also when they are used in combination, for the diagnosis of CTS.

This study had some limitations. Although CTS is common, recruitment of patients was slow for three main reasons; 1. A large number of patients referred to the clinic due to suspected CTS did not fulfill the inclusion criteria of having a fractionated sensory nerve conduction velocity across the wrist of 40 m/s or less. 2. A number of patients were unable to manage the PROMs due to language problems. 3. Many patients had the impression that CTS can only be treated with prompt carpal tunnel release, and knew people who were satisfied with this procedure, so they did not want to participate in any studies that could delay their operation.

Conclusions

The results of this study suggest that multi-frequency vibrometry could have a role in the diagnosis of CTS.

However, we do not consider that this method would be applicable to clinical routine, as a diagnostic tool, at this stage. Further studies are needed to identify the role of multi-frequency vibrometry in the diagnostic work-up of patients with suspected CTS. Of special interest is the possibility of detecting pathology in the peripheral receptors of the fingers, as seen for example in patients with sensory disturbances due to long-term exposure to hand-held vibrating tools. These patients can have symptoms that mimic the symptoms seen in patients with CTS. It is also well-known that patients can have clinical symptoms of CTS, a normal ENeG, and can improve after median nerve decompression. It would be interesting to investigate whether such patients have normal VPTs, or whether a normal multi-frequency vibrometry result can rule out CTS.

Acknowledgements
Thanks to Helena Erixson and Linda Linné for performing vibrometry examinations.

Funding
The authors received financial support from the Regional Research Fund of Region Skåne, Sweden; from Skåne University Hospital, Lund University, Sweden; and from VINNOVA, Sweden.

Authors' contributions
MF, AB, BR, GA, LD contributed to patient data acquisition, analysis and interpretation of data, preparation and review of the manuscript. TS contributed to statistical analysis of the data and review of the manuscript. All the authors have read and approved the final version of the manuscript.

Competing interests
The authors declare that they have no competing interests.

Author details
[1]Department of Hand Surgery, Skåne University Hospital, Jan Waldenströms gata 5, 20502 Malmö, SE, Sweden. [2]Departments of Neurophysiology, Skåne University Hospital, Malmö, Sweden. [3]Department of Clinical Studies Sweden – Forum South, Skåne University Hospital, Malmö, Sweden. [4]Department of Translational Medicine – Hand Surgery, Lund University, Malmö, Sweden. [5]Department of Clinical Sciences, Lund University, Lund, Sweden.

References
1. Chung KC. Current status of outcomes research in carpal tunnel surgery. Hand (N Y). 2006;1:9–13.
2. Papanicolaou GD, McCabe SJ, Firrell J. The prevalence and characteristics of nerve compression symptoms in the general population. J Hand Surg Am. 2001;26:460–6.
3. Schmid AB, Bland JD, Bhat MA, Bennett DL. The relationship of nerve fibre pathology to sensory function in entrapment neuropathy. Brain. 2014;137:3186–99.
4. Katz JN, Stirrat CR. A self-administered hand diagram for the diagnosis of carpal tunnel syndrome. J Hand Surg Am. 1990;15:360–3.
5. Bland JD. Carpal tunnel syndrome. BMJ. 2007;335:343–6.
6. Smith NJ. Nerve conduction studies for carpal tunnel syndrome: essential prelude to surgery or unnecessary luxury? J Hand Surg Br. 2002;27:83–5.
7. American Association of Electrodiagnostic Medicine AAoN, American Academy of Physical Medicine and Rehabilitation. Practice parameter for electrodiagnostic studies in carpal tunnel syndrome: summary statement. Muscle Nerve. 1993;16:1390-1.
8. Mainous AG, Nelson KR. How often are preoperative electrodiagnostic studies obtained for carpal tunnel syndrome in a Medicaid population? Muscle Nerve. 1996;19:256–7.
9. Stromberg T, Dahlin LB, Lundborg G. Vibrotactile sense in the hand-arm vibration syndrome. Scand J Work Environ Health. 1998;24:495–502.
10. Gin H, Rigalleau V, Baillet L, Rabemanantsoa C. Comparison between monofilament, tuning fork and vibration perception tests for screening patients at risk of foot complication. Diabetes Metab. 2002;28:457–61.
11. Thomsen NO, Cederlund R, Speidel T, Dahlin LB. Vibrotactile sense in patients with diabetes and carpal tunnel syndrome. Diabet Med. 2011;28:1401–6.
12. Dahlin E, Ekholm E, Gottsater A, Speidel T, Dahlin LB. Impaired vibrotactile sense at low frequencies in fingers in autoantibody positive and negative diabetes. Diabetes Res Clin Pract. 2013;100:e46–50.
13. Ellemann K, Nielsen KD, Poulsgaard L, Smith T. Vibrotactilometry as a diagnostic tool in ulnar nerve entrapment at the elbow. Scand J Plast Reconstr Surg Hand Surg. 1999;33:93–7.
14. Lundborg G, Lie-Stenström AK, Sollerman C, Strömberg T, Pyykkö J. Digital vibrogram: a new diagnostic tool for sensory testing in compression neuropathy. J Hand Surg. 1986;11A:693–9.
15. Dahlin LB, Granberg V, Rolandsson O, Rosen I, Dahlin E, Sundkvist G. Disturbed vibrotactile sense in finger pulps in patients with type 1 diabetes–correlations with glycaemic level, clinical examination and electrophysiology. Diabet Med. 2011;28:1045–52.
16. Keith MW, Masear V, Chung KC, Amadio PC, Andary M, Barth RW, et al. American Academy of Orthopaedic surgeons clinical practice guideline on the treatment of carpal tunnel syndrome. J Bone Joint Surg Am. 2010;92:218–9.
17. Management of Carpal Tunnel Syndrome Evidence-Based Clinical Practice Guidelines: [database on the Internet]. 2016;98:1750-54. Available from: www.aaos.org/ctsguideline.
18. Padua L, Lo Monaco M, Padua R, Gregori B, Tonali P. Neurophysiological classification of carpal tunnel syndrome: assessment of 600 symptomatic hands. Ital J Neurol Sci. 1997;18:145–50.
19. Dahlin LB, Guner N, Elding Larsson H, Speidel T. Vibrotactile perception in finger pulps and in the sole of the foot in healthy subjects among children or adolescents. PLoS One. 2015;10:e0119753.
20. Lele PP, Weddell G, Williams CM. The relationship between heat transfer, skin temperature and cutaneous sensibility. J Physiol. 1954;126:206–34.
21. Bell-Krotoski J, Weinstein S, Weinstein C. Testing sensibility, including touch-pressure, two-point discrimination, point localization and vibration. J Hand Ther. 1993;6:114–23.
22. Levine DW, Simmons BP, Koris MJ, Daltroy LH, Hohl GG, Fossel AH, et al. A self-administered questionnaire for yhe assessment of severity of symptoms and functional status in carpal tunnel syndrome. J Bone Joint Surg. 1993;75A:1585–92.
23. Ginanneschi F, Milani P, Rossi A. Anomalies of ulnar nerve conduction in different carpal tunnel syndrome stages. Muscle Nerve. 2008;38:1155–60.
24. Maeda Y, Kim H, Kettner N, Kim J, Cina S, Malatesta C, et al. Rewiring the primary somatosensory cortex in carpal tunnel syndrome with acupuncture. Brain. 2017;140:914–27.
25. Bland JDP. Do nerve conduction studies predict the outcome of carpal tunnel syndrom? Muscle Nerve. 2001;24:935–40.
26. Cartwright MS, Hobson-Webb LD, Boon AJ, Alter KE, Hunt CH, Flores VH, et al. Evidence-based guideline: neuromuscular ultrasound for the diagnosis of carpal tunnel syndrome. Muscle Nerve. 2012;46:287–93.

18

Nurse-work instability and incidence of sick leave – results of a prospective study of nurses aged over 40

Melanie Klein[1,2], Stefanie Wobbe-Ribinski[2], Anika Buchholz[3], Albert Nienhaus[1,4] and Anja Schablon[1*]

Abstract

Background: The Nurse Work Instability Scale (Nurse-WIS) is an occupation-specific instrument that ascertains "work instability," the interval before restricted work ability or prolonged sick leave occurs. The objective of the study was to assess if nurses with a high risk baseline-score in the Nurse-WIS take longer periods of sick leave due to musculoskeletal diseases and/or psychological impairments than other nurses.

Methods: A total of 4500 nurses randomly selected from one of the largest health insurance funds in Germany (DAK-Gesundheit) were invited by letter to participate in the study. The participants answered a questionnaire at baseline and gave consent to a transfer of data concerning sick leave during the twelve months following completion of the questionnaire from the health insurance to the study centre. Sensitivity, specificity and positive and negative predictive values (PPV and NPV) for long-term sick leave were calculated. In order to analyze the association between the Nurse-WIS and sick leave during follow-up, a multiple ordinal logistic model (proportional odds model) was applied.

Results: A total of 1592 nurses took part in the study (response 35.6%). No loss of follow-up occurred. The number of nurses with a high score (20–28 points) in the Nurse-WIS was 628 (39.4%), and 639 (40.1%) had taken sick leave due to musculoskeletal diseases or psychological impairment during the follow-up period. The odds ratio for sick leave in nurses with a high Nurse-WIS score was 3.42 (95%CI 2.54–4.60). Sensitivity for long-term sick leave (< 42 days) was 64.1%, specificity 63.4%, PPV 17.0% and NPP 93.8%.

Conclusion: The German version of the Nurse-WIS predicts long-term sick leave, but the PPV is rather low. Combining questionnaire data with secondary data from a health insurer was feasible. Therefore further studies employing this combination of data are advisable.

Keywords: Nurse-work instability scale, Nurses, Long-term sick leave, Secondary data of a health insurer

Background

Demographic transition will lead to an increase in the demand for nurses in many countries [1–3]. However, nurses frequently suffer from musculoskeletal diseases [4–10], psychological impairments, burnout, or poor general health [11–14]. According to the Health Report of one of the largest statutory health insurance funds in Germany, the DAK-Gesundheit, nurses more often take sick leave, and for longer periods than other insured

* Correspondence: a.schablon@uke.de
[1]Centre of Excellence for Epidemiology and Health Care Research for Health Care Workers (CVcare), University Medical Center Hamburg-Eppendorf (UKE), Martinistr. 41a, 20521 Hamburg, Germany
Full list of author information is available at the end of the article

groups [15]. Diseases of the musculoskeletal system and psychological impairments are the most frequent causes of long-term sick leave. Moreover, long-term sick leave is often an intermediate stage on the way to early retirement [16], which is frequent among nurses [17]. Therefore it is important to maintain nurses' work ability. In order to achieve this goal, it appears sensible to offer interventions that allow nurses to remain healthy and motivated in their profession until retirement age. The most effective approach toward achieving this goal is to use multimodal interventions [18] or interventions that include persons with the initial symptoms of musculoskeletal disease [19–22]. However, no effective screening instrument has been available for early recognition of nurses at risk. The Nurse-Work Instability Scale (Nurse-WIS) is a questionnaire that seems to fulfill this requirement [23]. Work instability is the interval before restricted work ability when the subject has increasing difficulty in performing his or her duties at work, and can be ascertained with this occupation-specific instrument for nurses. Interventions during this interval can prevent impending loss of work ability. Thus early identification of work instability is the key to preventing the subject's situation from deteriorating, with the resulting loss in work ability [24–26]. The development and validation of the German version of the scale, were performed using a cohort of geriatric care workers [27, 28]. The study showed that the German version of the scale is an easy, reliable and valid instrument with moderate prognostic ability to ascertain impending sick leave. The questionnaire has not yet been validated for nurses. Therefore one goal of the study presented here was to assess the performance of the Nurse-WIS in a cohort of nurses. In addition, the scale was updated because it is desirable to perform screening tests in populations with a high prevalence or increased risk of the disease [29, 30]. For this reason, the Nurse-WIS was complemented by an entry criterion so that the scale is mainly used for nurses who exhibit the first signs of musculoskeletal disease but have not yet sought medical help. In addition, a cohort of nurses aged 40+ was selected, as long-term sick leave occurs more frequently with increasing age [15].

In the first study on the German version of the Nurse-WIS, information about sick leave was provided by the nurses themselves [27, 28]. In cooperation with DAK-Gesundheit the scale has now been applied in a prospective study in nurses. Because of this cooperation, it was possible to use the health insurance fund's secondary data on sick leave with the corresponding diagnoses. Therefore an additional objective of the study was to investigate the predictive value of the Nurse-WIS for the duration of sick leave. The hypothesis is that nurses with high risk according to the Nurse-WIS at baseline take longer periods of sick leave due to musculoskeletal diseases and/or psychological impairments than other nurses. This aspect is interesting as the probability of early retirement increases with longer periods of sick leave [31, 32]. Moreover, the model was used to explore whether the duration of sick leave is influenced by other factors such as age, gender, or frequently long and irregular working hours or rotating shifts.

Methods
Study design
In cooperation with DAK-Gesundheit, a prospective cohort study was performed with employed nurses aged 40 years and above. The study combined questionnaires and secondary insurance data.

Setting
The cohort was examined at two different points in time. Baseline measurements were performed in autumn 2011, when the nurses completed a standardised questionnaire.

The DAK-Gesundheit prepared a pseudonymised secondary dataset for the follow-up one year later (2012) and also reported which subjects were still unable to work on 31 December 2012. Continuations of sick-leaves into 2013 cannot be ruled out.

Participants and data protection
In order to fulfill all the guidelines on data protection, the process of recruitment of the cohort was done as specified by Scharnetzky et al. 2013 [33] as described here.

Definition of the cohort
A total of 4500 nurses were selected randomly from the DAK-Gesundheit database of insured persons, based on the following criteria:

- The person was a certified and registered nurse or nursing assistant (DEÜV Social Insurance Code *Occupation* Key 853 and 854).
- The person was professionally active, i.e. not unemployed or unwaged.
- The person was aged ≥40 years and ≤ 65 years.

In addition to these inclusion criteria, the following exclusion criteria were defined:

- Now working in another professional field (e.g. secretary).
- Receiving a pension for reduced work capacity before the survey period.
- Looking for work or taking parental leave.
- Leaving the DAK or death during the survey period.

Baseline
In order to guarantee data protection, the data of the defined cohort of nurses was pseudonymised. For this purpose, DAK-Gesundheit randomly generated an identification number (ID) for each nurse of the cohort. This ID was printed on the declaration of consent and on the questionnaire. At Baseline these and other study documents (participant information, data protection information, prepaid return envelope) were posted by the DAK-Gesundheit to the defined cohort. The participating nurses then returned the signed declaration of consent and the completed questionnaire to an independent and confidential study centre (University Medical Centre Hamburg-Eppendorf, German Centre for Health Services Research in Dermatology) in the prepaid envelope. The declaration of consent (with the name and signature of the study participant) was separated from the questionnaire there and sent to the

DAK-Gesundheit. The completed questionnaires were sent to the researcher at the CVcare (Competence Centre for Epidemiology and Health Services Research for Healthcare Professionals, University Medical Center Hamburg-Eppendorf).

Follow-up

For the follow-up, CVcare compiled a list with the IDs printed on the questionnaires and transmitted this list to DAK-Gesundheit. For this defined group, DAK-Gesundheit prepared a pseudonymised dataset with the secondary data, replacing name, address and other identification characteristics by the corresponding ID. A non-responder analysis was not possible, as all data relating to not participating nurses were deleted for data protection reasons. The dataset was then combined with the baseline data based on the ID by the CVcare researchers. In this way the researchers had no access to the declaration of consent with the name or signature of the study participant and DAK-Gesundheit had no access to the completed questionnaires. For analysis, the data from the baseline questionnaire was linked to the secondary data from the follow-up. In December 2013, DAK-Gesundheit provided administrative data records to the researcher.

This procedure was checked and approved by the Hamburg Commissioner for Data Protection and Freedom of Information. In addition, the Ethics Committee of the Hamburg Medical Association approved the study (No. PV3869).

Variables and data sources
Exposure

As mentioned above, the hypothesis is that nurses with a high risk score at baseline of the Nurse-WIS take longer periods of sick leave due to musculoskeletal diseases and/ or psychological impairments. The German version of the Nurse-WIS is based on the original English questionnaire of Gilworth et al. [23] and its underlying concept of work instability as described by Harling et al. [27, 28]. In the present study, an inclusion criterion was added to the German version of the Nurse-WIS in order to identify nurses who had experienced recent signs of a musculoskeletal disease. Only subjects who reported significant musculoskeletal symptoms (lasting more than two hours at a time) in the previous three months were asked to complete the Nurse-WIS. For those who did not fulfill this criterion, the score of the Nurse-WIS was considered as zero. The German version of the scale consists of 28 items covering different aspects of work instability, such as musculoskeletal complaints caused by certain tasks and different psychosocial factors. The individual questions in the scale can be answered with "agree" (=1) or "disagree" (=0) [23, 27]. To calculate the cumulative scores, the points are added up. The greater the value of this cumulative score,

the greater the risk of work instability. The score ranges from zero to 28 and is grouped into four categories. With 0 points, there is no risk, or the scale was not applied because of the initial question. With 1 to 9 points, there is a slight risk, with 10 to 19 points a moderate risk, and with 20 to 28 points a high risk is assumed.

Outcome variable

For the outcome variables, secondary insurance data of the DAK-Gesundheit on sick leave was used. This dataset included at least one ICD Code (International Statistical Classification of Diseases and Related Health Problems) for each period of sick leave. As previously stated, the secondary dataset included data for the follow-up year (2012) and also reported which subjects were still unable to work on 31 December 2012.

In the data record of the health insurance fund, you can only differentiate between main and secondary diagnoses for inpatient diagnoses, whereby the main diagnosis was used to create the outcome variable. For data from the outpatient sector, it is possible that several diagnoses are specified on sick leave, but no distinction is made between main and secondary diagnoses. For this reason, all diagnoses for the formation of the outcome variable were selected for the outpatient data as soon as a musculoskeletal or mental illness was present.

As described in the literature [36–38] diseases of the back and the upper extremities are of particular interest as occupational risk factors. Moreover disorders in psychological wellbeing, stress disorders and impairments such as depression and burnout are often associated with acute and chronic musculoskeletal diseases [39–41].

Based on the ICD Code and the corresponding number of days of absence in each individual period of sick leave, diverse outcome variables for sick leave due to a musculoskeletal (ICD Code M40-M54) and/or psychological impairment (ICD Code F32-F48, Z73) were defined as explained below.

Potential confounders

In addition to the Nurse-WIS, the standardised questionnaire at baseline contained questions concerning sociodemographic characteristics (e.g. gender, age, occupational training) and the occupational situation (e.g. length of service in that occupation) as well as questions concerning sick leave over the previous 12 months before baseline (2011). Accordingly, the secondary data set also includes data on occupation [DEÜV-Social Insurance Code], date of birth and gender.

This information was used to construct the following variables, which were considered as potential confounders:

- age,
- gender,

- type of work (administrative, nursing, equal amounts of administrative and nursing work),
- shift (day duty, always at the same time, rotating shift excluding nights, rotating shift including nights, only night work),
- facility (clinic or hospital, old people's home, facility for the handicapped),
- training (diploma in nursing, nursing assistant, without training),
- absenteeism due to musculoskeletal disease and/or psychological impairment in the previous year before baseline (2011).

Statistical analysis

Assessment of the predictive characteristics of the nurse-WIS for long-term sick leave

The following parameters were used to assess the performance of the Nurse-WIS in relation to long-term sick leave during the follow-up period, i.e. 2012: sensitivity, specificity, PPV, NPP and likelihood ratios. Long-term sick leave was defined as a sick leave of more than six weeks (> 42 days) due to musculoskeletal diseases and/or psychological impairments in 2012.

Prognostic influence of the nurse-WIS on the duration of sick leave

As mentioned above, the hypothesis is that nurses with high risk according to the Nurse-WIS at baseline take longer periods of sick leave due to musculoskeletal diseases and/or psychological impairments. In order to consider the association between the Nurse-WIS and sick leave in the following year (2012) in a more differentiated manner, a multiple ordinal logistical model (proportional odds model) was used. For this purpose, the duration of sick leave was divided into the following categories:

- no sick leave (0 days),
- sick leave up to 6 weeks (1–42 days),
- sick leave from 6 weeks to 12 months (43 days to 364 days),
- sick leave of 12 months or more (≥365 days, still unable to work after 31 December 2012).

Aside from the Nurse-WIS, potential confounders as described above were considered. Based on these factors, step-wise backward selection using likelihood ratio tests at a significance level of 0.05 was performed. After each step, it was examined whether the respective factor was a confounder for the Nurse-WIS (defined as a change of ≥10% in the coefficients of the Nurse-WIS relative to the full model). Factors identified as confounders remained in the model. We checked the proportional odds assumption of the ordinal logistic model by performing a

likelihood ratio test (significance level 0.05) between the ordinal and the corresponding multinomial model.

For the final model, odds ratios (OR) with corresponding 95% confidence intervals (95%CI) and Wald p values are reported. In addition, for the Nurse-WIS the predicted marginal probabilities (as means over participants) are given with corresponding 95% confidence intervals (95%CI). The analyses were conducted with Stata 14.1 (StataCorp 2015, College Station, TX).

Results

Study population

A total of 1592 nurses took part in the baseline survey (response rate 35.6%). By using the ID at follow-up, the data of all the participants in the baseline survey could be linked to the sick leave data of the health insurance fund (loss to follow-up 0%) (Fig. 1). The characteristics of the study population are shown in Table 1. Most of the nurses were female (91.8%). About 30% of the study participants were 50–54 years old, 88.4% had received nursing training, 84.5% worked in a hospital and 55.5% had worked in nursing for more than 30 years. Most of the study participants were in full-time employment (55.0%) and either worked in rotating shifts excluding nights (30.6%) or including nights (45.2%). Most study participants (57.3%) performed equal amounts of nursing and administrative work. While 36.4% reported that they mainly performed nursing work, only 6.3% reported that they mainly performed administrative work. According to the Nurse-WIS, 19.7% have no risk, 7.7% a slight risk, 33.2% a moderate risk and 39.4% a high risk of a long-term sick leave (Table 1).

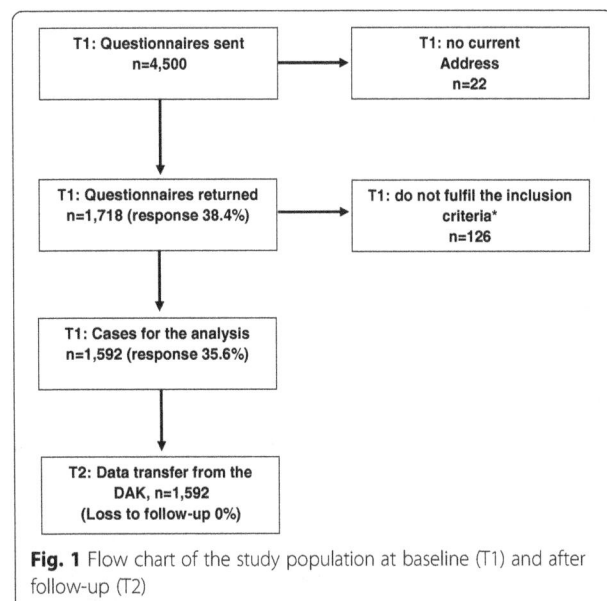

Fig. 1 Flow chart of the study population at baseline (T1) and after follow-up (T2)

Table 1 Description of the study population and the categories of the Nurse-WIS (n = 1592)

Variables	% (n)
Gender	
Female	91.8% (1462)
Male	8.2% (130)
Age	
40 to 44 years	18.0% (286)
45 to 49 years	26.1% (416)
50 to 54 years	29.0% (462)
55 to 59 years	21.0% (334)
> 60 years	5.9% (94)
Occupational training	
Qualified nurse or geriatric care worker	88.4% (1408)
Nursing assistant without nursing training	11.6% (184)
Facility	
Clinic or hospital	84.5% (1346)
Old people's home, nursing home, facility for the handicapped	15.5% (246)
Length of service	
0–20 years	9.7% (154)
21–30 years	34.9% (555)
More than 30 years	55.5% (883)
Scope of employment	
Full-time	55.0% (875)
Part-time (< 35 h a week)	45.0% (717)
Working hours	
Rotating shifts excluding nights	30.6% (487)
Rotating shifts including nights	45.2% (720)
Day duty, always at the same times	17.0% (271)
Only night work	7.2% (114)
Principal activity	
Nursing work	36.4% (579)
Administrative work	6.3% (100)
Equal parts of both	57.3% (913)
Nurse-WIS	
No risk (0 points)	19.7% (313)
Slight risk (1–9 points)	7.7% (123)
Moderate risk (10–19 points)	33.2% (528)
High risk (20–28 points)	39.4% (628)

Sick leave during the follow-up

Sick leaves of at least one day were most often due to other diseases. While 27.4% of sick leave periods were due to musculoskeletal diseases and 16.3% to psychological impairment. 40.1% of participants took sick leave of at least one day due to musculoskeletal diseases and/ or psychological impairments. As regards the duration

of sick leave, the proportion of persons who took less than 6 weeks' sick leave was greatest in the diagnostic group of other diseases. Sick leave of > 6 to 12 weeks was also most frequent in other diseases (10.1%). However, sick leave of more than 12 months was more frequently due to a musculoskeletal disease or a psychological impairment (Table 2).

Association between the nurse-WIS and the duration of sick leave

Of the potential prognostic factors examined, only the Nurse-WIS had a significant influence on the duration of sick leave ($p < 0.001$). The factors age, gender and shift work were identified as confounders of the Nurse-WIS and were therefore considered in the final regression model. The proportional odds ratio for a Nurse-WIS point value between 10 and 19 (moderate risk) relative to 0 points (no risk) for the duration of sick leave was 1.69 (95% CI [1.24, 2.30]; p < 0.001) (Fig. 2). In more detail, this means that the odds of taking sick leave of more than 1 day (i.e. for the combined categories of up to 6 weeks, 6 weeks to 12 months and more than 12 months) are 1.69 times higher than for nurses with a zero score in the Nurse-WIS. Because of the proportional odds assumption, the odds ratios for sick leave of more than 6 weeks versus less than 6 weeks, as well as (more than) one year versus less than one year, are also 1.69. The proportional odds ratio relative to no risk (0 points) increases for higher point values in the Nurse-WIS. At slight risk (1–9 points), the odds ratio in comparison to no risk was not increased (1.15 (95%CI [0.72, 1.84]; $p = 0.550$)). However, at high risk (20–28 points), the odds ratio increased to 3.42 (95%CI [2.54, 4.60] p < 0.001).

This relationship is also reflected in the predicted marginal probabilities (Fig. 3). With increasing risk according to the Nurse-WIS, the predicted probability for longer sick leave due to a musculoskeletal disease and/or a psychological impairment increases. With no, slight or moderate risk according to the Nurse-WIS, the predicted probabilities for no sick leave are 74.7% (96%CI [70.0%, 79.5%]), 71.9% ([64.0%, 79.9%]) and 63.7% ([59.7%, 67.7%]) respectively, while it was only 46.6% ([42.7%, 50.4%]) for 20 points and more (high risk). In contrast, the predicted probability for sick leave of up to 6 weeks was 20.1% for a Nurse-WIS of 0 points, 22.1% for 1–9 points, 27.8% for 10–19 points and 37.6% for 20–28 points. For a high risk of 20–28 points, the predicted probability of long-term sick leave of 6 weeks to 12 months was 11.4%, compared to 3.9% for no risk.

In the high risk group (Nurse-WIS 20–28 points) the sensitivity for long-term sick leave during the follow-up was 64.1% and the specificity was 63.4. The PPV was 17.0 and the NPV 93.8% (Table 3).

Table 2 Sick leave in the follow-up depending on the disease

	For other diseases	Due to a musculo-skeletal disease	Due to a psycho-logical impairment	Due to musculoskeletal disease and/or psychological impairment
Sick leave	% (n)	% (n)	% (n)	% (n)
No	54.1% (861)	72.6% (1155)	83.7% (1333)	59.9% (953)
Yes (at least 1 day)	45.9% (731)	27.4% (437)	16.3% (259)	40.1% (639)
Length of sick leave				
Up to 6 weeks (1–42 days)	34.9% (556)	21.8% (347)	11.6% (185)	29.6% (472)
> 6 weeks – 12 months (43–364 days)	10.1% (161)	4.1% (65)	3.4% (54)	7.6% (121)
> 12 months (≥365 days)	0.9% (14)	1.6% (25)	1.3% (20)	2.9% (46)

Discussion

To our knowledge, this is the first study to have analysed the prevalence of work instability in nurses and the predictive value of a high score with regard to long-term sick leave during follow-up by combining survey data with secondary data of a health insurance fund. The prevalence of a high risk of work instability was quite high (39.4%). One nurse out of ten took long-term sick leave due to musculoskeletal diseases and/or psychological impairment during follow-up. Even though the odds ratio for sick leave increased with a Nurse-WIS > 10 points, the sensitivity and specificity of the Nurse-WIS with regard to long-term sick leave during follow-up were rather modest, which is also reflected in a low PPV (17Compared with our previous study of geriatric care workers, sensitivity and specificity of the Nurse-WIS was lower (sensitivity 73.9 versus 64.1 specificity 76.7 versus 63.4) [27]. Therefore the attempt to improve predictive values by introducing an additional variable, pain during the previous three months, was not successful.

As the predictive value depends on the prevalence of the disease, only persons aged 40+ were surveyed, as the risk of sick leave increases with age [15]. In addition, an entry question was added to the questionnaire, so that only those persons who had suffered symptoms lasting longer than 2 h in their musculoskeletal system over the previous 3 months were requested to complete the questionnaire. The predictive characteristics of the updated version of the scale with the entry criterion were then compared with those of the geriatric care workers study. In the geriatric care workers study, 28.4% of the subjects reported a high risk in the Nurse-WIS. This was lower than the corresponding value for nurses (39.4%). This may be explained by the higher age of the cohort of nurses, as it has been shown that the probability of increased risk in the Nurse-WIS increases with age [27]. What was astonishing was that the proportion who had taken long-term sick leave due to a musculoskeletal disease and/or a psychological impairment was similar (about 10%) in both studies. A higher value had been

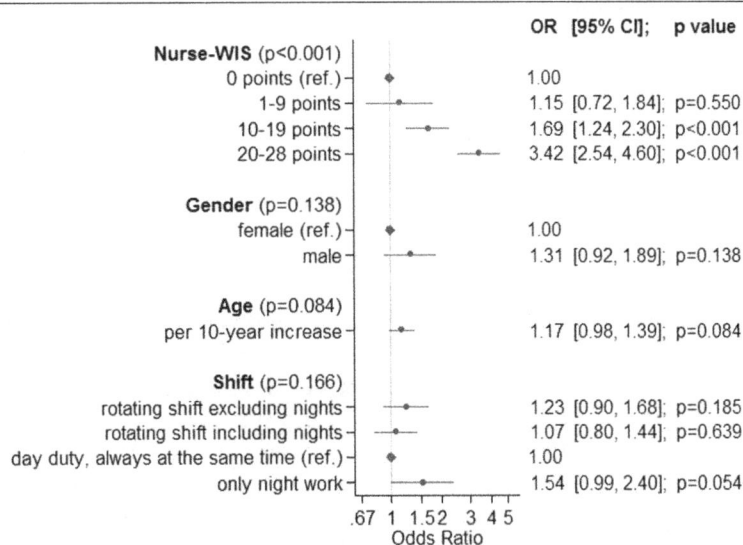

Fig. 2 Odds Ratio for sick leave due to musculoskeletal disease and /or psychological impairment depending on Nurse-WIS, Gender, Age and Shift Work

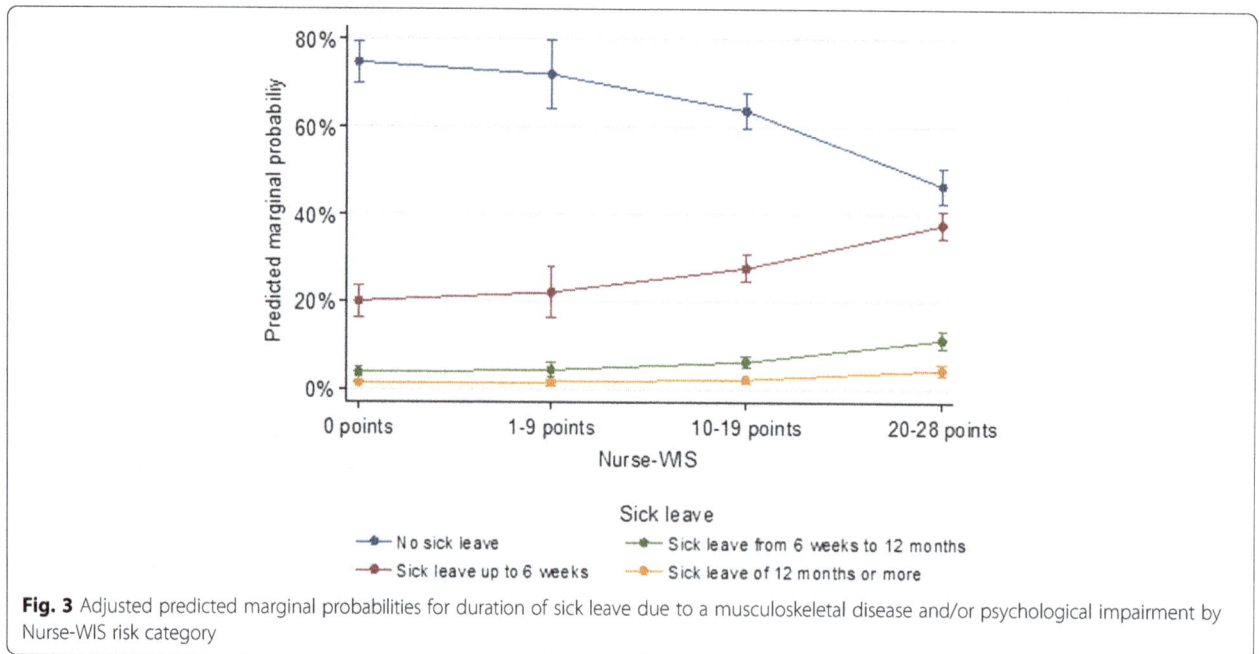

Fig. 3 Adjusted predicted marginal probabilities for duration of sick leave due to a musculoskeletal disease and/or psychological impairment by Nurse-WIS risk category

expected in the cohort of nurses which was restricted to older nurses. The two studies used the same definition of long-term sick leave, although the underlying data was quite different. In the geriatric care workers study, periods of sick leave were calculated based on information provided by the subject. They may be distorted by recall bias, particularly when the sick leave was some time earlier. In the nurse study this data was taken from the health insurance fund and had therefore been systematically collected and electronically recorded in the context of administration or cost reimbursement [42]. We assume that it is therefore more valid. Furthermore, different follow-up rates might be responsible for divergent results in the two studies.

Table 3 Sensitivity, specificity, likelihood ratio and predictive value of the Nurse-WIS for long-term sick leave[1] during follow-up

	% (n)
High risk according to Nurse-WIS	39.4 (628)
Long-term sick leave[1]	10.9 (173)
Sensitivity	64.1
Positive likelihood ratio[2]	1.75
Specificity	63.4
Negative likelihood ratio[2]	0.57
Positive predictive value (PPV)	17.0
Negative predictive value (NPV)	93.8

[1]Long-term sick leave > 42 days due to musculoskeletal diseases and/or psychological impairment (e.g. burn-out)
[2]No unit

Association between the nurse-WIS and the length of sick leave

A second objective of the study was to determine the prognostic influence of the Nurse-WIS in a multivariable model on the duration of sick leave (no sick leave, up to 6 weeks, > 6 weeks to 12 months, ≥12 months). Here, only the Nurse-WIS had a significant influence on the duration of sick leave during follow-up in 2012, with proportional odds of 3.42 for a Nurse-WIS score 20 to 28. This supports the hypothesis that nurses with an increased score in the Nurse-WIS have a higher risk of a longer sick leave [31, 32]. As the probability of early retirement increases with the length of a sick leave, the Nurse-WIS appears to be suited to detect persons at risk. For this reason, it is probable – even though the predictive values of the scale were poorer than in the geriatric care workers study [28] – that the Nurse-WIS can provide at least initial evidence that a person is at risk of a long sick leave and might benefit from intervention. It would also be conceivable to have the result of the Nurse-WIS confirmed by additional investigation by an occupational therapist, company doctor or other physician.

The factors age, gender, and shift work were identified as confounders. This means that age influences both the length of sick leave and the Nurse-WIS. This is well in line with the observation that the general state of health and length of sick leave change with age in several occupational groups, including nurses [34, 35]. It has also been suggested that frequently long and irregular working hours and rotating shifts may influence the development of disease [43, 44]. These factors could be considered when the Nurse-WIS is used in future, for example by inclusion in the questionnaire.

Cooperation with the health insurance fund and special features of the study design

The present study was performed in cooperation with DAK-Gesundheit, which has about 4.9 million members and 6 million insured persons. As the DAK was originally a health insurance fund for employees, it now typically insures employees in jobs typically done by women (e.g. in the health service, retail, office work and administration). The health service is an economic sector that employs particularly large numbers of DAK members [45]. Thus DAK-Gesundheit was a suitable partner in the study on validation of the Nurse-WIS. Moreover, this cooperation permitted the use of secondary data. One special feature of the study was the design. As in Scharnetzky et al. 2013 [33], this employed a procedure comprising interviews of insured persons followed by linkage of this data with the secondary health insurance fund's data for this cohort (with their consent). There was no loss of follow-up, which is a considerable advantage of this approach. Loss of follow-up might be an explanation of the divergent results of the nurses and geriatric care workers study [27]. It can be assumed that the sick leave data from the health insurance fund is more valid than the information obtained by means of a questionnaire. In addition, sick leave always corresponds to a restriction in working capacity as certified by a doctor and is not equivalent to the presence of a disease. It must therefore be assumed, that the sick leave data contains both underestimates ("presentism") and overestimates [46]. Furthermore, sick leave assessment on the basis of administrative data omits some short-term sick leave. In Germany, sick leave of up to three days does not usually require certification by a physician. Therefore, short-term sick leave was underestimated. This might have introduced some non- differential misclassification most likely diluting the effect estimates.

Nevertheless, it has been shown that data from the social insurance system is suitable for scientific analysis. For example, a Danish study used secondary data to show length of sick leave to be a predictor for receiving disability pension in future [31].

Limitations

Our study has some limitations. The response rate of 35.6% is low and therefore the results are not necessarily transferable to the total group of nurses. Furthermore, a selection bias cannot be excluded and may have led to an overestimation or underestimation. Because of the data collection by the DAK, as described in the method section, no non- responder analysis could be performed and we unfortunately have no information about the group of non-responders.

In this study an additional variable (pain during the last three months) was used to improve the predictive value compared to previous studies. Unfortunately, this attempt has not been successful. Due to the low positive predictive value, the question arises whether the Nurse-WIS is well suited as a screening tool. Even if the predictive values of the scale have deteriorated compared to the elderly care study, it is likely that the Nurse WIS can provide at least a first indication of persons who are at risk of a longer sick leave and who would possibly benefit from early intervention measures. However, it should be discussed whether the result of the nurse WIS should be confirmed by an additional examination by an occupational therapist, company physician or physician. The factors age, gender, and shift work were identified as confounders. However, we do not have information about occupational risk factors or live style factors so that controlling for confounding is limited in our analysis.

Conclusion

The German version of the Nurse-WIS predicts long-term sick leave. Introducing an entry criterion did not improve the predictive value of the score. Restricting the cohort to nurses aged 40 and over increased the proportion of those with a high risk score but did not improve prediction of long-term sick leave compared with the previous geriatric care worker study. Nevertheless, our data corroborates the hypothesis that the Nurse-WIS is a useful tool for assigning rehabilitation programmes to nurses. Combining questionnaire data with secondary data from a health insurance fund was feasible and successful in terms of follow-up. Therefore further studies employing this combination of data are recommended.

Abbreviations

DAK: Health Insurance FundBoard Manager for Health Care Research; DEÜV: Social Insurance Code Occupation Key; ICD Code: International Statistical Classification of Diseases and Related Health Problems; Nurse-WIS: Nurse-Work Instability Scale; OR: Odds Ratio; PPV: Positive predictive value; LR + : Positive likelihood ratio; LR- : negative likelihood ratio

Acknowledgements

We thank all nurses for participating in the study and devoting their time. At DAK-Gesundheit, we would like to thank Mrs. Schöwerding and Dr. Scharnetzky for their support in the study logistics.

Funding

No special funds were received for this study. However, the Centre of Excellence for Epidemiology and Health Care Research for Health Care Workers (CVcare) at the University Clinics Hamburg-Eppendorf (UKE) receives unrestricted funds from the Institution for Statutory Accident Insurance and Prevention in the Health and Welfare services (BGW) on an annual basis to maintain the working group at the UKE. The funds are provided by a non-profit organisation that is part of the social security system in Germany. The funder had no role in study design, data collection and analysis, the decision to publish, or preparation of the manuscript.

Authors' contributions

Conceived and designed the study: MK, AN, AS. Performed: MK, SW, AS. Analysed the data: MK, AB. Created figures and tables: MK, AB. Wrote the first draft of the paper: MK, AS. Made substantial critical comments on the draft: SW, AB, AN. All authors agreed to the final version of the manuscript.

Competing interests

The authors declare that no competing interests exist.

Author details

[1]Centre of Excellence for Epidemiology and Health Care Research for Health Care Workers (CVcare), University Medical Center Hamburg-Eppendorf (UKE), Martinistr. 41a, 20521 Hamburg, Germany. [2]DAK-Gesundheit (Health Insurance Fund, Board Manager for Health Care Research, Nagelsweg 27-31, 20097 Hamburg, Germany. [3]Institute of Medical Biometry and Epidemiology (IMBE), University Medical Center Hamburg-Eppendorf (UKE), Martinistr. 52, 20246 Hamburg, Germany. [4]Department of Occupational Health Research, German Social Accident Insurance Institution for the Health and Welfare Services, Pappelallee 33-37, 22089 Hamburg, Germany.

References

1. Demographic Transition in Germany. Wiesbaden: German National and State Statistical Offices; 2010.
2. Bickel H. Lebenserwartung und Pflegebedürftigkeit in Deutschland. (Life expectancy and need for care in Germany). Gesundheitswesen. 2001;63:9–14.
3. Dietz B. Entwicklung des Pflegebedarfs bis 2050: Kosten steigen schneller als erwartet. (Development of care needs to 2050: costs rise faster than expected). Soz Sicherh Z Arbeit Soz. 2001:2–9.
4. Byrns G, Reeder G, Jin G, Pachis K. Risk factors for work-related low back pain in registered nurses, and potential obstacles in using mechanical lifting devices. J Occup Environ Hyg. 2004;1:11–21.
5. Engkvist IL, Hjelm EW, Hagberg M, Menckel E, Ekenvall L. Risk indicators for reported over-exertion back injuries among female nursing personnel. Epidemiology. 2000;11:519–22.
6. Freitag S, Ellegast R, Dulon M, Nienhaus A. Quantitative measurement of stressful trunk postures in nursing professions. Ann Occup Hyg. 2007;51:385–95.
7. Freitag S, Fincke-Junos I, Nienhaus A. Analyse von belastenden Körperhaltungen bei Pflegekräften - Vergleich zwischen einer geriatrischen Station und anderen Krankenhausstationen. (Measurement-based analysis of stressful postures in care workers - comparison between a geriatric ward and other hospital wards.). In: Nienhaus A, editor. Gefährdungsprofile - Unfälle und arbeitsbedingte Erkrankungen in Gesundheitsdienst und Wohlfahrtspflege 2 edn. Landsberg/Lech: ecomed Medizin; 2010. p. 160–79.
8. Hignett S. Work-related back pain in nurses. J Adv Nurs. 1996;23:1238–46.
9. Jäger M, Jordan C, Theilmeier A, Wortmann N, Kuhn S, Nienhaus A, Luttmann A. Lumbar-load analysis of manual patient-handling activities for biomechanical overload prevention among healthcare workers. Ann Occup Hyg. 2013;57:528–44.
10. Stolt M, Suhonen R, Virolainen P, Leino-Kilpi H. Lower extremity musculoskeletal disorders in nurses: A narrative literature review. Scand J Public Health. 2016;44:106–15.
11. Garrett C. The effect of nurse staffing patterns on medical errors and nurse burnout. AORN J. 2008;87:1191–204.
12. Kromark K, Dulon M, Nienhaus A. Gesundheitsindikatoren und Präventionsverhalten bei älteren Beschäftigten in der Altenpflege. (Health indicators and preventive behaviour in older geriatric care workers). Gesundheitswesen. 2008;70:137–44.
13. McHugh MD, Kutney-Lee A, Cimiotti JP, Sloane DM, Aiken LH. Nurses' widespread job dissatisfaction, burnout, and frustration with health benefits signal problems for patient care. Health Aff (Millwood). 2011;30:202–10.

14. Siegrist J, Rödel A. Arbeitsbelastungen im Altenpflegeberuf unter besonderer Berücksichtigung der Wiedereinstiegsproblematik - Zusammenfassung der Ergebnisse der Literaturrecherche und bibliographische Hinweise. (Work-related stress in geriatric care with a special focus on re-entry problems - a summary of results of literature research and bibliographical notes.). In: Kowalski J, Pauli G, editors. Machbarkeitsstudie - Gesunder Wiedereinstieg in den Altenpflegeberuf. Köln: Institut für Betriebliche Gesundheitsförderung BGF GmbH; 2005. p. 1–36.
15. DAK-Unternehmen Leben. DAK-Gesundheitsreport 2010. (DAK Health Report 2010.). Berlin: DAK-Unternehmen Leben; 2010. p. 161.
16. Gjesdal S, Bratberg E. The role of gender in long-term sickness absence and transition to permanent disability benefits. Results from a multiregister based, prospective study in Norway 1990-1995. Eur J Pub Health. 2002;12:180–6.
17. Harling M, Schablon A, Nienhaus A. Abgeschlossene medizinische Rehabilitationen und Erwerbsminderungsrenten bei Pflegepersonal im Vergleich zu anderen Berufsgruppen. (Completed medical rehabilitation and disability pensions among nursing personnel compared with other occupational groups.). In: Rentenversicherung D, editor. Gesundheit, Migration und Einkommensgleichheit. Berlin: Bericht vom siebten Workshop des Forschungsdatenzentrums der Rentenversicherung (FDZ-RV) im Wissenschaftszentrum Berlin für Sozialforschung (WZB) - Band 55/2010; 2010. p. 72–85.
18. Hignett S. Intervention strategies to reduce musculoskeletal injuries associated with handling patients: a systematic review. Occup Environ Med. 2003;60:E6.
19. Linton SJ, Andersson T. Can chronic disability be prevented? A randomized trial of a cognitive-behavior intervention and two forms of information for patients with spinal pain. Spine (Phila Pa 1976). 2000;25:2825–31 discussion 2824.
20. Linton SJ, Nordin E. A 5-year follow-up evaluation of the health and economic consequences of an early cognitive behavioral intervention for back pain: a randomized, controlled trial. Spine (Phila Pa 1976). 2006;31:853–8.
21. van Oostrom SH, Driessen MT, de Vet HC, Franche RL, Schonstein E, Loisel P, van Mechelen W, Anema JR. Workplace interventions for preventing work disability. Cochrane Database Syst Rev. 2009:CD006955.
22. de Boer AG, van Beek JC, Durinck J, Verbeek JH, van Dijk FJ. An occupational health intervention programme for workers at risk for early retirement; a randomised controlled trial. Occup Environ Med. 2004;61:924–9.
23. Gilworth G, Bhakta B, Eyres S, Carey A, Anne Chamberlain M, Tennant A. Keeping nurses working: development and psychometric testing of the Nurse-Work Instability Scale (Nurse-WIS). J Adv Nurs. 2007;57:543–51.
24. Gilworth G, Chamberlain MA, Harvey A, Woodhouse A, Smith J, Smyth MG, Tennant A. Development of a work instability scale for rheumatoid arthritis. Arthritis Rheum. 2003;49:349–54.
25. Gilworth G, Emery P, Barkham N, Smyth MG, Helliwell P, Tennant A. Reducing work disability in Ankylosing Spondylitis: development of a work instability scale for AS. BMC Musculoskelet Disord. 2009;10:68.
26. Gilworth G, Carey A, Eyres S, Sloan J, Rainford B, Bodenham D, Neumann V, Tennant A. Screening for job loss: development of a work instability scale for traumatic brain injury. Brain Inj. 2006;20:835–43.
27. Harling M, Schablon A, Nienhaus A. Validation of the German version of the Nurse-Work Instability Scale: baseline survey findings of a prospective study of a cohort of geriatric care workers. J Occup Med Toxicol. 2013;8:33.
28. Harling M, Schablon A, Peters C, Nienhaus A. Predictive values and other quality criteria of the German version of the Nurse-Work Instability Scale (Nurse-WIS) - follow-up survey findings of a prospective study of a cohort of geriatric care workers. J Occup Med Toxicol. 2014;9:30.
29. Bender R. Interpretation von Effizienzmaßen der Vierfeldertafel für Diagnostik und Behandlung. (Interpretation of efficiency measures of the fourfold table for diagnostics and treatment.). Med Klin Intensivmed Notfallmed. 2001;96:116–21.
30. Akobeng AK. Understanding diagnostic tests 1: sensitivity, specificity and predictive values. Acta Paediatr. 2007;96:338–41.
31. Lund T, Kivimaki M, Labriola M, Villadsen E, Christensen KB. Using administrative sickness absence data as a marker of future disability pension: the prospective DREAM study of Danish private sector employees. Occup Environ Med. 2008;65:28–31.
32. Labriola M. Conceptual framework of sickness absence and return to work, focusing on both the individual and the contextual level. Work. 2008;30: 377–87.
33. Scharnetzky E, Busch H, Wobbe S, Rebscher H. Versorgungsforschung aus der Perspektive einer gesetzlichen Krankenkasse. (Healthcare research from the viewpoint of a statutory health insurance fund.). Gesundheitsökonmie Qualitätsmanagement. 2013;18:290–4.

34. Nübling M, Stößel U, Hasselhorn HM, Michaelis M, Hofmann F. Methoden zur Erfassung psychischer Belastungen - Erprobung eines Messinstrumentes (COPSOQ). Dortmund, Berlin, Dresden: Wirtschaftsverlag NW Verlag für neue Wissenschaften; 2005.

35. Nübling M, Stößel U, Hasselhorn HM, Michaelis M, Hofmann F. Measuring psychological stress and strain at work - Evaluation of the COPSOQ Questionnaire in Germany. Psychosoc Med. 2006;3:Doc05.

36. Bernard BP. Musculosceletal Disorders and Workplace Factors - A Critical Review of Epidemiologic Evidence for Work-Related Musculosceletal Disorders of the Neck, Upper Extremity, and Low Back. Cincinnati: DHHS (NIOSH); 1997.

37. Sluiter JK, Rest KM, Frings-Dresen MH. Criteria document for evaluating the work-relatedness of upper-extremity musculoskeletal disorders. Scand J Work Environ Health. 2001;27 Suppl 1:1–102.

38. Hartmann B, Spallek M. Arbeitsbezogene Muskel-Skelett-Erkrankungen - Eine Gegenstandsbestimmung. (Work-related musculoskeletal diseases - definition of the subject for study.). Arbeitsmed Sozialmed Umweltmed. 2009;44:423–36.

39. Flothow A, Zeh A, Nienhaus A. Unspezifische Rückenschmerzen – Grundlagen und Interventionsmöglichkeiten aus psychologischer Sicht (Non-specific back pain - bases and intervention options from the psychological viewpoint). Gesundheitswesen. 2009;71:845–56.

40. Seidler A, Liebers F, Latza U. Prävention von Low-Back-Pain im beruflichen Kontext. Bundesgesundheitsbl Gesundheitsforsch Gesundheitsschutz. 2008; 51:322–33.

41. Stadler P, Spieß E. Arbeit - Psyche - Rückenschmerzen. Einflussfaktoren und Präventionsmöglichkeiten. (Work - psyche - back pain. Influencing factors and preventive possibilities.). Arbeitsmed Sozialmed Umweltmed. 2009;44:68–76.

42. Hoffman F, Glaeske G. Analyse von Routinedaten. (Analysing routine data.). In: Pfaff H, Neugebauer EAM, Glaeske G, Schrappe M, editors. Lehrbuch Versorgungsforschung Systematik - Methodik - Anwendung. Stuttgart: Schattauer-Verlag; 2010. p. 317–22.

43. Caruso CC, Waters TR. A review of work schedule issues and musculoskeletal disorders with an emphasis on the healthcare sector. Ind Health. 2008;46:523–34.

44. Lipscomb JA, Trinkoff AM, Geiger-Brown J, Brady B. Work-schedule characteristics and reported musculoskeletal disorders of registered nurses. Scand J Work Environ Health. 2002;28:394–401.

45. DAK Gesundheit. DAK-Gesundheitsreport 2014. (DAK Health Report 2014.). Hamburg: DAK Gesundheit; 2014. p. 157.

46. March S, Iskenius M, Hardt J, Swart E. Methodische Überlegungen für das Datenlinkage von Primär- und Sekundärdaten im Rahmen arbeitsepidemiologischer Studien. (Methodological observations on linking primary and secondary data in the context of occupation-related epidemiological studies.). Bundesgesundheitsbl Gesundheitsforsch Gesundheitsschutz. 2013;56:571–8.

19

Noise exposure and auditory thresholds of military musicians: a follow up study

Reinhard Müller[1]* and Joachim Schneider[2]

Abstract

Background: Military musicians are working in a noisy environment with high sound exposure levels above the international standards. Aim of the current study is to find out, whether they develop the expected hearing impairments. Adherence to the regulations for prevention in musicians is more difficult than in other occupational fields.

Methods: In an interval of 13.3 years, 36 out of 58 male military musicians of a German army music corps were subjected twice to an audiometric audit. There were no exclusion criteria apart from acute ENT infections (three musicians). These results were compared with one another and evaluated by means of statistical methods for relationships with several factors.

Results: At frequencies below 3 kHz, the follow-up audiograms were up to 5 dB better than the preliminary examination. From 4 kHz up to 8 kHz the preliminary investigations showed less hearing impairment. Averaging all frequencies the improvement of hearing ability was around 1 dB. Above 1 kHz the average hearing of the right ear was up to 7 dB better than that of the left ear. Age-induced hearing loss was 3 to 8 dB lower than predicted by ISO standards over the entire frequency range. The side of the ear (right/left) and the frequency (3, 4, and 6 kHz) were significant ($p < 0.05$) in hearing loss, whereas the influence of the instrument and the acoustic traumata were not.

Conclusion: Despite the high noise levels, the average hearing ability of the 36 military musicians during the investigation period only slightly deteriorated in the noise-sensitive frequencies (3, 5 and 6 kHz). Music may be less harmful than industrial noise, or the long-term auditory training of the musicians leads to a delayed presbycusis.

Keywords: Military musicians, Audiometry, Hearing, Hearing loss, Noise exposure

Background

At the time of the old Israelites, trumpets are said to have been able to bring whole city walls to collapse, according to the relevant account in the Old Testament of the Bible, in Joshua 6. Even today, brass orchestras are able to produce a significant sound pressure, which may be felt in a larger radius. While lovers of military music appreciate these brass instruments and the sound, the usually excessive volume encounters refusal, especially with gentler natures. But not only military orchestras can produce high sound pressure levels but even ballet orchestras are suspected of hearing hazard [1].

The musicians as parts of the sound source themselves are more exposed to these sounds than the audience in some distance and should therefore take a greater risk to develop noise induced hearing loss. In order to determine these sonic loads, appropriate measurements were made in some studies. These relate predominantly to classical orchestras. Since the number of military musicians on the whole seems rather small, their hearing is rarely subject of published investigations. A search in PubMed with the search query: <"military musicians" AND "hearing"> provides only three matches. One of these articles [2] complains about the below-average poor health surveillance of military musicians without commenting on their hearing status, so that only two articles remain. Both were published in 2013. While a

* Correspondence: reinmu@gmx.net
[1]Justus-Liebig-Universität Giessen, Aulweg 123, 35392 Giessen, Germany
Full list of author information is available at the end of the article

Brazilian study [3] reports an approximately 15-fold increased risk of hearing loss of military musicians compared to an unimpaired population, Patil et al. [4] reports no increased risk of hearing damage in British Army musicians compared to military administrative personnel. In 1981 Axelsson and Lindgren [5] already described in a larger study the hearing ability of orchestral musicians, that military music poses no increased risk of developing hearing damage compared to orchestral music. For most musicians with noticeable hearing damage (> 80%), a connection could be established with the music practice. Sound measurements in orchestras performed during rehearsals and public performances predominantly indicate level margins and average values which exceed the upper exposure action value of 85 dB(A) on daily shift [6]. McBride et al. [7] report up to 160% of the allowed daily dose on an average day with rehearsals and concert. According to ISO 1999 [8], therefore, the effects of sound exposure on the ear should be found. Mostly, however, lower levels of hearing loss are found in musicians than the ISO 1999 [8] predicts [4, 9–15]. Female musicians heard equally well as their male counterparts of the same age group [11, 16]. Several authors reported a better hearing of the right ear compared to the left ear [5, 14, 16, 17]. Especially with violinists, the volume of their own instrument is a dominant factor [18]. The left ear near the instrument is averagely exposed to 4.6 dB more than the right ear, which is averted from the instrument. In a literature study on the sonic load and hearing of musicians Sataloff [19] comes to the conclusion that musicians can produce dangerous sound levels, but further investigations would be necessary with regard to the effect on the hearing. A German study [20] to the hearing status of orchestral musicians found more than 50% musicians with hearing loss ≥15 dB and equivalent sound exposure levels $L_{EX} > 90$ dB(A).

Overall, there is a rather heterogeneous picture regarding the hearing of musicians in the literature, which presents partly contradictory results and is not always comparable in terms of methodology. An important step towards standardization could be the application of a new parametric method by Bo et al. (2016) for the noise risk assessment of professional orchestral musicians [21]. The present longitudinal study examines military musicians who have been audited twice at intervals of more than 13 years. As the first examination [22] was carried out, sound measurements were also taken during rehearsals and concerts. A typical rehearsal with the musicians in a rehearsal room with corresponding sound measurements is shown in Fig. 1.

All microphone positions, with values up to 93 dB (A), show equivalent sound exposure well above the upper exposure action values [6].

The comparison of two audiograms to the same persons should enable to make reliable statements about the development of hearing or the development of a hearing damage in these persons under sound exposure far above the upper exposure action values [6].

Methods
Participants
Out of a total of 58 male military musicians of the army music corps in Bremerhaven 39 musicians could be tested a second time after about 13 years. Only complete data sets were evaluated. Three musicians who suffered from a cold were excluded. A total of 36 musicians could be evaluated in the present longitudinal study. Existing hearing damage was not an exclusion criterion, as only the development of hearing was of interest, whilst comparing the two hearing tests.

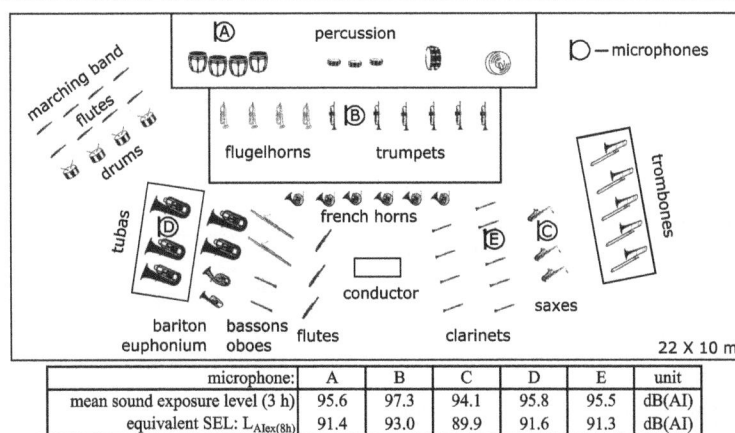

microphone:	A	B	C	D	E	unit
mean sound exposure level (3 h)	95.6	97.3	94.1	95.8	95.5	dB(AI)
equivalent SEL: $L_{AIex(8h)}$	91.4	93.0	89.9	91.6	91.3	dB(AI)

Fig. 1 Military musicians at a three hours rehearsal with sound measurements at 5 microphone positions a-e. Mean sound exposure levels within 3 h and recalculated Levels to one working shift: $L_{AIex(8h)}$ in dB(AI). (Illustration modified from F. Pfander, 1985) [22]

Instrumentation

For the audiometry 4 audiometers of the company Hortmann type CA540 and an audiometer of the company Maico type MA53 in connection with circum-aural transducers type HDA200 of the company Sennheiser were used. These transducers were calibrated according to ISO 389–8 [23] and ISO 389–5 [24]. Hearing tests were performed with pulsed sine tones. The data was displayed and stored with the software Avantgarde 2.0 of the company Nuess via the serial interface RS 232 in PCs.

The first audiometry tests were performed with audiometers from Siemens type T31 and Beomat 2005 SR with supra-aural transducers from Beyer type DT 48 with sinusoidal tones. The tranducers were calibrated according to ISO 389–1 [25]. The audiometers were not yet connected to computers, but the hearing thresholds were entered on cardboard forms of the manufacturers. For the evaluation, the threshold values were transferred individually into a database.

Acoustic measurements

The acoustic measurements during the rehearsal were carried out by the technicians of Pfander [22]. The measurements were performed with three ½ inch free-field microphones type 4165 (at A, B and C) and two ½ inch free-field microphones type 4133 (at D and E). All with preamps type 2619 and amplifier type 2606 of Brüel & Kjær (Danmark). The measure points A, B and C were recorded with a level statistics device type 4426 of Brüel & Kjær, and the points D and E with a PCM-recorder combination PCM-F1/SL-F1E from the company Sony (Japan).

Software und statistics

The data processing was carried out with the Office programs Access and Excel Microsoft Office 2010, whereby even simple T-tests were used. The age-related hearing loss from ISO 7029 (2nd and 3rd editions) [24, 25] was also calculated in Excel and included for comparison. A repetitive multivariate ANOVA was performed using SPSS 15 with 3 inner-subjects factors (repeat) audiogram, frequency and ear and 2 between-subjects factors instrument and acoustic trauma. The statistical evaluation addressed the frequencies 3, 4 and 6 kHz, in which all datasets were complete. Only at 10 kHz three musicians had missing data values. One of these musicians had no value on both ears and two only on the left ear.

Results

Hearing thresholds

At intervals of about 13.3 years (mean age of the groups 31.4 and 44.7 years) military musicians of the German Federal Armed Forces were checked twice by means of audiometry and questioning.

In Fig. 2 the average hearing ability of the musicians for both the right and left ear as well as at the time of the first measurement (Audio1) and 2nd measurement (Audio2) is shown separately. With the exception of the frequency at 125 Hz in the left ear, a hearing improvement was observed in both ears over all frequencies below 2 kHz over time, ranging from 1 to 4 dB. At 2 kHz, on average there was no change. At 3 kHz, the hearing thresholds behave differently in both ears. Over time, the right ear has improved by about 1 dB while the left ear has deteriorated by about 1 dB. Between 4 and 8 kHz the later audiometry shows a 2 to 5 dB worse hearing than the first examination. At 10 kHz, a slight improvement in hearing thresholds can be observed. Overall, the hearing of the right ear is slightly better than the left, which is shown in Fig. 3.

Figure 3 shows the averaged differences in auditory thresholds (Audio 2 minus Audio 1) for left and right ear seperately. These differences were compared to the current standard on hearing ISO 7029:2000 [26] and also to the new draft ISO 7029:2014 [27] for the age group between 31.4 and 44.7 years in the same diagram. It can be seen from this, that there are clear deviations between the expected and the measured hearing losses. Based on the new ISO standard (dashed black line in Fig. 3), the expected hearing loss is lower than for the still valid ISO from the year 2000 (solid black line in Fig. 3). The hearing loss differences in military musicians between both measurements across all frequencies is similar to the difference according to ISO aging. Almost across all frequencies, the military musicians show less age impaired hearing compared to the predicted aging

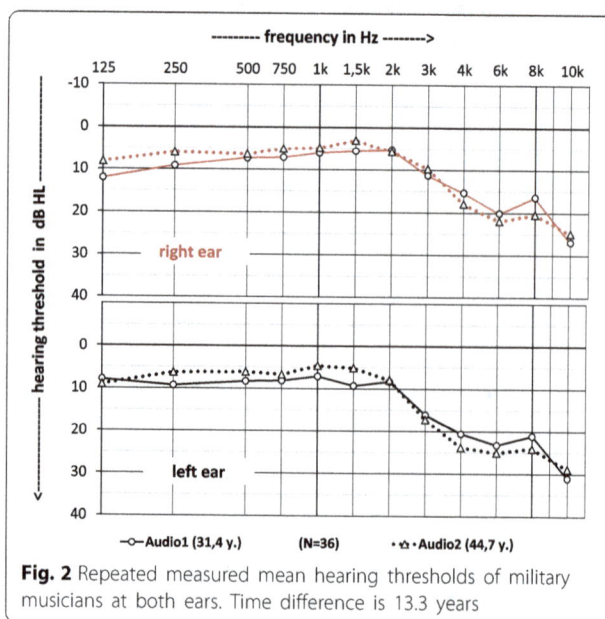

Fig. 2 Repeated measured mean hearing thresholds of military musicians at both ears. Time difference is 13.3 years

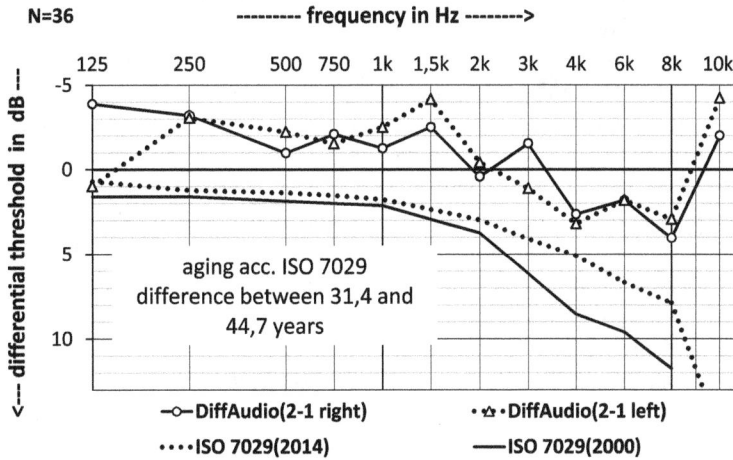

Fig. 3 Audiograms (difference between later audiogram (2) and first audiogram (1)) of military musicians taken within a 13.3 years time-span, thereby comparing both ears separately with the age-induced hearing loss according to the current ISO 7029:2000 [26] and the draft ISO 7029:2014 [27] at the same mean ages

according to the ISO standards with a deviation of about – 5 dB, which corresponds to an entire setting level in the audiometer. At 10 kHz, there is a slight improvement in the hearing thresholds of – 2 dB at the right ear and – 4 dB at the left ear. While ISO 7029:2000 [26] has no standard values at 10 kHz, the provisional new ISO standard (2014) [27] for this frequency predicts a hearing loss of 15.6 dB between the ages of 33.4 and 44.7 years. The difference in hearing thresholds between the two ears varies between 0 and 5 dB, with the curves crossing several times. Positive values indicate a deterioration in hearing.

The average differences between the hearing thresholds of the right and left ear are shown in Fig. 4. It can be seen that the asymmetry of the ears at frequencies below 1.5 kHz is in a range between 0.2 and – 1 dB. A clear exception is seen at 125 Hz (in the first audiometry), where the hearing of the right ear in comparison

to the other is 4 dB worse than that of the left ear. By subtracting the average hearing thresholds, the age-related, but also the noise-induced threshold differences are excluded, provided the effect is assumed to be the same for both ears. However, this does not seem to apply especially in the frequency range above 1 kHz. Between 2 and 7.5 dB we observe better hearing thresholds in the right ear. Averaged for 3, 4 and 6 kHz, the differences are about 5 dB. That this is a real effect is shown in the statistical significance for the ear factor at $p = 0.036$. A clear trend towards larger deviations at higher frequencies can be seen.

Statistics

The statistical verification of relationships was performed with a multifactorial analysis of variance (ANOVA) with repeated measurements based on 5 factors and their interactions. Three factors: the frequency with three

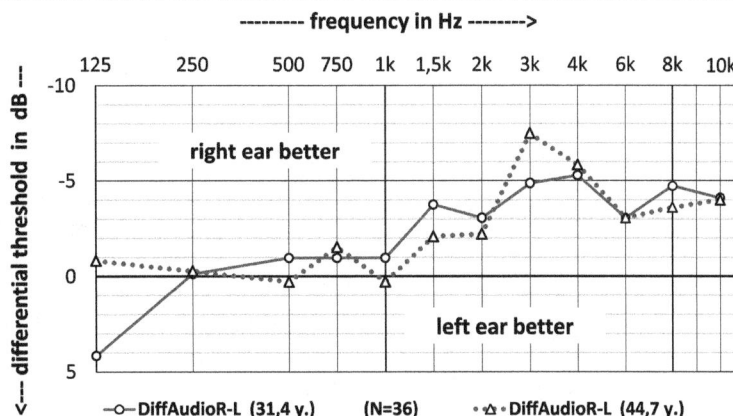

Fig. 4 Audiograms (difference between right and left ear) of military musicians taken within a 13.3 years time-span. Negative values show better hearing of the right ear and positive values of the left ear

measurement levels (3, 4 and 6 kHz, which are most sensitive to high sound levels!), The ear (right / left) and the audiogram (first and second) are the inner-subjects factors (repeated measures) and two factors: the musician's instrument ($N = 14$) and the history of the experienced acoustic shocks, both mentioned in the questionnaire, represent between-subjects factors.

Significant differences were only found for the within-subjects factors "frequency" and the "ear", while the auditory thresholds of audiograms 1 and 2 did not differ significantly for a time span of about 13 years. The *between subject* factor "instrument" with 7 trumpets, 6 clarinets, 5 trombones, 4 horns, 3 percussionists, 2 tubes and saxophones each and 1 baritone, conductor, electric bass, bassoon, transverse flute, keyboard and piano did not show any significant differences in the hearing thresholds ($p = 0.292$ as seen in Table 1). Also, the acoustic shocks mentioned in the questionnaire had no significant impact. All interactions of the individual factors were also not significant, as shown in Table 1, even those with the significant factors of frequency and ear. More interactions were calculated than indicated in Table 1, all of which were not significant.

Noise induced hearing loss

With the equation: $N50 = [u + v * \lg (t / t0)] * (L_{EX,8h} - L_0)^2$ from the ISO 1999 [8] the median of a hearing loss can be predicted. Here, u, v and L_0 are frequency-dependent table values of ISO 1999 [8]: **t** is the duration of the load, $\mathbf{t_0}$ 1 year and $\mathbf{L_{EX,8h}}$ the determined average sound load during the time period **t**.

Table 1 Results of a multifactorial analysis of variance (ANOVA) with repeated measurements. Two between-subjects factors: instrument and acoustic shocks and three within-groups factors: audiogram (first and second), frequency (3, 4 and 6 kHz) and the ear (right/left) with four interactions

between groups	df	F	p
Instrument	1	1.350	0.292
Acoustic Shock	1	0.748	0.402
within groups			
Audiogram	1	1.318	0.270
Frequency	**2**	**20.518**	**<0.001**
Ear	**1**	**5.353**	**0.036**
Audiogram * Frequency	2	1.779	0.187
Audiogram * Ear	1	0.035	0.855
Audiogram * Frequency * Ear	2	1.505	0.240
Frequency * Ear	2	0.547	0.585

Significant factors and interactions (*) are expressed **red bold**

The duration of sound exposure $t = 13.3$ years. The average sound load $L_{EX,8h} = 91.4$ dB(A) as well as determined at microphone position A (See Fig. 1).

This results in predicted hearing losses for the frequencies 3 kHz: 11.2 dB, for 4 kHz: 14.4 dB and for 6 kHz: 9.6 dB. These hearing losses are a rough estimate and are based on the assumption that the sonic load of 91.4 dB(A) persisted for each musician and every working day during the 13.3 years without using ear protection devices or any other protective measures.

Discussion

When comparing the two studies with an average interval of 13.3 years in Fig. 2, first of all the great similarity of the average audiograms stands out. At all frequencies below 2 kHz with the exception of 125 Hz in the left ear, the second audiometry is even better than the first examination. At 2 kHz, the hearing thresholds of both examinations are almost identical. The frequency at 3 kHz shows a different behaviour for both ears. For the right ear, the second audiogram is 1 dB better and for the left ear the first one is. At 4, 6, and 8 kHz frequencies, the auditory curves are parallel, with the auditory thresholds being better for the first audiogram than the second, as might be expected. Together with the 3 kHz frequency, this range is the most sensitive to the harmful effects of noise. The hearing threshold at 10 kHz behaves contrary to expectations. Although the presbyacusis is most pronounced at high frequencies, better thresholds are seen in the later study of military musicians. For clarification, these differences in the threshold values in Fig. 3 were highlighted and compared with the predicted age-impairment from ISO 7029 (2nd and 3rd editions) [26, 27]. The curves all have a similar course over the frequencies, but the ISO curves are clearly below the average threshold differences obtained from the measurements in the later and in the first audiogram (see legend to Fig. 2 called "DiffAudio"). These differences are greatest between the observed and the by ISO predicted thresholds at 10 kHz. Here, − 3 dB (both ears combined) contrasts with a value of 15.6 dB (ISO 7029:2014) [27]. The difference is therefore 18.6 dB and shows the opposite of a presbyacusis.

Musicians in classical orchestras (Chicago Symphony) [15] have high sound pressure levels with a mean of 90 dB(A) created by their instruments while practicing their profession for 15 h per week. Converted to a 40 h shift per week the mean levels are 85.5 dB(A). Impulse peaks reaches 143.5 dB, above the upper exposure action value of 137 dB(C) [6].

Finnish members of the National Opera are exposed to sound levels above the upper action exposure values of 85 dB (A) [28].

In an Australian study [29] mean L_{EX} levels for the brass section could be measured up to 90.7 dB(A) and peak levels for the percussion section reached 146,9 dB(C).

In a Canadian study [1], the average sound levels of wind players were between 88 dB(A) (oboe) and 94 dB(A) (trumpet) during 3 h. In comparison workers were exposed to industrial noise for about 2000 h per year, musicians for about 360 h per year. Thereby a correction value of – 7.4 dB was calculated and used.

In his measurements (Fig. 1) Pfander [22] uses the time constant "impulse" because of the high peak values, which occured especially in drums. Thus, the measured values are no longer directly comparable to the literature values. However, the burdens of military musicians may actually be higher than those of classical orchestra musicians, because of the over-proportionally large brass-section in comparison to the classical orchestra composition.

Nevertheless, the hearing thresholds at 3, 4 and 6 kHz with $p = 0.270$ (audiogram) are not significantly different between the two examinations over 13.3 years of exposure. ISO 1999 [8] predicts noise-induced permanent threshold shift (NIPTS) for sound levels of 91.4 dB in 13.3 years of 11.2 dB (3 kHz), 14.4 dB (4 kHz) and 9. 6 dB (6 kHz). This will by far not be confirmed by the second investigation: Here we observed neither hearing loss (positive threshold values in Fig. 3) at 3 kHz is ±1 dB, at 4 kHz 3 dB and 2 dB at 6 kHz, NIPTS (ISO 1999) [8] nor presbyacusis (ISO 7029) [26, 27]. The difference between expected and observed value is about 10 dB. In order to confirm the measured values by the ISO 1999 [8], average sound levels of about 83 dB would have to be assumed in the calculation.

In addition to the music played during working hours, additional exposure is added by playing music during leisure time and other noisy hobbies [20]. Further exposure is due to impulse noise in the regular military shooting practice. The dip in the audiogram between 2 and 8 kHz also shows these effects of the impulse noise. In the questionnaire, 13 musicians stated that they had suffered an acoustic trauma during their time as soldiers. There is no indication from the audiogram of 8 musicians, so that the temporary hearing loss has receded. 5 musicians with the indication of an acoustic trauma had a corresponding sink in the audiogram. On the other hand, a further 12 musicians showed clear traces of past hearing damage due to impulse noise in the audiogram, without having reported this event in the questionnaire. In two cases, the question of acoustic trauma was not answered. In conclusion, less than one third ($N = 5$) of all observed/suspected acoustic traumata ($N = 17$) are

identified by the survey. Therefore, the missing statistically significant correlation of the hearing thresholds with acoustic trauma (yes/no) ($p = 0.402$) can be explained. Sonic events that lead to clearly visible sinks in the audiogram are usually kept in mind by those affected, especially since their consequences can have an impact on the performance of the musicians. The discrepancy between the anamnestic questionnaire and the audiometric findings on acoustic trauma may well be the result.

The frequency-dependent differences at 3, 4 and 6 kHz, which statistically describe the observed drop in the hearing curve are highly significant ($p < 0.001$). Since the thresholds at 8 kHz are better than at 6 kHz, we can speak of a sink in the audiogram indicating a history of noise exposure.

In the current investigations, a significantly better hearing of the right than the left ear was found (see Table 1 and Fig. 3). That this is a real effect is shown in the statistical significance for the ear factor at $p = 0.036$.

This difference may be due to a generally greater vulnerability of the left ear in comparison to the right ear [30] or to an asymmetric impact of damaging sound [18, 22]. The latter would also be an indication of the origin of the hearing damage caused by impulse or shooting noise and especially not by the practice of music. Except for the flutes and horns most of the wind instruments radiate the sound symmetrically forward or upward.

he factor instrument also was not significant ($p = 0.292$), which is surprising in view of the large differences between the instruments in terms of maximum volume and their frequency spectrum. In the statistical review, the factor instrument had no significant influence nor possible interactions with the ear (not listed in Table 1). As early as 1985, Johnsson et al. [31] found that the instrument being played and the position in the orchestra did not lead to significant differences in hearing, which is confirmed by the current data.

Possible reasons for only small differences in the two investigations could be the different measurement techniques and the use of pulsed test tones in the second study with better measurement results, compared to continuous tones in the first study. However, there is no evidence in the literature, on the contrary, only marginal differences were found [32]. Similarly, the circumaural transducers of the second study have a better external noise attenuation than the supra-aural transducers of the first study and measurement results are more reliable [33]. Another limitation may be the relatively small number of 36 participants, which, however, is of less importance in longitudinal than in cross-sectional studies.

Conclusions

Overall, the musician's hearing has remained largely unchanged during the period under review, just over 13 years. The effect of noise on hearing remains far behind the predictions of ISO 1999 [8]. Similarly, the aging predicted by the ISO 7029 [26, 27] with progressive lowering of the thresholds in the collective of military musicians cannot be confirmed. In this sense we can speak of a delayed presbyacusis in musicians. This could be due to the highly selected collective of musicians with special training in hearing. By adaptation processes the practice of music with planned sound effect does not seem to be as damaging to the hearing due to the stapedius reflex, as unwanted pulsed industrial noise with the same sound levels. But this should not lead musicians to negligently deal with their hearing, but to ensure that special peak noise levels are avoided or mitigated with ear protection and to ensure adequate recovery of hearing during break-times.

Acknowledgements

Our thanks go to Gerald Fleischer for the idea of the study and the release of the datasets. Thanks also to Heinz Brinkmann, who provided us with the audiograms of the first investigation by Friedrich Pfander. Mr. Olaf Tech was kind enough to provide the report on the sound measurements of the Army Music Corps and the publication of Friedrich Pfander. Thanks also to Eckhard Hoffmann for his research and data collection for follow-up.

Funding

No funding.

Authors' contributions

Conception and design: RM and JS. Administrative support: RM. Provision of study materials and patients: RM. Collection and assembly of data: RM. Data analysis and interpretation: RM and JS. Manuscript writing: RM and JS. Final approval of manuscript: RM and JS.

Competing interests

The authors declare that they have no competing interests.

Author details

[1]Justus-Liebig-Universität Giessen, Aulweg 123, 35392 Giessen, Germany.
[2]Institut und Poliklinik für Arbeits- und Sozialmedizin am Universitätsklinikum Giessen und Marburg, Aulweg 129, Giessen 35392, Germany.

References

1. Qian CL, Behar A, Wong W. Noise exposure of musicians of a ballet orchestra. Noise Health. 2011;13(50):59–63.
2. Smith C, Beamer S, Hall S, Helfer T, Kluchinsky TA Jr. A preliminary analysis of noise exposure and medical outcomes for department of defense military musicians. US Army Med Dep J. 2015;3(Jul.-Sept.):76–82.
3. Gonçalves CG, Lacerda AB, Zeigelboim BS, Marques JM, Luders D. Auditory thresholds among military musicians: conventional and high frequency. Codas. 2013;25(2):181–7.
4. Patil ML, Sadhra S, Taylor C, Folkes SE. Hearing loss in British Army musicians. Occup Med. 2013;63(4):281–3.
5. Axelsson A, Lindgren F. Hearing in classical musicians. Acta Otolaryngol. 1981;91(Suppl 377):3–74.
6. EU Directive 2003/10/EC of the European Parliament and of the council, 2007.
7. McBride D, Gill F, Proops D, Harrington M, Gardiner K, Attwell C. Noise and the classical musician. BMJ. 1992;305:1561–3.
8. ISO 1999. Acoustics – estimation of noise induced hearing loss. Geneva: International Organization for Standardisation; 2013.
9. Brusis T. Akuter Hörverlust beim Orchestermusiker. HNO. 2010;59:664–73.
10. Karlsson K, Lundquist PG, Olaussen T. The hearing of symphony orchestra musicians. Scand Audiol. 1983;12:257–64.
11. Kähäri KR, Axelsson A, Hellström PA, Zachau G. Hearing assessment of classical orchestral misicians. Scand Audiol. 2001;30:13–23.
12. Kähäri KR, Axelsson A, Hellström PA, Zachau G. Hearing development in classical orchestral musicians. A follow-up study. Scand Audiol. 2001;30:141–9.
13. Obeling L, Poulsen T. Hearing ability in Danish symphony orchestra musicians. Noise Health. 1999;2:43–9.
14. Royster JD, Royster LH, Killion MC. Sound exposures and hearing thresholds of symphony orchestra musicians. J Acoust Soc Am. 1991;89(6):2793–803.
15. Toppila EM, Koskinen H, Pyykkö I. Hearing loss among classical-orchestra musicians. Noise Health. 2011;13:45–50.
16. Ostri B, Eller N, Dahlin E, Skylv G. Hearing impairment in orchestral musicians. Scand Audiol. 1989;18:243–9.
17. Reuter K, Hammershøi D. Distortion product otoacoustic emission of symphony orchestra musicians before and after rehearsal. J Acoust Soc Am. 2007;121(1):327–36.
18. Schmidt JH, Pedersen ER, Møller Juhl P, Christensen-Dalgaard J, et al. Sound exposure of symphony orchestra musicians. Ann Occup Hyg. 2011; 55:893–905.
19. Sataloff RT. Hearing loss in musicians. Am J Otol. 1991;12:122–7.
20. Emmerich E, Rudel L, Richter F. Is the audiologic status of professional musicians a reflection of the noise exposure in classical orchestral music? Eur Arch Otorhinolaryngol. 2008;265(7):753–8.
21. Bo M, Clerico M, Pognant F. Parametric method for the noise risk assessment of professional orchestral musicians. Noise Health. 2016;18(85):319–28.
22. Pfander F. Akustische Belastung der Bundeswehrmusiker und ihre arbeitsmedizinische Beurteilung. Wehrmedizinische Monatsschrift. 1985; 29(8):329–31.
23. ISO 389-8. Acoustics – reference zero for the calibration of audiometric equipment – part 8: reference equivalent threshold sound pressure levels for pure tones and circum-aural earphones. Geneva: International Organization for Standardization; 2004.
24. ISO 389-5. Acoustics – reference zero for the calibration of audiometric equipment – part 5: reference equivalent threshold sound pressure levels for pure tones in the frequency range 8 kHz to 16 kHz. Geneva: International Organization for Standardization; 1999.
25. ISO 389-1. Acoustics – reference zero for the calibration of audiometric equipment – part 8: reference equivalent threshold sound pressure levels for pure tones and supra-aural earphones. Geneva: International Organization for Standardization; 2000.
26. ISO 7029. Acoustics – statistical distribution of hearing thresholds as a function of age. Geneva: International Organization for Standardisation; 2000.
27. ISO 7029 (draft). Acoustics – statistical distribution of hearing thresholds as a function of age. Geneva: International Organization for Standardisation; 2014.
28. Laitinen HM, Toppila EM, Olkinuora PS, Kuisma K. Sound exposure among the Finnish National Opera personnel. Appl Occup Environ Hyg. 2003;18(3):177–82.

29. O'Brien I, Wilson W, Bradley A. Nature of orchestral noise. J Acoust Soc Am. 2008;124(2):926–39.
30. Pirilä T, Jounio-Ervasti K, Sorri M. Left-right asymmetries in hearing threshold levels in three age groups of a random population. Audiology. 1992;31:150–61.
31. Johnson DW, Sherman RE, Aldridge J, Lorraine A. Effects of instrument type and orchestral position on hearing sensitivity for 0.25 to 20 kHz in the orchestral musician. Scand Audiol. 1985;14:215–21.
32. Burk MH, Wiley TL. Continuous versus pulsed tones in audiometry. Am J Audiol. 2004;13(1):54–61.
33. Flamme GA, Geda K, Mcgregor KD, Wyllys K, Deiters KK, et al. Stimulus and transducer effects on threshold. Int J Audiol. 2015;54(Supl. 1):19–29.

20

Impact of shift work on the diurnal cortisol rhythm: a one-year longitudinal study in junior physicians

Jian Li[1][*] ⓘ, Martin Bidlingmaier[2], Raluca Petru[3], Francisco Pedrosa Gil [4], Adrian Loerbroks[1] and Peter Angerer[1]

Abstract

Background: Cumulative epidemiological evidence suggests that shift work exerts harmful effects on human health. However, the physiological mechanisms are not well understood. This study aimed to examine the impact of shift work on the dysregulation of the hypothalamic-pituitary-adrenal axis, i.e. diurnal cortisol rhythm.

Methods: Seventy physicians with a mean age 30 years participated in this one-year longitudinal study. Working schedules, either shift work or regular schedules with day shift, were assessed at baseline. Salivary cortisol samples were collected on two consecutive regular working days, four times a day (including waking, + 4 h, + 8 h, and + 16 h), at both baseline and the one-year follow-up. The diurnal cortisol decline (slope) and total cortisol concentration (area under the curve, AUC) were calculated.

Results: After adjusting for cortisol secretion at baseline and numerous covariates, shift work at baseline significantly predicted a steeper slope ($p < 0.01$) and a larger AUC ($p < 0.05$) of diurnal cortisol rhythm at follow-up in this sample of physicians. In particular, waking cortisol at follow-up was significantly higher among those engaged in shift work than day shift ($p < 0.01$).

Conclusions: Our findings support the notion that shift work changes the diurnal cortisol pattern, and is predictive of increased cortisol secretion consequently in junior physicians.

Keywords: Shift work, Cortisol, Hypothalamic-pituitary-adrenal axis, Longitudinal study, Occupational health

Background

Shift work is common in contemporary working life. In the United States, about 29% of the employees had their work time arrangements as shift work, according the 2010 National Health Interview Survey [1]; while the 2010 European Working Conditions Survey indicated that more than 20% workers in Europe were engaged in shift work [2]. In the past decades, several chronic health conditions have been identified to be related to shift work [3]. For example, in 2007 the World Health Organization International Agency for Research on Cancer announced the probable association between shift work and cancer risk [4], particularly breast cancer in women [5] and prostate cancer in men [6]; in addition, it has been observed that shift work increases risk of diabetes [7], myocardial infarction, all coronary events, and ischaemic stroke [8].

Some physiological mechanisms have been proposed to explain links between shift work and adverse health outcomes. Among others, shift work-caused disruption of the circadian time organization is one core explanation, which exerts far-reaching effects at the molecular and cellular levels. Exposure to shift work during one's occupational career, through the close physiological interaction of circadian clock-related and cell-cycle factors, may result in a variety of processes that initiate epigenetic modifications, with malignant potential. Supportively, expression and methylation of circadian genes, such as BMAL1 and PER1, are evident among shift workers in recent years [9–11]. Meanwhile, melatonin which is produced in the pineal gland and circulated during darkness has received significant attention

* Correspondence: jian.li@uni-duesseldorf.de
[1]Institute of Occupational, Social and Environmental Medicine, Centre for Health and Society, Faculty of Medicine, University of Düsseldorf, Universitätsstraße 1, 40225 Düsseldorf, Germany
Full list of author information is available at the end of the article

in shift work research. It exerts broad effects, via specific receptors or entry into cells directly as a small lipophilic molecule, playing a crucial role in regulating the circadian time organization. Commonly co-existing with circadian disruption, "melatonin hypothesis" was formulated in 1987 to link melatonin suppression and cancer risk [12]. To date, much evidence has been gained in the past three decades, on melatonin suppression due to shift work [13, 14]. In addition, shift work is closely related to sleep deprivation and disturbance, causing immune dysfunction as elevated concentrations of C-reactive protein and interleukin 6, and an increase in cellular stress in terms of an altered balance of pro-oxidative and anti-oxidative markers [15].

Regarding the cardiometabolic risk associated with shift work, circadian disruption represents a crucial pathway as well [16, 17]. It has been postulated that circadian disruption induced by shift work would impair the functioning of the hypothalamic-pituitary-adrenal (HPA) axis which regulates the biological response to stressful stimuli [18], while abnormal HPA axis activity increases the risk of subsequent cardiometabolic conditions [19–21]. Cortisol is the most widely studied biomarker of the HPA axis, and it is usually assayed from saliva, serum, urine, or hair [22]. Cortisol shows a strong diurnal rhythm. In the morning cortisol peaks during awakening, then it declines gradually over the day till bedtime [23, 24]. In general, different features of the cortisol diurnal pattern have been frequently examined as indicators of HPA axis function, including the waking cortisol response which is superimposed on the circadian cycle of cortisol release [25], the slope of cortisol decline over the day and the total cortisol concentration over the day such as area under the curve (AUC) [26].

So far, epidemiological studies on shift work and cortisol have found inconsistent, even contrasting, results. For instance, two French studies found that serum cortisol in the evening was increased among workers in night shift [27, 28]. Using urinary or hair cortisol, two studies from the US and the Netherlands respectively observed that shift workers had significantly higher cortisol levels [29, 30]. Also, a British study showed that shift work was associated with higher waking cortisol as well as total AUC in saliva [31]. By contrast, Hung et al. reported lower cortisol AUC in shift workers [32]. In addition, five studies indicated negative associations between shift work and waking salivary cortisol [13, 33–36]. Regarding the decline rate of cortisol rhythm over the day, a flatter slope was demonstrated by three studies from the UK, US, and Canada, respectively [31, 32, 37]. By contrast, a Canadian study among paramedics did not find any relationships between shift work and cortisol secretion [38]. Nevertheless, we need to bear it in mind that the studies mentioned above were all with cross-sectional design.

Due to the simultaneous assessment of shift work and cortisol it remains impossible to draw any causal inference based on such studies. In the past decade, only few longitudinal studies on shift work and cortisol trends over time have been published. Four studies examined recovery of cortisol diurnal pattern after shift work. Two Norwegian studies among offshore oil rig workers found that cortisol diurnal profiles were not recovered on day 7 and day 11 after 2-week 12-h night-shifts [39, 40]; while cortisol diurnal profile was recovered on day 5 after 5-day 8-h night-shifts among Chinese nurses [41], and it was recovered on day 7 after 7-day 8-h night-shifts among Danish police officers [42]. When the follow-up period is prolonged, the findings seem to become mixed. Kudielka et al. followed up a sample of German workers in an electronic manufacturing plant for 2 months, and they reported that AUC of salivary cortisol was significantly increased in the group of night shift [43]; similarly, a Dutch study in police officers suggested waking salivary cortisol began to rise from baseline to significantly higher levels at one-year follow-up after they started shift duty, then declined slightly at two-year follow-up [44]. However, Copertaro et al. did not confirm any significant association of shift work with serum cortisol among Italian nurses with one-year follow-up [45]. Overall, most of studies on shift work and cortisol had a major limitation in terms of their small sample sizes (usually < 50 subjects).

We therefore carried out a longitudinal study with one-year follow-up, in order to investigate the impact of shift work on the dysregulation of the HPA axis in terms of diurnal cortisol rhythm, in a sample of hospital physicians during residency who were at high risk of circadian disruption due to shift work schedule arrangement.

Methods

Study sample

At baseline, 1000 junior physicians in their 2nd or 3rd year of specialty training (residency) working in the wider area of Munich, Germany, were randomly selected to participate in a questionnaire survey, based on registration data of the Bavarian Chamber of Medical Doctors. A total of 621 completed questionnaires were returned (response rate 62.1%). Among the 1000 invited physicians, one third random sample, i.e., 334 subjects were also invited to participate in a series of saliva tests. Saliva samples were collected on 2 consecutive working days (which were not during or on the days after night shift), 4 times a day, including time points at waking (0 h), + 4 h, + 8 h, and + 16 h. Questionnaires were usually answered 1–3 days before saliva sampling. Of the 334 participants, 146 returned saliva samples (response rate: 43.7%). However, 57 samples had to be excluded due to steroid treatment, sampling error, low volume of saliva, or missing data on any 4 times of samples, which left valid saliva samples 99 subjects at baseline. After one year we followed up those 146 physicians who had previously responded both questionnaire survey and saliva samples. Among them, 91 physicians (response rate 62.3%) returned two-day saliva samples (same procedure as baseline). From those, 21 were excluded from further analysis due to the above mentioned reasons. Thus, valid cortisol measurements at both baseline and follow-up were available from 70 participants.

The study was approved by the Committee on Ethics of Human Research of the Medical Faculty, Ludwig-Maximilians University Munich (No. 016/04), and participants signed a letter of informed consent.

Measures

In the baseline questionnaire, the physicians were asked "Do you take shift work (which is regular work outside normal daily working hours)?" with two response categories of "No" and "Yes".

Saliva samples were collected using a small cotton swab with no additives (Salivette®, Sarstedt, Numbrecht, Germany). Participants were instructed to chew on the swab for 3 min, put the swab into the Salivette, note the time of sampling, keep the samples at ambient temperature and return them to the lab within 1 week. Cortisol remains stable for this period of time. Participants were asked to collect samples on 2 days. All saliva samples were stored in the laboratory at -20 °C until cortisol analysis. Cortisol concentrations were determined employing a highly sensitive chemiluminescence immunoassay (Cortisol Saliva LIA, IBL, Hamburg, Germany). Endpoint detection was done using a chemiluminescence reader (Victor, Perkin Elmer, Rodgau, Germany). The assay shows a relevant cross reaction with the following steroids: Prednisolone (57%), 11-deoxycortisol (12%), corticosterone (2.5%), cortisone (2%) and prednisolone (1%). The lower detection limit of this assay is less than 0.16 ng/ml. To reduce error variance caused by interassay imprecision, all samples from one subject were assayed in the same run. In our hands, within-assay coefficient of variation was 7.2 and 5.4% at 0.8 and 5.0 ng/ml, respectively. Between-assay coefficient of variation at the same concentrations was 9.45 and 6.6%, respectively. Since cortisol data from two consecutive working days were available, we calculated the mean values to represent cortisol levels for the four sampling time points, waking (0 h), + 4 h, + 8 h, and + 16 h, respectively. Diurnal slope was produced by regressing cortisol values on sampling time, with anchorage on the waking point, to generate a mean rate of reduction in cortisol per hour [26, 31]. Total cortisol concentration over the day (AUC, ng/ml × hours) was calculated using a formula for area under the curve with respect to ground, based on all the four sampling time points [46].

In addition, information on age, gender, professional tenure, working hours, partnership, children, smoking, risky alcohol use, physical activity, overweight and obesity was also collected at baseline.

Data analysis

Firstly, descriptive statistics were performed. Means and standard deviations (SD) were calculated for continuous variables, and relative frequencies for categorical variables. Due to the fact we draw on a subsample to investigate cortisol research, we also compared the baseline characteristics between cortisol-involved participants in the current analyses ($N = 70$) and cortisol-involved non-participants ($N = 551$) within the whole study population, using Student's t-test for continuous variables or Chi-square test for categorical variables. Secondly, we further tested the differences of baseline characteristics and cortisol secretion levels between the groups without or with shift work. Thirdly, differences of cortisol levels on four sampling time points (waking (0 h), + 4 h, + 8 h, and + 16 h) at follow-up were examined by analysis of covariance adjusting for age, gender, professional tenure, working hours, partnership, children, smoking, risky alcohol use, physical activity, overweight and obesity at baseline; more importantly, we also controlled for cortisol levels at baseline to account for potential ceiling effect (i.e., upward change less likely for higher baseline scores) and floor effect (i.e., downward change less likely for lower baseline scores). Fourthly, multivariate linear regression was applied to examine longitudinal associations between shift work levels at baseline (independent variable) and diurnal cortisol pattern (slope and AUC) at follow-up (dependent variables). The results are shown as regression coefficients (β) with 95% confidence intervals (CI). These analyses were adjusted for biological factors (age and gender), work factors (professional tenure and working hours), family factors (partnership and children), and behavioral factors (smoking, risky alcohol use, physical activity, overweight and obesity) at baseline as well as baseline cortisol values, in order to assess robustness of associations. Finally, considering the nature of repeated measures in longitudinal studies, particularly when correlations at different time-points within-subjects need to be addressed, we also used mixed regression modeling to examine the longitudinal associations between shift work at baseline and repeated measures of cortisol levels over the one-year period of follow-up [47]. All analyses were conducted with SAS 9.4 SAS Institute Inc., North Carolina, US).

Results

Table 1 shows the characteristics of the study samples (with valid cortisol data) at baseline ($N = 70$). The mean age equaled nearly 30 years, and 57% were women. Seventy-six percent were living with partners, and 83% had no children. Regarding health-related behaviors, the majority did not smoke, did not have risky alcohol use, were engaged in regular physical activity, and the vast majority had normal body weight. Half of the participants were in their first 2 years of medical residency, and mean working time was nearly 51 h/week. The cortisol-involved subjects ($N = 70$) were fairly comparable to the others who did not participate in corisol collection or did not have valid cortisol data ($N = 551$) with respect to socio-demographic, work-related, or behavioral characteristics.

Out of 70 study subjects, 19 (27%) physicians were engaged in shift work at baseline. Typical diurnal cortisol rhythm was observed, i.e., the cortisol level was highest at waking, and then declined gradually over the day. The overall cortisol slope was − 0.39, and AUC was 42.38. However, none of the study characteristics including all cortisol indicators was significantly different between physicians without and with shift work (Table 2).

Figure 1 illustrates diurnal cortisol rhythm at follow-up for the shift work group vs. the non-shift work group. After adjustment for socio-demographic, behavioral, work and family factors, as well as cortisol levels at baseline, waking cortisol was found to be significantly higher among physicians engaged in shift work ($p < 0.01$), whereas cortisol levels at the other three time points (+ 4 h, + 8 h, and + 16 h) did not differ by shift work status (details not shown).

The results of linear regression are shown in the Table 3. Throughout the adjustment procedure from models I to V, the associations remained stable. In the fully (final) adjusted model, shift work at baseline was associated with increased cortisol slope negatively by 0.12 ($p < 0.01$) and elevated total cortisol AUC positively by 6.64 ($p < 0.05$) 1 year later, indicating steeper slope and larger AUC over the day. Notably, mixed regression modeling, while taking the correlations of cortisol at baseline and at follow-up into account, exerted very similar findings (Table 4).

Discussion

The aim of our study was to examine the longitudinal impact of shift work on diurnal cortisol rhythm. Drawing on a sample of junior physicians from Germany, we found

Table 1 Characteristics of cortisol-involved participants and non-participants at baseline

Variables		Cortisol-involved participants $N = 70$	Cortisol-involved non-participants $N = 551$	p
Age (years)	(mean ± SD)	30.61 ± 2.63	30.51 ± 2.72	0.7777
Working hours per week	(mean ± SD)	50.86 ± 9.46	51.18 ± 9.66	0.7903
Gender	Men	30, 42.86%	273, 49.55%	0.2916
	Women	40, 57.14%	278, 50.45%	
Partnership	No	17, 24.29%	132, 23.96%	0.9515
	Yes	53, 75.71%	419, 76.04%	
Children	No	58, 82.86%	462, 83.85%	0.8325
	Yes	12, 17.14%	89, 16.15%	
Professional tenure	≤ 2 years	34, 48.57%	239, 43.38%	0.4094
	> 2 years	36, 51.43%	312, 56.62%	
Shift work	No	51, 72.86%	375, 68.06%	0.4151
	Yes	19, 27.14%	176, 31.94%	
Smoking	No	59, 84.29%	448, 81.31%	0.5442
	Yes	11, 15.71%	103, 18.69%	
Risky alcohol use	No	63, 90.00%	486, 88.20%	0.6583
	Yes	7, 10.00%	65, 11.80%	
Physical activity	Inactive	18, 25.71%	157, 28.49%	0.6263
	Active	52, 74.29%	394, 71.51%	
Overweight and obesity	No	60, 85.71%	446, 80.94%	0.3331
	Yes	10, 14.29%	105, 19.06%	

Difference determined by Student's t-test or Chi-square test

Table 2 Characteristics of study subjects at baseline

Variables		Shift work: No N = 51	Shift work: Yes N = 19	p	Total (N = 70)
Age (years)	(mean ± SD)	30.57 ± 2.48	30.74 ± 3.05	0.8138	30.61 ± 2.63
Working hours per week	(mean ± SD)	50.82 ± 10.27	50.95 ± 7.08	0.9616	50.86 ± 6.46
Gender	Men	25, 49.02%	5, 26.32%	0.0878	30, 42.86%
	Women	26, 50.98%	14, 73.68%		40, 57.14%
Partnership	No	12, 23.53%	5, 26.32%	0.8090	17, 24.29%
	Yes	39, 76.47%	14, 73.68%		53, 75.71%
Children	No	43, 84.31%	15, 78.95%	0.5963	58, 82.86%
	Yes	8, 15.69%	4, 21.05%		12, 17.14%
Professional tenure	≤ 2 years	27, 52.94%	7, 36.84%	0.2307	34, 48.57%
	> 2 years	24, 47.06%	12, 63.16%		36, 51.43%
Smoking	No	42, 82.35%	17, 89.47%	0.4666	59, 84.29%
	Yes	9, 17.65%	2, 10.53%		11, 15.71%
Risky alcohol use	No	45, 88.24%	18, 94.74%	0.4201	63, 90.00%
	Yes	6, 11.76%	1, 5.26%		7, 10.00%
Physical activity	Inactive	13, 25.49%	5, 26.32%	0.9440	18, 25.71%
	Active	38, 74.51%	14, 73.68%		52, 74.29%
Overweight and obesity	No	45, 88.24%	15, 78.95%	0.3234	60, 85.71%
	Yes	6, 11.76%	4, 21.05%		10, 14.29%
Cortisol at waking, 0 h (ng/ml)	(mean ± SD)	7.90 ± 4.82	8.36 ± 3.55	0.7003	8.02 ± 4.50
Cortisol at +4 h	(mean ± SD)	2.90 ± 2.34	2.84 ± 1.46	0.9029	2.88 ± 2.13
Cortisol at + 8 h	(mean ± SD)	1.98 ± 1.19	1.59 ± 0.98	0.2078	1.87 ± 1.15
Cortisol at + 16 h	(mean ± SD)	0.91 ± 0.70	0.83 ± 0.65	0.6567	0.89 ± 0.68
Cortisol slope	(mean ± SD)	−0.38 ± 0.24	− 0.41 ± 0.17	0.6137	− 0.39 ± 0.22
Total cortisol AUC (ng/ml × hours)	(mean ± SD)	42.91 ± 20.55	40.95 ± 14.30	0.7037	42.38 ± 18.98

Difference determined by Student's t-test or Chi-square test

that shift work at baseline significantly changed the diurnal cortisol pattern at follow-up, in terms of higher waking cortisol, steeper slope and larger AUC, thereby predicting increased cortisol secretion at follow-up.

To date, cross-sectional studies generated contrasting evidence on the relationships between shift work and cortisol. As we mentioned above, in order to enable causal inference, longitudinal design is preferable. Therefore, the three longitudinal studies in the past decade deserve a close look. The Dutch study found an increase in waking salivary cortisol when police officers commenced duty of shift work 1 year later, and the effect was maintained for almost 2 years [44], while the German study, among industrial workers, suggested more cortisol secretion in saliva as larger AUC by changing work schedule from day shift to night shift for 2 months [43]. However, these two studies did not set an external reference group, that is, pre-and-post comparisons were actually conducted within subjects. The research design of the third study, conducted among Italian nurses, was quite similar to ours, with an external reference group

(daytime work), with a one-year follow-up, and with adjustment for baseline cortisol values to take ceiling and floor effect into account [45]. Unfortunately, that study did not suggest any significant associations between shift work at baseline and cortisol levels at follow-up. Potential explanations might pertain to the approach to cortisol measurement, i.e., serum cortisol, because blood sampling itself represented acute stress reaction; and sampling point was one time only, i.e., 8:30–9:30 in the morning, resulting that the diurnal cortisol rhythm was impossible to be investigated [45].

Strengths of our study include its longitudinal study design to explore the potential causal association of baseline shift work and future changes in diurnal cortisol pattern which requires multiple sampling time points over the day. Furthermore, we recruited relatively larger sample size empowering our ability to detect fairly modest associations with statistical significance compared to most of earlier studies. To our knowledge, our study also produced first evidence of a longitudinal link between shift work and the cortisol slope, in addition to existing

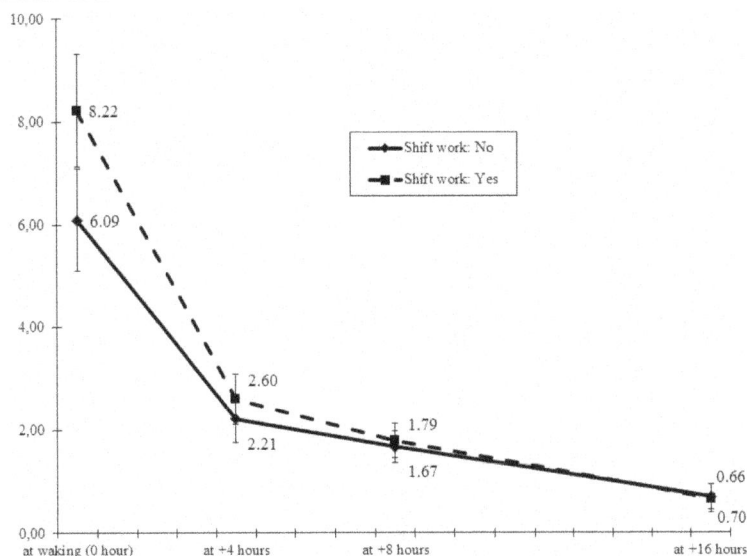

Fig. 1 Diurnal pattern of cortisol secretion at follow-up according to shift work at baseline. (Solid line represents cortisol pattern at follow-up for physicians with shift work status "no" at baseline ($N = 51$); dashed line represents cortisol pattern at follow-up for physicians with shift work status "yes" at baseline ($N = 19$); Error bars represent standard errors of adjusted means (ng/ml) of four time points cortisol levels at follow-up)

longitudinal findings on waking cortisol and total cortisol AUC [43, 44]. Nevertheless, our study also suffered several limitations. Firstly, just like in many previous studies on shift work, our assessment of shift work was not comprehensive enough [48]. In our study, participants only reported whether they were engaged into shift work. Additional information of interest had related to, (i) shift system on rotating or permanent schedule, regular or irregular arrangement; (ii) cumulative length of exposure; and (iii) shift intensity with time off (recovery days) between shifts [48]. Secondly, we need to mention the age difference and its effect on circadian impact of shift work. Both our study and one prior longitudinal study [44] identified higher waking cortisol by shift work, but many studies found shift work was associated with lower levels of waking cortisol [13, 33–36]. Also, we observed shift work steepened the decline rate of cortisol rhythm, whereas flatter slope was reported by

other studies [31, 32, 37]. Age might serve as one potential explanation. The mean age was 30 years in our study and 27 years in the study by Lammers-van der Holst et al., respectively [44]. However, the mean age of most other studies was around 40 years or even older. Plenty of research has testified that, compared to younger people, waking cortisol is relatively lower and evening cortisol is relative higher in older people [49, 50]. This may imply that the pattern of shift work-caused diurnal cortisol change may differ in younger workers from ageing workers. The HPA axis is activated quickly in the morning and recovers in the evening (i.e., steeper cortisol slope) among young workers exposed to shift work; whereas the effect of shift work is obvious on evening cortisol but not on waking cortisol (i.e., flatter slope) among older workers. Certainly, future research on age, shift work, and HPA axis regulation is warranted. Thirdly, in our study, a cortisol sample was collected

Table 3 Longitudinal associations between shift work at baseline and diurnal cortisol pattern at follow-up ($N = 70$)

Cortisol slope	Model I	Model II	Model III	Model IV	Model V
Shift work: No	0	0	0	0	0
Shift work: Yes	−0.09 (− 0.18, − 0.01)*	−0.11 (− 0.20, − 0.02) *	−0.11 (− 0.20, − 0.02)*	−0.12 (− 0.21, − 0.04)**	−0.12 (− 0.21, − 0.03)**
Total cortisol AUC	Model I	Model II	Model III	Model IV	Model V
Shift work: No	0	0	0	0	0
Shift work: Yes	5.36 (0.20, 10.52) *	6.19 (1.13, 11.25) *	6.33 (1.25, 11.41) *	6.71 (1.55, 11.86) *	6.64 (1.48, 11.79) *

Linear regression, β (95% CI), *$p < 0.05$, **$p < 0.01$
Model I: adjustment for biological factors (age and gender)
Model II: Model I + additional adjustment for work factors (professional tenure and working hours) at baseline
Model III: Model II + additional adjustment for family factors (partnership and children) at baseline
Model IV: Model III + additional adjustment for behavioral factors (smoking, risky alcohol use, physical activity, overweight and obesity) at baseline
Model V: Model IV + additional adjustment for cortisol secretion at baseline

Table 4 Longitudinal associations between shift work at baseline and diurnal cortisol pattern over one-year period of follow-up (N = 70)

	Cortisol at waking	Cortisol at +4 h	Cortisol at +8 h	Cortisol at +16 h
Shift work: No	0	0	0	0
Shift work: Yes	2.02 (0.68, 3.36)**	0.30 (−0.28, 0.88)	−0.01 (−0.38, 0.36)	0.02 (−0.26, 0.29)
	Cortisol slope		Total cortisol AUC	
Shift work: No	0		0	
Shift work: Yes	−0.10 (−0.17, −0.03)**		5.84 (1.36, 10.32)*	

Mixed regression, β (95% CI), *$p < 0.05$, **$p < 0.01$
Adjustment for biological factors (age and gender), work factors (professional tenure and working hours), family factors (partnership and children), behavioral factors (smoking, risky alcohol use, physical activity, overweight and obesity) at baseline

only on a single occasion in the morning, i.e., at waking. In psychoneuroendocrinological research, data on two sampling time points in the morning is generally preferred. If appropriately timed, those two assessments reflect the so-called "cortisol awakening response", which is conceptualized as "a sharp increase in cortisol levels across the first 30-45 min following morning awakening" [51]. However, sampling accuracy and participants' adherence are the major challenges in practice. Lacking data of cortisol awakening response is one main limitation regarding the research of diurnal cortisol rhythm. For future research, the consensus guidelines by an expert panel from the International Society of Psychoneuroendocrinology would be of great help [51]. Finally, as the current findings are restricted to young working people and one single occupation only, the ability of generalization to other age categories and occupations is limited. More longitudinal studies with larger sample size covering wider age range and various occupations are urgently needed in future.

As stated in a recent report from the US National Toxicology Program's workshop on shift work at night, artificial light at night, and circadian disruption, "Understanding potential mechanisms and characteristics of light or shift work that are related to circadian disruption or biomarkers of disease may help identify interventions to protect public health." [52] The available research evidence on shift work and diurnal cortisol rhythm would provide meaningful information to future interventions regarding work schedule management. For instance, according to a handful studies with respect to recovery of cortisol diurnal pattern after shift work, it would be desirable to allow for sufficient time periods off between shifts, such as 2 consecutive night shift days + 2 consecutive recovery days, or 5 + 5, 7 + 7, 14 + 14 arrangements [39–42]. Moreover, a review published in 2014 identified 44 intervention studies on health improvement among shift workers. In general, results support the benefits of fast-forward rotating shift schedules, i.e., morning-evening-night [53]. Specifically, compared to fast-backward rotating shifts, fast-forward rotating shifts exerted lower cortisol levels during the morning and night shifts [54].

Conclusions

In conclusion, our longitudinal study, among junior physicians from Germany, supports the notion that shift work at baseline detrimentally affects the diurnal cortisol pattern 1 year later, specifically, higher waking cortisol, steeper slope and increased total cortisol secretion.

Funding

This study was funded in part by the German Medical Association and supported by the Bavarian Chamber of Doctors, Marburger Bund, and Munich Center of Health Sciences.

Authors' contributions

JL and PA developed the study conception; RP collected the data; MB prepared the cortisol measurement protocol and conducted the cortisol assay; JL performed the statistical analyses; MB, RP, FPG, AL, PA, and JL critically interpreted the results; JL prepared a first draft of the manuscript; AL and PA contributed substantially to the argumentation and revision. All authors read and approved the final version of the manuscript.

Competing interests

The authors declare that they have no competing interests.

Author details

[1]Institute of Occupational, Social and Environmental Medicine, Centre for Health and Society, Faculty of Medicine, University of Düsseldorf, Universitätsstraße 1, 40225 Düsseldorf, Germany. [2]Endocrine Research Unit, Medizinische Klinik und Poliklinik IV, Ludwig-Maximilians-University, Munich, Germany. [3]Institute and Outpatient Clinic for Occupational, Social and Environmental Medicine, WHO Collaborating Centre for Occupational Health, Ludwig-Maximilians-University, Munich, Germany. [4]Clinic for Psychiatry, Psychotherapy and Psychosomatics, Helios Vogtland Clinical Center, Plauen, Germany.

References

1. Alterman T, Luckhaupt SE, Dahlhamer JM, Ward BW, Calvert GM. Prevalence rates of work organization characteristics among workers in the U.S.: data from the 2010 National Health Interview Survey. Am J Ind Med. 2013;56:647–59.
2. Slany C, Schütte S, Chastang JF, Parent-Thirion A, Vermeylen G, Niedhammer I. Psychosocial work factors and long sickness absence in Europe. Int J Occup Environ Health. 2014;20:16–25.
3. Kecklund G, Axelsson J. Health consequences of shift work and insufficient sleep. BMJ. 2016;355:i5210.
4. Straif K, Baan R, Grosse Y, Secretan B, El Ghissassi F, Bouvard V, et al. Carcinogenicity of shift-work, painting, and fire-fighting. Lancet Oncol. 2007;8:1065–6.
5. Lin X, Chen W, Wei F, Ying M, Wei W, Xie X. Night-shift work increases morbidity of breast cancer and all-cause mortality: a meta-analysis of 16 prospective cohort studies. Sleep Med. 2015;16:1381–7.
6. Rao D, Yu H, Bai Y, Zheng X, Xie L. Does night-shift work increase the risk of prostate cancer? A systematic review and meta-analysis. Onco Targets Ther. 2015;8:2817–26.
7. Gan Y, Yang C, Tong X, Sun H, Cong Y, Yin X, et al. Shift work and diabetes mellitus: a meta-analysis of observational studies. Occup Environ Med. 2015;72:72–8.
8. Vyas MV, Garg AX, Iansavichus AV, Costella J, Donner A, Laugsand LE, et al. Shift work and vascular events: systematic review and meta-analysis. BMJ. 2012;345:e4800.
9. Reszka E, Peplonska B, Wieczorek E, Sobala W, Bukowska A, Gromadzinska J, et al. Circadian gene expression in peripheral blood leukocytes of rotating night shift nurses. Scand J Work Environ Health. 2013;39:187–94.
10. Reszka E, Wieczorek E, Przybek M, Jabłońska E, Kałużny P, Bukowska-Damska A, et al. Circadian gene methylation in rotating-shift nurses: a cross-sectional study. Chronobiol Int. 2018;35:111–21.
11. Samulin Erdem J, Skare Ø, Petersen-Øverleir M, Notø HØ, Lie JS, Reszka E, et al. Mechanisms of breast Cancer in shift workers: DNA methylation in five Core circadian genes in nurses working night shifts. J Cancer. 2017;8:2876–84.
12. Stevens RG. Electric power use and breast cancer: a hypothesis. Am J Epidemiol. 1987;125:556–61.
13. Bracci M, Ciarapica V, Copertaro A, Barbaresi M, Manzella N, Tomasetti M, et al. Peripheral skin temperature and circadian biological clock in shift nurses after a day off. Int J Mol Sci. 2016;17:E623.
14. Hunter CM, Figueiro MG. Measuring light at night and melatonin levels in shift workers: a review of the literature. Biol Res Nurs. 2017;19:365–74.
15. Faraut B, Bayon V, Léger D. Neuroendocrine, immune and oxidative stress in shift workers. Sleep Med Rev. 2013;17:433–44.
16. Rüger M, Scheer FA. Effects of circadian disruption on the cardiometabolic system. Rev Endocr Metab Disord. 2009;10:245–60.
17. Reutrakul S, Knutson KL. Consequences of circadian disruption on cardiometabolic health. Sleep Med Clin. 2015;10:455–68.
18. Nader N, Chrousos GP, Kino T. Interactions of the circadian CLOCK system and the HPA axis. Trends Endocrinol Metab. 2010;21:277–86.
19. Rosmond R, Bjorntorp P. The hypothalamic-pituitary-adrenal axis activity as a predictor of cardiovascular disease, type 2 diabetes and stroke. J Int Med. 2000;247:188–97.
20. Vogelzangs N, Beekman AT, Milaneschi Y, Bandinelli S, Ferrucci L, Penninx BW. Urinary cortisol and six-year risk of all-cause and cardiovascular mortality. J Clin Endocrinol Metab. 2010;95:4959–64.
21. Kumari M, Shipley M, Stafford M, Kivimaki M. Association of diurnal patterns in salivary cortisol with all-cause and cardiovascular mortality: findings from the Whitehall II study. J Clin Endocrinol Metab. 2011;96:1478–85.
22. Miller GE, Chen E, Zhou ES. If it goes up, must it come down? Chronic stress and the hypothalamic-pituitary-adrenocortical axis in humans. Psychol Bull. 2007;133:25–45.
23. Van Cauter E. Diurnal and ultradian rhythms in human endocrine function: a minireview. Horm Res. 1990;34:45–53.
24. Czeisler CA, Klerman EB. Circadian and sleep-dependent regulation of hormone release in humans. Recent Prog Horm Res. 1999;54:97–130.
25. Kudielka BM, Gierens A, Hellhammer DH, Wust S, Schlotz W. Salivary cortisol in ambulatory assessment – some dos, some don'ts, and some open questions. Psychosom Med. 2012;74:418–31.
26. Adam EK, Kumari M. Assessing salivary cortisol in large-scale, epidemiological research. Psychoneuroendocrinology. 2009;34:1423–36.
27. Touitou Y, Motohashi Y, Reinberg A, Touitou C, Bourdeleau P, Bogdan A, et al. Effect of shift work on the night-time secretory patterns of melatonin, prolactin, cortisol and testosterone. Eur J Appl Physiol Occup Physiol. 1990;60:288–92.
28. Weibel L, Spiegel K, Follenius M, Ehrhart J, Brandenberger G. Internal dissociation of the circadian markers of the cortisol rhythm in night workers. Am J Phys. 1996;270:E608–13.
29. Mirick DK, Bhatti P, Chen C, Nordt F, Stanczyk FZ, Davis S. Night shift work and levels of 6-sulfatoxymelatonin and cortisol in men. Cancer Epidemiol Biomark Prev. 2013;22:1079–87.
30. Manenschijn L, van Kruysbergen RG, de Jong FH, Koper JW, van Rossum EF. Shift work at young age is associated with elevated long-term cortisol levels and body mass index. J Clin Endocrinol Metab. 2011;96:E1862–5.
31. Bostock S, Steptoe A. Influences of early shift work on the diurnal cortisol rhythm, mood and sleep: within-subject variation in male airline pilots. Psychoneuroendocrinology. 2013;38:533–41.
32. Hung EW, Aronson KJ, Leung M, Day A, Tranmer J. Shift work parameters and disruption of diurnal cortisol production in female hospital employees. Chronobiol Int. 2016;33:1045–55.
33. Hennig J, Kieferdorf P, Moritz C, Huwe S, Netter P. Changes in cortisol secretion during shiftwork: implications for tolerance to shiftwork? Ergonomics. 1998;41:610–21.
34. Lac G, Chamoux A. Biological and psychological responses to two rapid shiftwork schedules. Ergonomics. 2004;47:1339–49.
35. Machi MS, Staum M, Callaway CW, Moore C, Jeong K, Suyama J, et al. The relationship between shift work, sleep, and cognition in career emergency physicians. Acad Emerg Med. 2012;19:85–91.
36. Fekedulegn D, Burchfiel CM, Violanti JM, Hartley TA, Charles LE, Andrew ME, et al. Associations of long-term shift work with waking salivary cortisol concentration and patterns among police officers. Ind Health. 2012;50:476–86.
37. Charles LE, Fekedulegn D, Burchfiel CM, Hartley TA, Andrew ME, Violanti JM, et al. Shiftwork and diurnal salivary cortisol patterns among police officers. J Occup Environ Med. 2016;58:542–9.
38. Wong IS, Ostry AS, Demers PA, Davies HW. Job strain and shift work influences on biomarkers and subclinical heart disease indicators: a pilot study. J Occup Environ Hyg. 2012;9:467–77.
39. Harris A, Waage S, Ursin H, Hansen AM, Bjorvatn B, Eriksen HR. Cortisol, reaction time test and health among offshore shift workers. Psychoneuroendocrinology. 2010;35:1339–47.
40. Merkus SL, Holte KA, Huysmans MA, Hansen ÅM, van de Ven PM, van Mechelen W, et al. Neuroendocrine recovery after 2-week 12-h day and night shifts: an 11-day follow-up. Int Arch Occup Environ Health. 2015;88:247–57.
41. Niu SF, Chung MH, Chu H, Tsai JC, Lin CC, Liao YM, et al. Differences in cortisol profiles and circadian adjustment time between nurses working night shifts and regular day shifts: a prospective longitudinal study. Int J Nurs Stud. 2015;52:1193–201.
42. Jensen MA, Hansen ÅM, Kristiansen J, Nabe-Nielsen K, Garde AH. Changes in the diurnal rhythms of cortisol, melatonin, and testosterone after 2, 4, and 7 consecutive night shifts in male police officers. Chronobiol Int. 2016;33:1280–92.
43. Kudielka BM, Buchtal J, Uhde A, Wüst S. Circadian cortisol profiles and psychological self-reports in shift workers with and without recent change in the shift rotation system. Biol Psychol. 2007;74:92–103.
44. Lammers-van der Holst HM, Kerkhof GA. Individual differences in the cortisol-awakening response during the first two years of shift work: a longitudinal study in novice police officers. Chronobiol Int. 2015;32:1162–7.
45. Copertaro A, Bracci M, Gesuita R, Carle F, Amati M, Baldassari M, et al. Influence of shift-work on selected immune variables in nurses. Ind Health. 2011;49:597–604.
46. Pruessner JC, Kirschbaum C, Meinlschmid G, Hellhammer DH. Two formulas for computation of the area under the curve represent measures of total hormone concentration versus time-dependent change. Psychoneuroendocrinology. 2003;28:916–31.
47. Detry MA, Ma Y. Analyzing repeated measurements using mixed models. JAMA. 2016;315:407–8.
48. Stevens RG, Hansen J, Costa G, Haus E, Kauppinen T, Aronson KJ, et al. Considerations of circadian impact for defining "shift work" in cancer studies: IARC working group report. Occup Environ Med. 2011;68:154–62.

49. Veldhuis JD, Sharma A, Roelfsema F. Age-dependent and gender-dependent regulation of hypothalamic-adrenocorticotropic-adrenal axis. Endocrinol Metab Clin N Am. 2013;42:201–25.

50. Roelfsema F, van Heemst D, Iranmanesh A, Takahashi P, Yang R, Veldhuis JD. Impact of age, sex and body mass index on cortisol secretion in 143 healthy adults. Endocr Connect. 2017;6:500–9.

51. Stalder T, Kirschbaum C, Kudielka BM, Adam EK, Pruessner JC, Wüst S, et al. Assessment of the cortisol awakening response: expert consensus guidelines. Psychoneuroendocrinology. 2016;63:414–32.

52. Lunn RM, Blask DE, Coogan AN, Figueiro MG, Gorman MR, Hall JE, et al. Health consequences of electric lighting practices in the modern world: a report on the National Toxicology Program's workshop on shift work at night, artificial light at night, and circadian disruption. Sci Total Environ. 2017;607-608:1073–84.

53. Neil-Sztramko SE, Pahwa M, Demers PA, Gotay CC. Health-related interventions among night shift workers: a critical review of the literature. Scand J Work Environ Health. 2014;40:543–56.

54. Vangelova K. The effect of shift rotation on variations of cortisol, fatigue and sleep in sound engineers. Ind Health. 2008;46:490–3.

21

Knowledge of first aid methods and attitude about snake bite among medical students

Nuwadatta Subedi[1]* ⓘ, Ishwari Sharma Paudel[2], Ajay Khadka[3], Umesh Shrestha[3], Vipul Bhusan Mallik[3] and K. C. Ankur[3]

Abstract

Background: Snake bite is a neglected public health problem in tropical and subtropical region. The study was conducted with objectives to determine the knowledge of first aid methods in snake bite and the perception of snake bite among the medical students of Gandaki Medical College, Pokhara, Nepal.

Methods: We conducted a cross sectional survey among 302 (231 preclinical and 71 clinical) Bachelor of Medicine and Bachelor of Surgery (MBBS) students of Gandaki Medical College using a pretested questionnaire to assess the knowledge of first aid of snake bite based on WHO protocol and perception of snakebite. The study duration was from January to May 2018. The total score of the knowledge was obtained and compared among variables using Mann-Whitney U test. Chi square test was used for comparing the responses with the level of students. P value of < 0.05 was considered as significant.

Results: Among 302 respondents, 193(63.9%) were from Mountain districts. The families of 25 (8.3%) respondents were bitten by snakes. The correct responses were significantly higher from the 71 (23.5%) clinical students for most of the questions and the knowledge score of clinical students was significantly higher than the 231 (76.5%) preclinical students. Twenty eight (9.27%) students believed that the snake should be killed after it bites the victim and 25 (8.28%) believed that the snake will capture the image of the offender who teases it and takes revenge later. School books were the commonest source of such knowledge among the preclinical students.

Conclusion: Most of the preclinical students had inadequate knowledge of first aid of snake bite. The common source of the knowledge was school books which often provide faulty knowledge. Only a few students had negative perception about snakes. Incorporation of proper first aid measures in the textbooks of various levels is essential.

Keywords: First aid, Medical students, Public health, Snake bite

Background

Snakebite is a common and neglected public health problem in tropical and subtropical region affecting people mostly of lower socioeconomic group. It mostly affects the farmers and those who work in the fields and thus one of the occupational injury. The public health issues of snakebite is neglected globally [1], and it has only been added to WHO's list of neglected tropical diseases in June 2017. The annual incidence of snake bites in Nepal is 15,000 and 10% of them are with envenomation with 10% mortality rate among the bite by poisonous snakes. There might be under reporting of the snakebite cases from Nepal and in the latest time, the actions have been taken by increasing supervisory visit to the reporting sites to overcome it [2].

The public of Nepal have many misconceptions about snakes and snake bite, that can deleteriously affect the treatment and its prognosis [3]. The patients of snake bite

* Correspondence: drndsubedi@gmail.com
[1]Department of Forensic Medicine, Gandaki Medical College, Pokhara 33700, Nepal
Full list of author information is available at the end of the article

often seek traditional healers [4] and get faulty first aid measures before presenting to the hospital as reported from Nepal [3, 5–8] India [8–11], and even in China [12]. Improper first aid in snake bites causes more harm rather than improvement [13]. The textbooks mentioning the first aid measures of snake bite published from Nepal advocate up to 100% different than the published guidelines, omitting the indicated ones and recommending faulty and deleterious methods [14, 15]. This can lead to deep rooted false knowledge about first aid of snake bite to the people, deleteriously affecting the prognosis of the snake bitten victims if such techniques are used. This study can be useful to determine the existing knowledge among the MBBS students of Gandaki Medical College who are the future health care providers.

Methods
Objectives of the study
The study was conducted with objectives to determine the knowledge of first aid methods in snake bite and the perception of snake bite among the medical students of Gandaki Medical College.

Study design and population
It is a cross sectional study conducted among the MBBS students of Gandaki Medical College, Pokhara from January to May 2018. All the students present at the time of collection of the questionnaire and consenting for participation were included in the study. The students were approached by the authors after the end of their regular class and explained about the objectives of the study and the way to answer the questionnaire. They were encouraged to fill up the questionnaire to the best of their knowledge and perception. They were also informed that the responses would be confidential, and no any identifiers were used in the forms while filling up the questions so that the students were encouraged to answer confidently.

We had chosen the MBBS students as most of the talented students are enrolled in medical education in our country and their responses about the knowledge of snake bite would reflect the highest possible correct responses from the students if other streams are considered. They are also exposed to the formal education of snake bite treatment, the types of snake and the myths and truth about snakes during the third year MBBS in Forensic medicine and Toxicology. So, we could compare the knowledge of students before and after the such formal education.

A questionnaire including the participants' knowledge about the first aid methods for snake bite was prepared based on the WHO protocol of management of snake bite [16]. The sex, district of upbringing and information whether their immediate family members were bitten by snakes were recorded. Two questions were added to assess the perception of the students about snakes and snake bite.

We also included a question asking the respondents about the source of the knowledge that they had acquired. The questionnaire was pretested among 33 MBBS students of another medical college who were not included in the main study. The discrepancies were corrected, and the final questionnaire was administered to the participants.

At the college, the students are categorised as clinical from third year MBBS. But as the students were just admitted to the third year and had not got the formal clinical education, moreover in the snake bite management and first aid protocols, they were included among the preclinical students in our analysis.

The responses for the knowledge-based questions were "true", "false" and "do not know". For the questions assessing the knowledge of first aid of snake bite and its management issues, a score of one was given for each correct response and zero for the incorrect response and for "do not know" response. The total score was calculated with a minimum of zero and maximum nine. The overall knowledge was considered inadequate if the score was less than 70% (score of six and less) and adequate if more than 70% (score of seven and more) as done by Michael et al. [17].

Statistics
The data was collected and entered in MS Excel and further analysis done using SPSS version 16.0. To check whether the data was normally distributed, Kolmogorov Smirnov test was used. Non-parametric tests were used for the not normally distributed data. The level of knowledge was compared among sex, level of students, region of upbringing and whether their family members were bitten by snakes using Mann-Whitney U test. Chi square test was used for comparing the responses with the level of students (Preclinical and clinical) P value of < 0.05 was considered as significant.

Ethical consideration
Consent was obtained from the study participants before administering the questionnaire. We had adhered to the Declaration of Helsinki in enrolling our participants. The study was ethically approved by the Institutional Review Committee of Gandaki Medical College before commencing the study.

Results
There were a total of 395 MBBS students at Gandaki Medical College during the study period among which 302 (76.46%) were present at the time of data collection. Among 302 questionnaires distributed to the students, all of them were filled and returned. (Response rate, 100%). Among a total of 302 MBBS students participating in the study, 153 (50.7%) were males and 149 (49.3%) were females. The students with formal exposure to snake bite

management were categorized as clinical students while those without the exposure as preclinical students. There were 71 (23.5%) clinical students participating in the study. A total of 193(63.9%) of the students were from Mountain districts and 109 (36.1%) from Terai districts. Most of the students; 275 (91.1%) were educated from private schools and 27 (8.9%) from government schools up to secondary education. The families of 25 (8.3%) respondents were bitten by snakes. (Table 1).

The responses of the students for the knowledge questions are shown in Table 2. A total of 235(77.8%) responded that tight bands (tourniquets) should be applied around the limb proximal to the bite site, which is not correct. One hundred and seventy (56.29%) students were aware of pressure immobilization bandages to be applied around the bite site, 299 (99.01%) responded that the snake bite patient should be transported to the hospital soon and 261 (86.42%) knew that envenomation be cured by anti-venom therapy. When the knowledge of the students was categorized as adequate (Score more than 70%, or seven and more) and inadequate, it was explored that 29 out of 231 (12.6%) preclinical and 49 out of 71 (69%) clinical students had adequate knowledge about first aid of snake bite.

The knowledge of first aid and treatment of snake bite categorized as current and incorrect responses and comparison among the level of students is shown in Table 3. The correct responses were significantly higher from the clinical students for most of the questions except for transportation of the snakebite patient to the hospital as soon as possible. ($\chi^2 = 0.931$, $p = 0.446$, df = 1).

A total of 29 (12.6%) preclinical and 49 (69%) clinical students had adequate knowledge (score of seven and more) about the knowledge of snake bite. The total score

Table 1 Demographics of the participants

Variables	Number	Percent
Sex		
Males	153	50.7
Females	149	49.3
Level		
Preclinical	231	76.5
Clinical	71	23.5
School up to secondary level		
Government	27	8.9
Private	275	91.1
Region of upbringing		
Mountain	193	63.9
Terai	109	36.1
Family members bitten by snake		
Yes	25	8.3
No	277	91.7

of knowledge was not normally distributed as analyzed by Kolmogorov Smirnov test ($p < 0.001$, df = 302). The median score was five, minimum two and maximum nine. The comparison of the score of knowledge among the variables using Mann-Whitney U test is shown in Table 4. The knowledge score of clinical students was significantly higher (U = 2015.5, $p < 0.001$) than the preclinical students. The knowledge was not significantly associated with sex (U = 10,039, $p = 0.69$), region of upbringing (U = 9633, $p = 0.218$), school up to secondary level (U = 3299, $p = 0.333$), and family members bitten by snake or not (U = 41,232, $p = 0.075$).

We had collected some responses about the perception of snakes which is displayed in Table 5. A total of 17 (7.35%) preclinical and 11 (15.49%) clinical students believed that the snake should be killed as far as possible after it bites the victim. Twenty (8.66%) preclinical and five (7.04%) clinical student believed that the snake will capture the image of the offender who teases it and takes revenge later.

We had asked the source of information of knowledge about snake bite to the preclinical students. The common sources were school books as responded by 127 (54.98%), television (122, 52.81%) and school teacher (88, 38.09%), newspapers (69, 29.87%), radio (52, 22.51%) and others (27, 11.69%).

Discussion

The present study is a cross sectional questionnaire-based study conducted among the 302 first to final year MBBS students of Gandaki Medical College. The responses from the participants would reflect the knowledge and perception of snake bite of the knowledgeable graduate level students of Nepal. Moreover, as they undergo a formal training of the snake bite treatment, myths and misconceptions associated with snake bite, we could compare the knowledge of the students who had been formally trained and not.

Considerable number of students, mostly at the preclinical level still opt for obsolete and traditional means of first aid associated with snake bite. Some of the obsolete, traditional and deleterious measures still thought to be true first aid measures of snake bite are: making local incisions or pricks/punctures over the bite site, sucking the venom out of the wound by a healthy volunteer and tying tight bands (tourniquets) around the limb proximal to the bite site. These are performed with a belief that the venom would be taken out of the site of bite and prevent the spread of venom. Similar findings were presented in other studies [8–12, 18]. In a study among 39 patients with signs of snake bite envenomation in central Nepal, none of them had adopted WHO recommended first aid measures; pressure immobilization bandaging or local compression pad immobilization rather many of them had

Table 2 Respondents' knowledge of first aid of snake bite

Variables	Yes n (%)	No n (%)	I don't know n (%)
Should local incisions or pricks/punctures be made over the bite site?	99 (32.78)	142 (47.02)[a]	61 (20.12)
Should healthy volunteer suck the venom out of the wound?	86 (28.48)	204 (67.55)[a]	12 (3.97)
Should tight bands (tourniquets) be applied around the limb proximal to the bite site?	235 (77.81)	59 (19.54)[a]	8 (2.65)
Should pressure immobilization bandages be applied around the bite site?	170 (56.29) [a]	47 (15.56)	85 (28.15)
Is electric at the site of bite useful?	13 (4.30)	215 (71.19)[a]	74 (24.50)
Is topical instillation or application of herbs beneficial?	115 (38.08)	83 (27.48)[a]	104 (34.44)
Should the snakebite patient be transported to the hospital soon after the bite?	299 (99.01)[a]	2 (0.66)	1 (0.33)
Can envenomation be cured by anti-venom therapy?	261 (86.42)[a]	1 (0.33)	40 (13.24)
Are all snake bites associated with envenomation?	56 (18.54)	176 (48.34)[a]	70 (23.18)

[a]Denotes correct responses

Table 3 Knowledge categorized as current and incorrect responses and comparison among the level of students

SN	Knowledge on snake bite and First Aid and treatment Measures	Correct Response n (%)	Incorrect response n (%)	$\chi 2$	P Value
1	Should local incisions or pricks/punctures be made over the bite site?				
	Preclinical	81 (35.07)	150 (64.93)	56.372	< 0.001
	Clinical	61 (85.92)	10 (14.08)		
2	Should healthy volunteer suck the venom out of the wound?				
	Preclinical	137 (59.31)	94 (40.69)	25.490	< 0.001
	Clinical	65 (91.55)	6 (8.45)		
3	Should tight bands (tourniquets) be applied around the limb proximal to the bite site?				
	Preclinical	19 (8.22)	212 (91.78)	79.097	< 0.001
	Clinical	40 (56.34)	31 (43.66)		
4	Should pressure immobilization bandages be applied around the bite site?				
	Preclinical	118 (51.08)	113 (48.92)	10.836	0.001
	Clinical	52 (73.24)	19 (26.76)		
5	Is electric current at the site of bite useful?				
	Preclinical	155 (67.10)	76 (32.90)	8.024	0.005
	Clinical	60 (84.51)	11 (15.49)		
6	Is topical instillation or application of herbs beneficial?				
	Preclinical	54 (23.38)	177 (76.62)	8.315	0.004
	Clinical	29 (40.85)	42 (59.15)		
7	Should the snakebite patient be transported to the hospital soon after the bite?				
	Preclinical	228 (98.70)	3 (1.30)	0.931	0.446[a]
	Clinical	71 (100.00)	0 (0.00)		
8	Can envenomation be cured by anti-venom therapy?				
	Preclinical	191 (82.68)	40 (17.31)	11.713	0.001
	Clinical	70 (98.59)	1 (1.410		
9	Are all snake bites associated with envenomation?				
	Preclinical	115 (49.78)	116 (50.22)	29.159	< 0.001
	Clinical	61 (85.92)	10 (14.08)		

[a]Fisher Exact test

Table 4 Comparison of knowledge score among the variables

Variables	N	Rank average	Sum of ranks	U	Z	p-value
Sex						
Male	153	160.39	24,539.00	10039.00	−1.818	0.69
Female	149	142.38	21,214.00			
Level of students						
Preclinical	231	124.73	28,811.50	2015.50	−9.753	< 0.001
Clinical	71	238.61	16,941.50			
Region of upbringing						
Mountain	193	156.09	30,215.00	9633.00	−1.233	0.218
Terai	109	143.38	15,628.00			
School up to secondary level						
Private	275	153.00	42,076.00	3299.00	−0.969	0.333
Government	27	3677.00	3677.00			
Family member bitten by snake						
Yes	25	180.84	4521.00	41232.00	−1.780	0.075
No	277	148.85	41,232.00			

practiced traditional measures before getting admitted to the hospital [8]. More than half among 180 patients of snake bite had presented with application of tourniquet in an Indian study [19].

In a review about snake bite in South Asia, eight out of 15 studies showed that more than half of snake bite patients had used inappropriate and deleterious methods of first aid, among which tourniquets were used by a maximum number of patients [18]. The faulty and inappropriate first aid methods mentioned in the textbooks from primary to the bachelor's level [14, 15] can be an important contributing factor that has caused such deep rooted faulty knowledge.

In contrast to our study, Sri Lankan farmers were against the faulty first aid methods like incising the bite site and application of tourniquets, though it was not practiced perfectly [20]. Even the medical practitioners of Nigeria [17, 21] did not have adequate knowledge of snake bite envenomation and only few doctors of Hong Kong were confident of snake bite treatment [22].

The only evidence based first aid technique of snake bite which delays the spread of venom is the pressure immobilization technique. The other first aid measures like tourniquet application are harmful and should be avoided [23]. The interference of the wound of snake bite would by incising, rubbing, vigorously cleaning, applying chemicals and herbs etc. can cause infection, increased absorption of the snake venom and increment of local bleeding. The use of tight (arterial) tourniquets, if applied around the proximal portions of the limb, these can cause severe pain as there will be gradual development of ischaemia on the limbs and can lead to gangrene of left in place for a long time [16].

The source of such knowledge could have passed on from generations. The main reason behind this faulty knowledge to the students could be due to the incomplete and inappropriate first aid methods mentioned in the textbooks of primary to university level. Such textbooks published from Nepal provide incorrect information up to 100% errors [14, 15]. It is very important to provide updated and accurate information in the textbooks so that the students will acquire proper information of first aid of snake bite and they can also disseminate the information to the public in society. The author NS had witnessed a television program from a National television where the outdated and deleterious first aid measures of snake bite

Table 5 Perception of snake bite and snakes

SN	Perception of Snake bite	True n (%)	False n (%)	Do not know n (%)
1	The snake should be killed as far as possible after it bites the victim			
	Preclinical	17 (7.35)	201 (87.01)	13 (5.63)
	Clinical	11 (15.49)	59 (83.10)	1 (1.41)
2	The snake will capture the image of the offender who teases it and takes revenge later			
	Preclinical	20 (8.66)	183 (79.22)	28 (39.44)
	Clinical	5 (7.04)	57 (80.28)	9 (12.67)

were telecasted only a few years back. The concerned authorities should be very serious in this matter. The guideline of first aid of snake bite published by WHO recommends that at least no harm should be done to the victims of snake bite in an attempt to perform first aid measures in them [16]. The correct and updated information of first aid measures of snake bite has to be disseminated using newspapers, radio, television, internet etc.

The knowledge of the students about the first aid of snake bite was not significantly different in comparison with the variables like sex, type of school up to secondary level, district of upbringing and the status of family member bitten by snake. This indicates that the curriculum in private and public schools both of Nepal does not significantly include appropriate information which is supported by studies using textbooks from primary to university level [14, 15]. Almost all the students were positive about the transfer of the snakebite patients to the hospital soon after the bite. Most people know that definitive treatment of snake bite envenomation can be done at hospitals. Rapid transport of victims to a snake bite treatment center had decreased the mortality rate in a study from southeastern Nepal [3].

The knowledge of the clinical students was significantly higher than compared to the preclinical students. The third year MBBS curriculum of Forensic Medicine and Toxicology includes identification of snakes, management of snake bite including the established first aid methods, and myths and misconceptions associated with snakes and snake bite. The students are also practically demonstrated various types of poisonous and nonpoisonous snakes common in Nepal and South Asian region. The higher knowledge of the clinical students indicates that formal training can significantly correct the misconceptions about the deleterious first aid methods of snake bite. The potential medical personnel involved in the management of snake bite patients should be regularly updated of the advances and protocols. The increment in knowledge of snakes and competencies about the snake bite management by trainings and community education has also been demonstrated earlier [3, 4, 21].

Only 15% of all the 3000 species of snakes found globally are venomous [24] and the rest are non-venomous. When the snake bite is associated with envenomation, the definitive treatment is antivenom therapy and it should be administered when indicated [16]. The people have tendency to kill the snakes when they see them and more often when the snakes bite [25]. The snakes are important creatures to maintain ecological harmony and should preserved. In the attempt to kill the snakes, the people may be further bitten by it may be grievous. In our study, 28 (9.27%) respondents perceived that the snakes should be killed after it bites and 25 (8.28%) had the misconception that the snakes capture image of the offender who teases it and takes revenge later.

The later could be one of the reasons that people would like to kill the snakes when they encounter them.

Conclusion

Most of the preclinical students had inadequate knowledge of first aid of snake bite and many of them opted for obsolete and deleterious methods. The common source of the knowledge was school books which often provide faulty knowledge. Only a few students had negative perception about snakes. The students should be taught correct and updated methods of first aid of snake bite from the early stage of their education. If faulty technique is included in their curriculum, they might have deep rooted wrong knowledge which can ultimately affect the society.

Acknowledgements

We would like to acknowledge all the MBBS students of Gandaki Medical College who had participated in the study. Many thanks to Dr. Rajesh Gyawali, Associate Professor of BPKIHS for technical helps. We acknowledge Mr. Krishna Kanta Adhikari of Gandaki Medical College for helping us in data entry. We thank the management of Gandaki Medical College for the necessary stationary supports.

Authors' contributions

Conception and design of the work: NS. Acquisition of the data: NS, AK, US, VBM, and AKC. Analysis and interpretation of the data, drafting and critical revision of the manuscript for important intellectual content, accountable for all aspects of the work and approval of the final manuscript: NS, ISP, AK, US, VBM and AKC. All authors read and approved the final manuscript.

Competing interests

The authors declare that they have no competing interests.

Author details

[1]Department of Forensic Medicine, Gandaki Medical College, Pokhara 33700, Nepal. [2]Department of Community Medicine, Gandaki Medical College, Pokhara, Nepal. [3]Gandaki Medical College, Pokhara, Nepal.

References

1. Williams D, Gutiérrez JM, Harrison R, Warrell DA, White J, Winkel KD, Gopalakrishnakone P. The global snake bite initiative: an antidote for snake bite. Lancet. 2010;375(9708):89–91.
2. Department of Health Services, Government of Nepal, Ministry of Health Department of Health Services. Annual Report, 2072/73 (2015/2016). Kathmandu: The Department; 2017. p. 120. https://phpnepal.org.np/publication/current-issue/recently-released/136-annual-report-of-department-ofhealth-services-2072-73-2015-2016.
3. Sharma SK, Chappuis F, Jha N, Bovier PA, Loutan L, Koirala S. Impact of snake bites and determinants of fatal outcomes in south eastern Nepal. Am J Trop Med Hyg. 2004;71(2):234–8.
4. Pandey DP, Thapa CL, Hamal PK. Impact of first aid training in Management of Snake Bite Victims in Madi Valley. J Nepal Health Res Counc. 2010;8(1):5–9.
5. Sharma SK, Koirala S, Dahal G, Sah C. Clinico-epidemiological features of snakebite: a study from eastern Nepal. Trop Dr. 2004;34(1):20–2.
6. Pandey DD. Epidemiology of snakebites based on field survey in Chitwan and Nawalparasi districts. Nepal J Med Toxicol. 2007;3(4):164–8.
7. Chaudhary S, Singh S, Chaudhary N, Mahato SK. Snake-Bite in Nepal. J Universal Coll Med Sci. 2014;2(3):45–53.

8. Pandey DP, Vohra R, Stalcup P, Shrestha BR. A season of snakebite envenomation: presentation patterns, timing of care, anti-venom use, and case fatality rates from a hospital of southcentral Nepal. J Venom Res. 2016;7:1–9.

9. Kumar A, Dasgupta A, Biswas D, Sahoo SK, Das S, Preeti PS. Knowledge regarding snake bite in rural Bengal – are they still lingering on myths and misconceptions? Int Arch Integr Med. 2015;2(7):36–41.

10. Pandve HT, Makan A, Kulkarni TA. Assessment of awareness regarding snakebites and its related issues among rural communities. Scifed J Public Health. 2017;1:1.

11. Pathak I, Metgud C. Knowledge, attitude and practice regarding snakes and snake bite among rural adult of Belagavi, Karnataka. Int J Community Med Public Health. 2017;4(12):4527–31.

12. Chen C, Gui L, Kan T, Li S, Qiu C. A Survey of Snakebite Knowledge among Field Forces in China. Int J Environ Res Public Health. 2016;14(1):15. pii: E15. https://doi.org/10.3390/ijerph14010015.

13. Yanamandra U, Yanamandra S. Traditional first aid in a case of snake bite: more harm than good. BMJ Case Rep. 2014;2014. pii: bcr2013202891 https://doi.org/10.1136/bcr-2013-202891.

14. Tenzing D, Acharya G, Sherpa G. An evaluation of training texts regarding first aid measures for snakebite and rates of performance. World Acad. Res Environ Protect Sustain Dev. 2016;2(6):24–31.

15. Pandey DP, Khanal BP. Inclusion of incorrect information on snakebite first aid in school and university teaching materials in Nepal. J Toxicol Environ Health Sci. 2013;5(3):43–51.

16. World Health Organization. Guidelines for the management of snakebites. 2nd ed. New Delhi: World Health Organization; 2010.

17. Michael GC, Grema BA, Aliyu I, Alhaji MA, Lawal TO, Ibrahim H, et al. Knowledge of venomous snakes, snakebite first aid, treatment, and prevention among clinicians in northern Nigeria: a cross-sectional multicentre study. Trans R Soc Trop Med Hyg. 2018;112(2):47–56.

18. Alirol E, Sharma SK, Bawaskar HS, Kuch U, Chappuis F. Snake bite in South Asia: a review. PLoS Negl Trop Dis. 2010;4(1):e603.

19. Halesha BR, Harshavardhan L, Lokesh AJ, Channaveerappa PK, Venkatesh KB. A study on the Clinico-epidemiological profile and the outcome of snake bite victims in a tertiary care Centre in southern India. J Clin Diagn Res. 2013;7(1):122–6.

20. Silva A, Marikar F, Murugananthan A, Agampodi S. Awareness and perceptions on prevention, first aid and treatment of snakebites among Sri Lankan farmers: a knowledge practice mismatch? J Occup Med Toxicol. 2014;9:20.

21. Inthanomchanh V, Reyer JA, Blessmen J, Phrasisombath K, Yamamoto E, Hamajima N. Assessment of knowledge about snakebite management amongst healthcare providers in the provincial and two district hospitals in Savannakhet Province, Lao PDR. Nagoya J Med Sci. 2017;79(3):299–311.

22. Fung HT, Lam SK, Lam KK, Kam CW, Simpson ID. A survey of snakebite management knowledge amongst select physicians in Hong Kong and the implications for snakebite training. Wilderness Environ Med. 2009;20(4):364–70.

23. Avau B, Borra V, Vandekerckhove P, De Buck E. The treatment of snake bites in a first aid setting: a systematic review. PLoS Negl Trop Dis. 2016;10(10):e0005079. https://doi.org/10.1371/journal.pntd.0005079.

24. Gold BS, Dart RC, Barish RA. Bites of venomous snakes. N Engl J Med. 2002;347(5):347–56.

25. Alves RR, Silva VN, Trovao DM, Oliveira JV, Mourão JS, Dias TL. Students' attitudes toward and knowledge about snakes in the semiarid region of northeastern Brazil. J Ethnobiol Ethnomed. 2014;10:30.

22

Employment status and changes in working career in relation to asthma

Saara Taponen[1,3]* ⓘ, Lauri Lehtimäki[2,3], Kirsi Karvala[4], Ritva Luukkonen[5] and Jukka Uitti[3,4]

Abstract

Background: Asthmatics confront inconveniences in working life that make it more difficult to pursue a sustainable career, such as unemployment and work disability. Ways of dealing with these inconveniences may be career changes. More needs to be known about the backgrounds and consequences of career changes among asthmatics, especially their relation to asthma or a change in asthma symptoms. The aim of this study was to compare earlier career changes of adults with asthma who are working full time to those who have drifted away from active working life because of work disability, unemployment or early retirement. The frequency of having changed tasks, work place or occupation, whether the changes had been driven by asthma and furthermore, whether the changes had affected their asthma symptoms were investigated.

Methods: In this population-based survey study, all patients with reimbursement rights for asthma aged 20–65 years in the city of Tampere (total population 190,000), Finland ($n = 2613$) were recruited. The questionnaire was sent in October 2000 and the response rate was 79%. The questionnaire included questions e.g. on changing tasks, work place and occupation, whether these changes were driven by asthma or associated with change of asthma symptoms. The respondents were divided into four groups: working full-time, work disability, unemployed and retired due to age. We applied ANOVA with Dunnet's post-test (variances were not equal between the groups) for a continued variable age and Chi-squared tests for categorical variables. Logistic regression models were built using unemployed vs. full-time work or work disability vs. full-time work as an outcome variable. A p-value of <.05 was considered statistically significant.

Results: Adults with asthma working full time had more often made changes in their career, but not as often driven by asthma as those with current work disability. The reason for changing work place compared to full-time workers (24.9%) was more often mainly or partly due to asthma among those with work disability (47.9%, $p < 0.001$) and the unemployed (43.3%, $p = 0.006$). Of those who made career changes because of asthma, a major proportion (over 67%) reported relief in asthma symptoms. Changing tasks (OR 5.8, 95% CI 1.9–18.0, for unemployment vs. full-time work), work place (OR 2.8, 95% CI 1.1–7.0, for work disability vs. full-time work and OR 2.6, 95% CI 1.3–5.4, for unemployment vs. full-time work) or occupation (OR 2.7, 95% CI 1.2–6.0, for unemployment vs. full-time work) mainly because of asthma was associated with an elevated risk for undesirable employment status even after adjusting for age, gender, smoking and professional status.

Conclusions: Career changes that were made mainly because of asthma were associated with undesirable employment status in this study. However, asthma symptoms were relieved after career changes especially among those who reported asthma to be the reason for the change. In addition to proper treatment and counselling of asthma patients towards applicable area of work or study, it may be beneficial to support early career changes in maintaining sustainable working careers among adults with asthma.

Keywords: Work ability, Asthma, Job change, Career change

---

* Correspondence: saara.taponen@finla.fi
[1]Finla Occupational Health, Satakunnankatu 18 B, 33210 Tampere, Finland
[3]Faculty of Medicine and Life Sciences, University of Tampere, 33014 Tampere, Finland
Full list of author information is available at the end of the article

Background

Sustainable work has been set as a main goal by European Union countries, meaning that 'living and working conditions are such that they support people in engaging and remaining in work throughout an extended working life'[1]. For an employee with asthma, maintaining a sustainable working career may be a significant challenge. Selective exclusion from work as a consequence of asthma is observed in childhood asthmatics already at the beginning of their working life and for current adult-onset asthmatics at the end of their working life [2]. Throughout working life, adults with asthma commonly change jobs due to respiratory problems at work [3], they often deal with sickness absence [4], delayed return to work [5] or complete cessation of employment due to respiratory problems [6]. When work ability is reduced due to other health conditions, having asthma makes it even more difficult to return to work. For example, a large cohort study by Ervasti et al. [7] showed that return to work after sickness absence because of depression is delayed in the presence of asthma. In a study of public sector employees, asthma increased the risk of all-cause long-term work disability 1.8-fold compared to controls with no asthma. [8]

Work-related asthma symptoms may have a considerable socio-economic impact, job change or work loss due to asthma [9]. Work-exacerbated asthma (WEA) is common (medium prevalence 21.5% among adults with asthma) and occasionally supporting job change is needed to manage WEA when reducing exposures and optimizing treatment is not enough [10].

As these earlier studies have shown, adults with asthma may struggle with inconveniences in working life that make it more difficult to pursue a sustainable career. Changing jobs is common among employees with asthma and it may be one way of coping in working life with asthma. However, more needs to be known about the backgrounds and consequences of changing jobs among adults with asthma in order to focus on effective support of their working careers.

We have found in our earlier study that among adults with asthma, full-time workers are on average younger, more frequently nonmanual workers, they smoke less and have less asthma symptoms both at work and at leisure time despite of using less asthma medication than those who are unemployed, have work disability or are retired [11]. Full-time work was interpreted as an indicator of successful coping in working life. Now we wanted to analyze further, if changes in working career in relation to asthma could explain the better success in coping in working life of some adults with asthma.

The aim of this study was to compare earlier career changes of adults with asthma who are working full time to those who have drifted away from active working life because of work disability, unemployment or early retirement. We studied the frequency of having changed tasks, work place or occupation, whether the changes had been driven by asthma and furthermore, whether the changes had affected their asthma symptoms.

Methods

This cross-sectional survey study recruited all patients with reimbursement rights for asthma medication ($n = 2613$) aged 20–65 years and living in the city of Tampere (total population 190,000), Finland. The cases were identified from the Medication Reimbursement Register of the Finnish Social Insurance Institution. All those who had been granted special reimbursement rights for asthma medication until the end of 1997 and were alive in October 2000 were selected. To be granted reimbursement rights by the Finnish Social Insurance Institution, the disease must fulfill the diagnostic and severity criteria of asthma, including objective data of reversible/variable bronchial obstruction and a need for regular treatment with inhaled glucocorticoids for at least 6 months after the diagnosis. Among those granted special reimbursement rights for asthma medication, the reliability of the asthma diagnosis is high [12]. The questionnaire was sent in October 2000 and the response rate was 79%. Ninety-eight subjects were excluded from the analyses because they responded not having been diagnosed for asthma indeed by a physician (some individuals with reimbursement may have had e.g. asthma-COPD overlap) or because the employment status information was missing. For this study, the respondents were divided into five groups according to their working life status. There were 967 subjects working full-time, 197 unemployed subjects, 334 subjects with work disability (including all-cause sickness absence, disability pension, and disability pension applied but not yet granted) and 159 subjects retired due to age (in Finland, age-related pension starts at age of approximately 60–68 years depending on occupation and personal preferences). The fifth group consisting of subjects outside of full-time work for other reasons (e.g. housewives, students, part-time workers, maternity leave, etc.) were excluded from this study ($n = 309$).

Questionnaire

The self-administered questionnaire included questions on employment status, changes of work tasks, work places and occupation, whether the changes were driven by asthma and whether they affected asthma symptoms (Table 2).

Statistical analyses

We compared career changes in relation to asthma between different groups of working life status and we were especially interested whether full-time workers differ from the subjects in other three groups (unemployed, those with work disability and those retired). Our data set consisted of both continuous and categorical variables. When comparing the differences between groups we applied ANOVA with Dunnet's post-test (variances were not equal between the groups) for a continued variable age and Chi-squared tests for categorical variables. Among those who had made career changes we were interested whether asthma was mainly or partly the reason for those changes ("mainly" or "partly" or "none") and how a possible change affected asthma symptoms ("aggravated" or "no change" or "relieved"). The results are presented in Table 2. We computed the same results by limiting the data for those who had answered that asthma was mainly or partly the reason for career changes. Those results are presented in Table 3.

After these preliminary studies we built logistic regression models using unemployed vs. full-time work or work disability vs. full-time work as an outcome variable. Change of tasks within the same employer, change of work place, and change of occupation and whether the changes were driven by asthma ("mainly" or "partly" vs. "none"), and relief or aggravation of asthma symptoms after the changes were used as independent variables one at a time. In our data there were only very few persons who had answered that a career change aggravated the symptoms. Therefore, we combined the categories "aggravated" and "no change" before modeling. Our model building strategy was as follows: at first we estimated crude models and then adjusted models with age, gender, smoking, and professional status. The odds ratios (OR) with 95% confidence intervals (95% CI) are presented in Table 4. A p-value of <.05 was considered statistically significant. All analyses were carried out using SPSS (version 24) program.

Results
Characteristics of the five groups are presented Table 1 [11].

Work and career changes in different employment status groups are presented in Table 2.

Changing tasks
Changing tasks within the same employer after asthma diagnosis was similar in all groups (about 20% had changed tasks). 4.5% of full-time workers, 7.5% of the unemployed, 7.6% of the work disability group and 8.8% of the retired had changed tasks mainly because of asthma. Of those who had changed tasks, 43.5% of full-time workers compared to over 71% of all other groups reported that asthma was mainly or partly the reason for the change. It was most common to have been done the change mainly because of asthma in the retired group (44.4%), and more common in the work disability group (33.9%) and the unemployed group (39.4%) than in the full-time working group (22.3%).

Changing work place
The change of work place after asthma diagnosis was more common among full-time workers (39.9%) and the unemployed (39.9%) compared to the work disability group (19.8%) and to the retired group (14.4%). 5.5% of full-time workers, 10.3% of the unemployed, 6.8% of the

work disability group and 3.7% of the retired had changed work place mainly because of asthma. The reason for changing work place was more often mainly or partly due to asthma among those with work disability (47.9%) and the unemployed (43.3%) compared to full-time workers (24.9%).

Changing occupation
Changing occupation after asthma diagnosis was less common than changing work place. Full-time workers reported changing occupation more frequently (25.8%) than subjects with work disability (18.9%) or the retired (10.9%). 6.4% of full-time workers, 11.6% of the unemployed 8.8% of the work disability group and 7.3% of the retired had changed occupation mainly because of asthma. Making the change because of asthma was overall more common in changing occupation than in changing work place. Of those who had changed occupation, making the change mainly or partly because of asthma was more likely among those with work disability (60.4%) than among full-time workers (43.9%).

Career changes and asthma symptoms
After all work and career changes, it was common to report that the symptoms were relieved, especially after occupation change (> 50%). Noticeable is that in the work disability group, aggravation of symptoms after all career changes was more frequently reported than in other groups.

Retirement
Of those who had retired after asthma diagnosis (80.6% of the work disability group and 72.2% of the retired group), a significantly greater proportion of those retired because of work disability (39.4%) compared to those retired for old age (9.3%) reported that asthma was the main reason for their retirement. Among those retired for old age, 53.7% reported that asthma was not the reason for their retirement whereas 23.6% of those retired for work disability reported the same. However, after retirement, asthma symptoms were alleviated in both groups (60.7% in work disability group and 66.3% in retired group).

Changes of asthma symptoms in those adults with asthma who reported making work or career changes because of asthma are presented in Table 3. Among those who made the change due to asthma, relief of asthma symptoms after changing tasks was significantly more common among full-time workers than among the work disability group. Of those who changed work place because of asthma, relief of asthma symptoms was more common (85–90%) in all other groups than the work disability group, of whom 68% reported relief of asthma symptoms. Of those who had changed occupation, relief of asthma symptoms was reported frequently (90–100%) among full-time workers and the retired and less frequently (72–76%) among the unemployed and the work disability group.

Table 1 Characteristics according to working life status

	Full-time work n = 967	Unemployed n = 197	Work disability n = 334	Retired n = 159	p-value 1 vs. 2	p-value 1 vs. 3	p-value 1 vs. 4
Age, mean years (SD)	44.1 (10.2)	46.2 (11.0)	57.9 (8.2)	62.9 (3.8)	0.064	<.001	<.001
Gender							
Women	568 (58.7)	136 (69.0)	206 (61.7)	108 (67.9)	0.007	0.346	0.028
Men	399 (41.3)	61 (31.0)	128 (38.3)	51 (32.1)			
Smoking status							
Never smoker	432 (45.0)	70 (36.1)	132 (40.0)	92 (58.2)	0.004	0.002	<.001
Ex-smoker	217 (22.6)	40 (20.6)	98 (29.7)	38 (24.1)			
Current smoker	155 (16.1)	52 (26.8)	66 (20.0)	20 (12.7)			
Occasional smoker	157 (16.3)	32 (16.5)	34 (10.3)	8 (5.1)			
Professional status							
Self-employed	98 (10.2)	10 (5.2)	25 (8.0)	7 (4.6)	<.001	<.001	0.001
Upper level nonmanual worker	199 (20.7)	11 (5.8)	21 (6.7)	24 (15.9)			
Lower level nonmanual worker	284 (29.5)	50 (26.2)	59 (18.8)	35 (23.2)			
Manual worker	353 (36.7)	113 (59.2)	195 (62.1)	79 (52.3)			
Working from home, student, other	28 (2.9)	7 (3.7)	14 (4.5)	6 (4.0)			

Data is presented as n (%) unless otherwise stated

Table 2 Earlier changes in working career according to current employment status

		Full-time workers n = 951 – 954	Unemployed n = 176	Work disability n = 246 – 256	Retired n = 139	p-value 1 vs.2	p-value 1 vs. 3	p-value 1 vs. 4
Change of tasks within the same employer after asthma diagnosis	No	755 (79.4)	141 (80.1)	198 (77.3)	110 (79.1)	0.827	0.476	0.945
	Yes	196 (20.6)	35 (19.9)	58 (22.7)	29 (20.9)			
If yes, was asthma the reason for changing tasks?	Mainly	43 (22.3)	13 (39.4)	19 (33.9)	12 (44.4)	<.001	0.001	0.008
	Partly	41 (21.2)	14 (42.4)	21 (37.5)	8 (29.6)			
	No	109 (56.5)	6 (18.2)	16 (28.6)	7 (25.9)			
If yes, how did change of tasks affect asthma symptoms?	Aggravated	7 (3.9)	3 (9.4)	8 (16.0)	1 (4.2)	0.073	0.001	0.211
	No change	86 (48.0)	9 (28.1)	13 (26.0)	7 (29.2)			
	Relieved	86 (48.0)	20 (62.5)	29 (58.0)	16 (66.7)			
Change of work place after asthma diagnosis	No	373 (60.1)	107 (60.1)	202 (80.2)	119 (85.6)	0.991	<.001	<.001
	Yes	381 (39.9)	71 (39.9)	50 (19.8)	20 (14.4)			
If yes, was asthma the reason for changing work place?	Mainly	52 (13.8)	18 (26.9)	17 (35.4)	5 (27.8)	0.006	<.001	0.249
	Partly	42 (11.1)	11 (16.4)	6 (12.5)	2 (11.1)			
	No	283 (75.1)	38 (56.7)	25 (52.1)	11 (61.1)			
If yes, how did change of work place affect asthma symptoms?	Aggravated	8 (2.4)	2 (3.4)	3 (7.0)	1 (5.9)	0.052	0.058	0.361
	No change	206 (62.6)	27 (45.8)	20 (46.5)	8 (47.1)			
	Relieved	115 (35.0)	30 (50.8)	20 (46.5)	8 (47.1)			
Change of occupation after asthma diagnosis	No	708 (74.2)	122 (70.5)	202 (81.1)	122 (89.1)	0.310	0.024	<.001
	Yes	246 (25.8)	51 (29.5)	47 (18.9)	15 (10.9)			
If yes, was asthma the reason for changing occupation?	Mainly	61 (23.3)	20 (35.7)	22 (41.5)	10 (45.5)	0.086	0.020	0.069
	Partly	54 (20.6)	13 (23.2)	10 (18.9)	3 (13.6)			
	No	147 (56.1)	23 (41.1)	21 (39.6)	9 (40.9)			
If yes, how did change of occupation affect asthma symptoms?	Aggravated	6 (2.7)	2 (4.4)	4 (9.5)	1 (6.7)	0.781	0.015	0.004
	No change	100 (45.7)	20 (44.4)	11 (26.2)	1 (6.7)			
	Relieved	113 (51.6)	23 (51.1)	27 (64.3)	13 (86.7)			

Data is presented as n (%)

Table 3 Asthma symptom changes in those who had made career changes because of asthma

		Full-time workers (1) n = 951–954	Unemployed (2) n = 176	Work disability (3) n = 246–256	Retired (4) n = 139	p-value 1 vs.2	p-value 1 vs. 3	p-value 1 vs. 4
Change of tasks within the same employer after asthma diagnosis								
Was asthma the reason for changing tasks?	Mainly	43 (51.2)	13 (48.1)	19 (47.5)	12 (60.0)	<.783	<.701	0.478
	Partly	41 (48.8)	14 (51.9)	21 (52.5)	8 (40.0)			
How did change of tasks affect asthma symptoms?	Aggravated	2 (2.5)	2 (8.0)	3 (8.3)	0 (0.0)	0.182	0.036	0.978
	No change	11 (13.6)	5 (20.0)	9 (25.0)	3 (15.8)			
	Relieved	68 (84.0)	18 (72.0)	24 (66.7)	16 (84.2)			
Change of work place after asthma diagnosis								
Was asthma the reason for changing work place?	Mainly	52 (55.3)	18 (62.1)	17 (73.9)	5 (71.4)	0.521	0.104	0.465
	Partly	42 (44.7)	11 (37.9)	6 (26.1)	2 (28.6)			
How did change of work place affect asthma symptoms?	Aggravated	1 (1.1)	0 (0.0)	0 (0.0)	0 (0.0)	0.497	0.017	0.549
	No change	8 (9.0)	4 (14.8)	7 (31.8)	1 (14.3)			
	Relieved	80 (89.9)	23 (85.2)	15 (68.2)	86 (85.7)			
Change of occupation after asthma diagnosis								
Was asthma the reason for changing occupation?	Mainly	61 (53.5)	20 (60.6)	22 (71.0)	10 (76.9)	0.470	0.082	0.107
	Partly	53 (46.5)	13 (39.4)	9 (29.0)	3 (23.1)			
How did change of occupation affect asthma symptoms?	Aggravated	0 (0.0)	0 (0.0)	1 (3.4)	0 (0.0)	0.013	0.042	0.600
	No change	10 (9.7)	8 (27.6)	6 (20.7)	0 (0.0)			
	Relieved	93 (90.3)	21 (72.4)	22 (75.9)	13 (100)			

Data is presented as n (%)

Associations between employment status and changes in working career and their relation to asthma

Associations between employment status and earlier career changes: changing tasks, work place or occupation, and associations between employment status and whether the career change was made due to asthma or was associated with a change in asthma symptoms, were calculated using logistic regression models and are presented in Table 4. After adjusting for age, gender, smoking and professional status, those who had changed tasks mainly because of asthma, were more likely to be unemployed than work full-time (OR 5.8, 95% CI 1.9–18.0) but between work disability group and full-time working group the difference was not statistically significant. Those who had changed work place mainly because of asthma were more likely to have work disability than work full-time (OR 2.8, 95% CI 1.1–7.0) and more likely to be unemployed than full-time workers (OR 2.6, 95% CI 1.3–5.4). Those who had changed occupation mainly because of asthma, were more likely to be unemployed than full-time workers (OR 2.7, 95% CI 1.2–6.0) but between work disability group and full-time working group the difference was not statistically significant. Relief or aggravation of asthma symptoms after changing tasks, work place or occupation was not associated with employment status.

Discussion

Our cross-sectional study among adults with asthma shows that those who are currently full-time workers have made changes more often in their career than adults with asthma with current work disability. However, asthma was more seldom the reason for these changes among full-time workers than among those with work disability. Particularly among those who made one because of asthma, symptoms alleviated after a career change. On the other hand, when asthma was mainly the reason for the career change, it was associated with undesirable employment status, work disability or unemployment, compared to full-time workers. The risk for undesirable employment status was 2–6 -fold even after adjusting for age, gender, smoking and professional status.

Earlier studies concerning job changes have mostly dealt with job changes due to respiratory work-related symptoms and work disability or occupational asthma [6, 13–16]. In a study of 196 patients with asthma, as many as 39% believed that asthma had adversely affected their career by causing them to: not pursue a desired career, not get promoted due to absenteeism, change to a worse job, or be perceived as incapable. Changing jobs, work hours or duties was associated with less education, not wanting to work, more co-morbidity and more use of asthma medication [16]. In our study, we investigated adults with asthma identified from a

Table 4 Associations between changes in working career and employment status. Crude logistic regression models and models adjusted for age, gender, smoking, and professional status

		Unemployed vs. full-time work		Work disability vs. full-time work	
		Crude OR (95% CI)	Adjusted OR (95% CI)	Crude OR (95% CI)	Adjusted OR (95% CI)
Was asthma the reason for changing tasks?	Mainly vs. No	7.8 (2.7–22.6)	5.8 (1.9–18.0)	6.2 (2.5–15.2)	2.5 (0.8–7.7)
	Partly vs. No	6.1 (2.2–17.4)	4.7 (1.6–14.4)	5.4 (2.3–12.6)	2.9 (1.0–8.4)
How did change of tasks affect asthma symptoms?	Aggravated or No change vs. Relieved	0.4 (0.2–1.0)	0.6 (0.3–1.6)	0.7 (0.4–1.4)	1.6 (0.7–3.9)
Was asthma the reason for changing work place?	Mainly vs. No	3.1 (1.6–6.0)	2.6 (1.3–5.4)	3.6 (1.7–7.7)	2.8 (1.1–7.0)
	Partly vs. No	2.1 (1.0–4.5)	1.9 (0.9–4.3)	1.5 (0.5–4.1)	1.8 (0.6–5.8)
How did change of work place affect asthma symptoms?	Aggravated or No change vs. Relieved	0.5 (0.3–0.8)	0.6 (0.3–1.1)	0.7 (0.3–1.4)	1.2 (0.5–2.8)
Was asthma the reason for changing occupation?	Mainly vs. No	3.1 (1.5–6.6)	2.7 (1.2–6.0)	2.8 (1.3–5.9)	1.6 (0.6–3.9)
	Partly vs. No	2.0 (0.9–4.5)	1.7 (0.7–4.2)	1.4 (0.6–3.4)	1.4 (0.5–3.8)
How did change of occupation affect asthma symptoms?	Aggravated or No change vs. Relieved	0.9 (0.4–1.7)	1.0 (0.5–2.1)	0.6 (0.3–1.1)	0.9 (0.4–2.0)

general population. Our previous study showed that having frequent asthma symptoms or nightly wake-ups because of asthma is associated with less desirable employment status such as unemployment and work disability. Among individuals with asthma, full-time workers are on average younger, more frequently nonmanual workers, they smoke less and have less asthma symptoms both at work and at leisure time despite of using less asthma medication [11].

In this study, the main purpose was to analyze the career changes adults with asthma had made earlier in their working life and to compare them in current employment status groups. We were able to investigate whether the change had been driven by asthma and furthermore, whether it alleviated or aggravated asthma symptoms. This addresses the question of how much having asthma forces individuals to make changes in their working careers.

Occupation change may be considered a bigger step to take in one's working career than changing work place or tasks within the same, familiar employer. Changing occupation was less common in our study groups than changing task or work place, but asthma was more often the reason for change in occupation than change in work place. This reflects that the change of occupation is not made on a light basis but it may be that those who change occupation have a more difficult asthma to control. All groups (> 50%) experienced alleviation of asthma symptoms after occupation change and the relief was strongest in the eldest groups, retired and work disability groups.

Of those who had made career changes driven by asthma, the relief of asthma symptoms was most common among full-time workers and more common among other groups than the work disability group. Among the work disability group, aggravation of symptoms after making career changes driven by asthma was more common than in other groups. This suggests that if the subjects can alleviate

asthma symptoms by making changes in career, it predicts a favorable career outcome. Still, there is contradiction between the potential beneficial effect of career change on health which is seen as alleviation of asthma symptoms, and the potential deleterious impact of career change at socio-economical level seen in employment status. Even in those who had retired for old age, asthma often seemed to be a reason not to continue in working life and asthma symptoms tended to alleviate in a significant proportion of adults with asthma after retirement.

Full-time workers stand out from the other adults with asthma with having made changes in their earlier working career, whether it is a task change, work place change or occupation change, mostly for other reasons and less frequently driven by their asthma. Our earlier study showed that working full-time was associated with younger age, nonmanual work, less smoking and less symptomatic asthma despite of less asthma medication [11]. Their socio-economical status with younger age and nonmanual work probably also favors changes in their careers because of other reasons than their asthma. It is possible that full-time workers may be overall healthier with less comorbidities which may also enable better flexibility and changes in working life not driven by asthma.

It has been studied earlier that with severe asthma, workers tend to move to jobs involving lower level of exposure [14]. Known as the healthy worker effect, sicker individuals may choose work environments in which exposures are low, they may be excluded from being hired or once hired, they may seek transfer to less exposed jobs or leave work. [17]. In a longitudinal study of adults with occupational asthma, factors associated with individuals staying in their jobs included higher education and income, longer tenure with the company, having children to support and older age [15]. It is common among adults with asthma to change jobs throughout working life due to respiratory problems at work [3].

We studied if asthma was perceived by the subjects to be the reason for retirement and found out that it was significantly more common to retire because of asthma among those with work disability than among those retired for age. However, retirement seemed to similarly relieve asthma symptoms in over 60% of those who had retired regardless of the reason for the retirement. In this study, 90% of the retirement group did not see asthma as a main reason for their retirement, but a great proportion of them reported that asthma symptoms were alleviated after retirement. It may be that alleviation of asthma symptoms is related to lack of job-related stress in addition to less physical strain and exposures. A causal association between chronic psychosocial stress and asthma morbidity has been suggested in studies [18].

In our study, relief of asthma symptoms due to task change was reported by almost half or over half of subjects (48–67%) in all groups which encourages both the employer and occupational health units to support task changes due to asthma. Change of tasks seems to matter and efforts of collaboration between workplace and occupational health units are worthwhile in finding a suitable task, well-being at work and preventing early exit from work.

The strength of our study is the study population which is well representative of asthmatics at working age in Tampere. The response rate was 79%. We recruited all working-age adults with asthma in Tampere city with established asthma and special reimbursement and diagnosis based on lung function criteria. However, as a questionnaire-based study this lacks information on clinical measures and details of treatments on individual level. As a limitation of the study, we had data on all-cause sickness absence and lacked asthma-specific data. One weakness of the study was that in the original questionnaire the subjects were asked if they had made each type of career change after the diagnosis of asthma, but the number of such changes was not asked. It may be that some of the subjects had made several changes of each type, but this cannot be taken into account in the current analysis. Also, there are limitations in the cross-sectional study design. As in all questionnaire-based studies, selection bias is possible and we do not know whether those who answered this questionnaire have e.g. more severe asthma or vice versa. There may also be report bias among those with unfavorable working status. It may be that e.g. asthma was recalled and reported as the reason for a career change more often when the change or the result of the change was undesirable. Our material was collected in year 2000 and some aspects in asthma treatment or working life may have changed. In Finland, our national asthma guidelines and asthma program have stressed active treatment with inhaled corticosteroids (ICS) since early 1990's [19] and the use of ICS has not changed significantly since the collection of our data. Long-acting beta2-agonists (LABA)

were introduced in mid- 1990's but the use of this class of drugs has probably increased after year 2000 since the introduction of fixed ICS-LABA combinations. Finland has for long had a high level of social security and insurance system that has not significantly changed during the last decades and therefore our results from 2000 are still valid. The economic structure in Finland is typical for countries in Western Europe and has not changed fundamentally after the year 2000.

Conclusions

Those who were working full time, had most often made changes in their working career, which seem to be supported by younger age, nonmanual work and less asthma symptoms. Being driven to make career changes because of asthma was associated with undesirable employment status, suggesting that symptomatic asthma may accentuate the challenges in working life for adults with asthma. However, career changes especially because of asthma had potential beneficial effect on health seen as alleviation of asthma symptoms after the change. These highlight the importance of proper treatment of asthma, counselling of asthma patients towards applicable area of work or study, and possibly early, proactive support of career changes in maintaining sustainability in working life.

Acknowledgements
Not applicable.

Funding
The Finnish Work Environment Fund and Jalmari and Rauha Ahokas Foundation.

Authors' contributions
ST was the main author of the manuscript and contributed by analyzing and interpreting the data. LL and KK contributed by planning the study design, analyzing and interpreting data and writing the manuscript. RL contributed by planning and performing the statistical analyses and planning the design of this study. JU contributed as the leader of the study group, by planning the study design, analyzing and interpreting data and writing the manuscript. All authors read and approved the final manuscript.

Competing interests
The authors declare that they have no competing interests.

Author details
[1]Finla Occupational Health, Satakunnankatu 18 B, 33210 Tampere, Finland. [2]Allergy Centre, Tampere University Hospital, PO Box 2000, 33521 Tampere, Finland. [3]Faculty of Medicine and Life Sciences, University of Tampere, 33014 Tampere, Finland. [4]Finnish Institute of Occupational Health, PO Box 40, 00251 Helsinki, Finland. [5]Clinicum, Faculty of Medicine, University of Helsinki, PO Box 63, 00014 Helsinki, Finland.

References

1. Budginaitė I, Barcevičius E, Espasa J, Spurga S, Tsutskiridze L. Eurofound (2016), Sustainable work throughout the life course: National policies and strategies. Luxembourg: Publications Office of the European Union; 2016.

2. Thaon I, Wild P, Mouchot L, Monfort C, Touranchet A, Kreutz G, Derriennic F, Paris C. Long-term occupational consequences of asthma in a large French cohort of male workers followed up for 5 years. Am J Ind Med. 2008;51(5):317–23.

3. Blanc PD, Burney P, Janson C, Toren K. The prevalence and predictors of respiratory-related work limitation and occupational disability in an international study. Chest. 2003;124(3):1153–9.

4. Hansen CL, Baelum J, Skadhauge L, Thomsen G, Omland O, Thilsing T, Dahl S, Sigsgaard T, Sherson D. Consequences of asthma on job absenteeism and job retention. Scand J Public Health. 2012;40(4):377–84.

5. Peters J, Pickvance S, Wilford J, Macdonald E, Blank L. Predictors of delayed return to work or job loss with respiratory ill-health: a systematic review. J Occup Rehabil. 2007;17(2):317–26.

6. Toren K, Zock JP, Kogevinas M, Plana E, Sunyer J, Radon K, Jarvis D, Kromhout H, d'Errico A, Payo F, Anto JM, Blanc PD. An international prospective general population-based study of respiratory work disability. Thorax. 2009;64(4):339–44.

7. Ervasti J, Vahtera J, Pentti J, Oksanen T, Ahola K, Kivekas T, Kivimaki M, Virtanen M. Return to work after depression-related absence by employees with and without other health conditions: a cohort study. Psychosom Med. 2015;77(2):126–35.

8. Hakola R, Kauppi P, Leino T, Ojajarvi A, Pentti J, Oksanen T, Haahtela T, Kivimaki M, Vahtera J. Persistent asthma, comorbid conditions and the risk of work disability: a prospective cohort study. Allergy. 2011;66(12):1598–603.

9. Larbanois A, Jamart J, Delwiche JP, Vandenplas O. Socioeconomic outcome of subjects experiencing asthma symptoms at work. Eur Respir J. 2002;19(6):1107–13.

10. Henneberger PK, Redlich CA, Callahan DB, Harber P, Lemiere C, Martin J, Tarlo SM, Vandenplas O, Toren K. ATS Ad Hoc committee on work-exacerbated asthma: an official american thoracic society statement: work-exacerbated asthma. Am J Respir Crit Care Med. 2011;184(3):368–78.

11. Taponen S, Lehtimaki L, Karvala K, Luukkonen R, Uitti J. Correlates of employment status in individuals with asthma: a cross-sectional survey. J Occup Med Toxicol. 2017;12:19. 017–0165-6. eCollection 2017

12. Saarinen K, Karjalainen A, Martikainen R, Uitti J, Tammilehto L, Klaukka T, Kurppa K. Prevalence of work-aggravated symptoms in clinically established asthma. Eur Respir J. 2003;22(2):305–9.

13. Fell A, Abrahamsen R, Henneberger PK, Svendsen MV, Andersson E, Toren K, Kongerud J. Breath-taking jobs: a case-control study of respiratory work disability by occupation in Norway. Occup Environ Med. 2016;73(9):600–6.

14. Dumas O, Varraso R, Zock JP, Henneberger PK, Speizer FE, Wiley AS, Le Moual N, Camargo CA Jr. asthma history, job type and job changes among US nurses. Occup Environ Med. 2015;72(7):482–8.

15. Moscato G, Dellabianca A, Perfetti L, Brame B, Galdi E, Niniano R, Paggiaro P. Occupational asthma: a longitudinal study on the clinical and socioeconomic outcome after diagnosis. Chest. 1999;115(1):249–56.

16. Mancuso CA, Rincon M, Charlson ME. Adverse work outcomes and events attributed to asthma. Am J Ind Med. 2003;44(3):236–45.

17. Le Moual N, Kauffmann F, Eisen EA, Kennedy SM. The healthy worker effect in asthma: work may cause asthma, but asthma may also influence work. Am J Respir Crit Care Med. 2008;177(1):4–10.

18. Rosenberg SL, Miller GE, Brehm JM, Celedon JC. Stress and asthma: novel insights on genetic, epigenetic, and immunologic mechanisms. J Allergy Clin Immunol. 2014;134(5):1009–15.

19. Haahtela T, Klaukka T, Koskela K, Erhola M, Laitinen LA. Working Group Of the asthma Programme in Finland 1994-2004: asthma programme in Finland: a community problem needs community solutions. Thorax. 2001; 56(10):806–14.

23

Indoor concentrations of VOCs in beauty salons; association with cosmetic practices and health risk assessment

Mostafa Hadei[1], Philip K Hopke[2,3], Abbas Shahsavani[4,5*], Mahbobeh Moradi[4], Maryam Yarahmadi[6], Baharan Emam[4] and Noushin Rastkari[6,7]

Abstract

Background: The use of cosmetic products in beauty salons emits numerous kinds of toxic air pollutants. The objectives of this study were to measure the concentrations of benzene, toluene, ethylbenzene, xylene, formaldehyde, and acetaldehyde in 20 large beauty salons in Tehran and relate the observed concentrations to environmental and occupational characteristics of the salons.

Methods: Samples were collected from inside and outside air of 20 selected salons located in different areas of the city. Several additional parameters were recorded during the sampling process including surface area, number of active employees, type of ventilation, type of ongoing treatments, temperature, humidity. Deterministic and stochastic health risk assessment of the compounds were performed.

Results: Indoor concentrations of each pollutant were significantly higher than its outdoor concentrations. Health risk assessment showed that benzene, formaldehyde and acetaldehyde represent a possible cancer risk in the beauty salons. In addition, toluene, ethylbenzene, and xylene had negligible non-carcinogenic risks. Ventilation with air purifier, and fan with open window were more effective than using just a fan. Concentrations of benzene and toluene were affected by the number of hair dying treatments. The concentration of xylene was affected by the number of hair styling. The concentration of formaldehyde was affected by the number of hair styling and number of nail treatments.

Conclusion: With improved ventilation and requirements for reformulated cosmetic, concentrations of toxic air pollutants in beauty salons could be reduced.

Keywords: Benzene, Formaldehyde, Toluene, Xylene, Air pollution, Hairdressing

Background

Numerous chemical cosmetic products are used in hairdressing and beauty salons [1]. These products are used in facial cleansing, skin, nails and body hydrotherapy and care, anti-wrinkle treatments, pigmentation and acne treatment, make up, body and face massage, reflexology, aromatherapy, face and body hair removal, and hair styling and coloring services [2, 3]. These chemicals release volatile organic compounds (VOCs), including methacrylates,

phthalates, formaldehyde, etc. and pollutants like ozone and carbon monoxide [4]. People who work in beauty salons and even their customers can be exposed to high concentrations of these compounds.

Skin and respiratory disorders, carcinogenicity, and reproductive and genotoxic effects have been associated with compounds released in beauty salons [5–8]. Salon personnel often complain about eye, nose, throat, lung, and skin irritation [9–11]. Thus, such high-risk environments need to be assessed for the types and concentrations of toxic air pollutants that result in human exposure.

Benzene, toluene, ethylbenzene, and xylene (BTEX) have adverse health effects such as cancer and probable

* Correspondence: ashahsavani@gmail.com
[4]Environmental and Occupational Hazards Control Research Center, Shahid Beheshti University of Medical Sciences, Tehran, Iran
[5]Department of Environmental Health Engineering, School of Public Health and Safety, Shahid Beheshti University of Medical Sciences, Tehran, Iran
Full list of author information is available at the end of the article

neurological responses like weakness, loss of appetite, fatigue, confusion, and nausea [12]. The acute and chronic effects of formaldehyde include sensory irritation, reduced lung function, nasopharyngeal cancer, and myeloid leukemia [13]. Benzene, toluene, ethylbenzene, and xylene have been considered to be human carcinogen (group A), having inadequate information to assess carcinogenic potential, not classifiable as to human carcinogenicity (group D), and having inadequate data for carcinogenic potential, respectively [14–17]. Formaldehyde has been classified as a probable human carcinogen (group B1) by IRIS and as a human carcinogen (Group 1) by the International Agency for Research on Cancer (IARC) [18, 19]. Acute exposure to acetaldehyde causes irritation of the eyes, skin, and respiratory tract. Acetaldehyde is also considered as a probable human carcinogen (Group B2) by IRIS [20].

Several studies have been conducted to investigate indoor air quality in hairdressing and beauty salons. Goldin et al. (2014) measured total VOC (TVOC) concentrations, particulate matter with aerodynamic diameter less than 2.5 μm ($PM_{2.5}$), and carbon dioxide (CO_2) in nail salons in Boston, United States. They found that performing tasks increased the air pollutant concentrations, and ventilation improved indoor air quality [21]. In another study, concentrations of VOCs, formaldehyde, CO_2, and phthalate esters were measured at hairdressing salons in Taipei [22]. They detected a wide range of concentrations in various salons. Tsigonia et al. (2010) measured VOCs and formaldehyde in beauty salons. The main VOCs found in the salons were aromatics (toluene, xylene), esters and ketones (ethyl acetate, acetone, etc.) used as solvents, and terpenes (pinene, limonene, camphor, menthol) to provide desired odors [4].

These studies have reported measurements, but there remain uncertainties as to the relationships between the toxic air pollutant concentrations and the different various cosmetic practices. Investigating these relationships will determine the high-risk treatments and at-risk workers and customers. The use of mitigation methods have also not been adequately examined. The effects of different types of ventilation and air purifiers needs to be studied. The results of these studies can support the design of strategies for reducing exposure in these occupational environments. This aims of this study were to measure the concentrations of benzene, toluene, ethylbenzene, xylene, formaldehyde, and acetaldehyde in 20 large beauty salons and to relate these concentrations to the different environmental and occupational characteristics of salons.

Methods
Study design
Tehran is the capital of Iran, and have about 9 million residents. This city is faced with serious problems in

case of ambient air pollution [23–26]. There are reports of heavy use of cosmetics by Iranian women [27, 28]. Conventional cosmetics in Iran are imported mainly from China, Turkey, Korea, and England [29, 30].

Benzene, toluene, ethylbenzene, xylene (BTEX), formaldehyde and acetaldehyde were sampled from the indoor and outdoor air of 20 beauty salons during winter 2016–2017 in Tehran, Iran. The selected salons were located in different areas of the city. A questionnaire was completed by each salon owner to record the basic characteristics of salons, such as area (m^2), number of active employees, type of ventilation, working hours, type of ongoing treatments, etc. Smoking was prohibited in each monitored beauty salon. Three samples each were collected from both the inside and outside air of each salon using active sampling methods during mornings. To assess human exposure, the samplers were placed in the height of 1.5 m of active salons, near the working area. In total, 360 samples were collected, 180 each for inside and outside spaces (3 × 60 for BTEX, formaldehyde and acetaldehyde). After sampling, the sampling cartridges were sealed with plastic or brass end caps, placed in a sealed plastic box at 4 °C, and then transported to the laboratory. All sampling and analysis were completed during a 3 month period.

Services with potential emission of VOC were categorized in three main groups; hair coloring (dyes, bleaches, etc.), nail treatment (lacquers, polishes, etc.), and hair styling (oils, ointments, brilliantines, creams, gels, products for waving and straightening, etc.). The number of customers receiving each of these three services was recorded during sampling interval. The ventilations system of each salon can be categorized into three groups; 1) fan and closed window, 2) fan and open window, and 3) air purifier. Two salons used air purifiers. The models used were AIRMEGA 300 (COWAY, Korea) and IQAir HealthPro Plus - New Edition (IQAir, Switzerland) that have an activated carbon filter and a gas phase filter to remove gaseous pollutants, respectively. The air purifiers were placed in the center of salons.

Sampling and analysis
For BTEX, active sampling was performed using a pump (Universal 224-44MTX, SKC, USA) with a flow rate of 200 mL/min, and a solid sorbent tube (coconut shell charcoal, 100 mg/50 mg, 226–01 – SKC, USA) for 30 min. Three samples (each for 30 min) were collected sequentially indoors and outdoors. The sorbent from each tube was extracted using 1 mL CS_2 (76.13 g/mol, Merck, Germany) and 30 min sonication. Gas chromatography/ flame ionization detector (GC-FID: Agilent 7890B, Agilent Technologies, Waldbronn, Germany) was used to quantify the concentrations of BTEX. The sampling and analysis procedure implemented NIOSH method 1501 [31]. One

µL samples were injected to the glass column with a 5:1 split ratio. Injection and detector temperature were 250 °C and 300 °C, respectively. The column temperature was held at 40 °C for 10 min, and then increased by 10 °C/min to 230 °C. The carrier gas was helium with a flow of 2.6 mL/min. The results of sequential samplings were averaged to obtain a single value for each salon.

Formaldehyde samples were taken using a cartridge containing XAD-2 coated with (2-hydroxymethyl) piperdine (226–118 – SKC, USA), and a pump with flow rate of 50 mL/min for 30 min. Formaldehyde was desorbed from the cartridge with 10 mL of carbonyl-free acetonitrile (41.05 g/mol, Merck, Germany) and 30 min sonication. Gas chromatography/flame ionization detector (GC-FID: Agilent 7890B, Agilent Technologies, Waldbronn, Germany) was used to measure the formaldehyde concentrations. The procedure fully implemented NIOSH method 2541 [31]. One µL of the samples were injected into the capillary column in splitless mode, and with split vent time of 30 s. Injection and detector temperature were 250 °C and 300 °C, respectively. Column temperature was held at 70 °C for 1 min, and then increased by 15 °C/min to 240 °C, and held for 10 min. Carrier gas was helium with flow of 1 mL/min, with makeup flow of 29 mL/min.

Acetaldehyde was sampled using a solid sorbent tube 2-(hydroxymethyl) piperidine (2-HMP) on XAD-2, (450 mg/225 mg, 226–27 – SKC, USA) and a pump with flow rate of 50 mL/min for 30 min. Desorption was done with 5 mL toluene (92.14 g/mol, Merck, Germany) and 60 min ultrasonic. Gas chromatography/flame ionization detector (GC-FID: Agilent 7890B, Agilent Technologies, Waldbronn, Germany) was used to measure the acetaldehyde concentrations. The procedure fully implemented NIOSH method 2538 [31]. One µL splitless injections were made into the fused-silica capillary. Injection and detector temperature were 250 °C and 300 °C, respectively. The column temperature was increased from 70 °C by 6 °C/min to 110 °C, and then by 30 °C to 260 °C. The carrier gas was helium with flow of 1 mL/min, with makeup flow of 29 mL/min.

Quality control/quality assurance

The pump flowrate was calibrated before each sampling with a gas flow meter (Model 4140, TSI Inc., USA). Analytical instruments were calibrated using analytical grade reagents before each set of samples in reasonable concentration ranges for BTEX (1–50 µg/m^3), formaldehyde (1–100 µg/m^3), and acetaldehyde (1–100 µg/m^3). For quality assurance, in 10% of samplings, two sets of equipment were placed at the place simultaneously, and duplicate samples taken to estimate instrument precision. Replicate samples were recorded in two beauty salons. This analysis showed good agreement between sampling devices and replicate samples (Pearson's $r >$

0.97). Quality assurance procedures also included field, laboratory and solvent blanks to check for contamination. Blank samples showed negligible BTEX contamination.

Risk assessment

The cancer risks from exposure to benzene, formaldehyde, and acetaldehyde and non-cancer risk of toluene, ethylbenzene, and xylene were estimated. The Additional file 1 provides the details of the health risk assessments. Body weight and inhalation rate values recommended by US EPA are 70 kg and 20 m^3/day, respectively [32]. Considering 8-h working shifts per day and 30 vacation in each year, EF can be calculated ($=52 \times 6/3-30$) to be 74 days. Also, ED was assumed to be 30 years. In addition, averaging time for 70 years were obtained 25,500 days.

Deterministic risk assessment considers worst case or conservative scenarios. Alternatively, stochastic risk assessments estimate the probability distributions of toxic compounds' risk. Stochastic calculations treat some variables as random variables drawn from known probability distributions. ModelRisk (Vose Software) was used to simulate the distribution of risk based on the distribution of parameters used in the risk calculations by Monte Carlo analysis. The concentrations of the air pollutants were assumed to have log-normal distributions. Exposure frequency and exposure duration were considered to be distributed normally with the mean values of 74 days and 30 years, respectively. The minimum and maximum values were considered as 52 and 96 days for EF and 25 and 35 years for ED. CSFs for benzene and Reference concentrations (RfCs) for non-carcinogens were obtained from integrated risk information system (IRIS). According to this database, CSF for benzene, formaldehyde, and acetaldehyde are 0.029, 0.045, and 0.0077 1/(mg/kg.day), respectively. RfCs for chronic inhalation exposure of TEX and acetaldehyde compounds are 5.0, 1.0, and 0.1 mg/m^3, respectively. These values were converted to mg/kg.day as the dose unit. Therefore, the doses of toluene, ethylbenzene, and xylene were calculated to be 1.43, 0.29, and 0.029 mg/kg.day, respectively. The number of random samples were set at 1000. The outcome of the analysis for each compound was a histogram, and the 95% CI were calculated for each probability distribution.

Statistical analysis

All statistical analyses were performed using Sigma Plot 12. Kolmogorov-Smirnov and Levene tests were used to check the normality of data, and equality of variances, respectively. To compare indoor and outdoor concentrations of each pollutant, paired t-test was used for data with normal distributions and equal variances. The effect of ventilation type was investigated using one-way ANOVA and Holm-Sidak test. The correlations between the concentrations of the measured pollutants were assessed with Pearson's correlations. Multiple regression analysis was used to assess the effect of number of customers receiving different services (hair coloring, nail treatment, and hair styling) on the indoor VOC concentrations. Insignificant variables were removed from the model backward stepwise, and only the significant independent variable(s) are reported. The relationships between surface area of salons, temperature, relative humidity, and pollutant concentrations were analyzed separately using simple linear regression. The detailed results of statistical analyses are presented in the Additional file 1.

Results

Concentrations of BTEX, formaldehyde, and acetaldehyde were measured in 20 beauty salons, and several environmental and occupational factors were recorded simultaneously. The average air temperature and relative humidity were 21.8 °C and 29%, respectively. Table 1 presents some basic characteristics of BSs, number of cosmetologists, and number of customers receiving treatments with high VOCs potential during sampling.

Figure 1 presents box and whisker plots displaying the distributions of the pollutants inside and outside the beauty salons. Indoor concentrations of each pollutant were significantly higher than its outdoor concentrations ($p < 0.05$). The indoor to outdoor ratios for benzene, toluene, ethylbenzene, xylene, formaldehyde, and acetaldehyde were 2.04, 1.73, 2.01, 2.46, 2.11, and 2.21, respectively.

Concentrations of compounds in salons with different building characteristics were compared and the results are presented in Supplemental Material. The comparison between 3 types of ventilation mode showed that ventilations with air purifier, and fan and open window were more effective than just the fan ($p < 0.05$). No significant relationship was found between ventilation with air purifier, and fan and open window. In addition, floor area of salons did not affect the air pollutant concentrations ($p > 0.05$). Significant correlations were found between the concentrations of total VOCs (sum of all the measured compounds) and temperature ($R^2 = 0.71$) and humidity ($R^2 = 0.74$).

Table 2 presents the results of multiple regression about the relationship between the number of ongoing processes in beauty salons and concentrations of air pollutants. The results of multiple regression showed that concentrations of benzene and toluene

Table 1 Characteristics of 20 beauty salons used in this study

Salon No.	Area (m²)	Working hour (h)	No. of cosmetologists	Hair coloring[a]	Nail treatment[a]	Hair styling[a]	Ventilation[b]
1	120	8	8	5	3	7	F
2	130	9	7	7	3	12	F
3	120	9	5	4	5	10	F
4	130	7	9	2	7	4	F + W
5	160	8	15	7	4	6	F
6	105	9	3	3	2	2	F + W
7	125	10	9	8	4	4	AP
8	110	8	9	5	8	2	F + W
9	95	9	7	7	5	7	F
10	100	7	8	8	6	5	F
11	95	9	8	7	9	6	F
12	95	11	8	9	6	4	F
13	100	8	10	8	8	9	F
14	110	10	12	5	4	8	F
15	105	8	10	5	5	6	F + W
16	105	8	11	8	4	7	F + W
17	130	9	14	7	3	6	AP
18	100	11	10	6	7	9	F
19	115	7	12	4	3	7	F + W
20	95	9	9	6	6	8	F

[a]Each comprises all the activities related to hair coloring, nail treatment, and hair styling
[b]F fan, F + W fan plus open window, AP air purifier

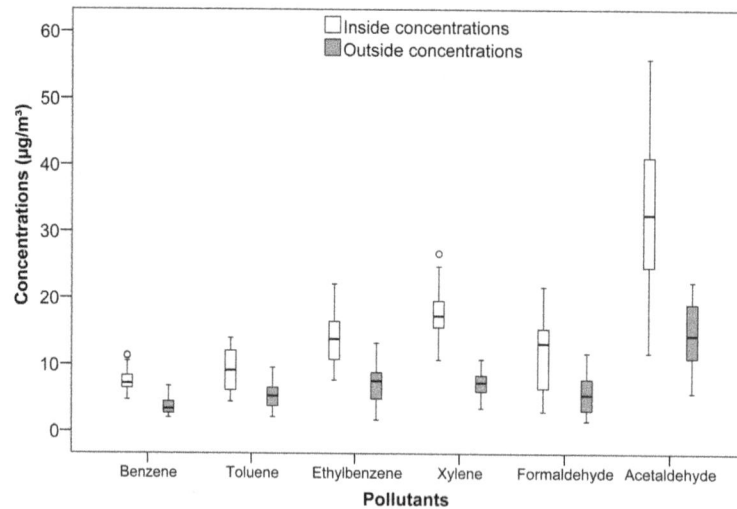

Fig. 1 Descriptive statistics of inside and outside concentrations of air pollutants. Legend: The median, quartiles, minimum and maximum (whiskers), outliers (circles) and extreme values (asterisks) are shown in this Figure

were affected only by the number of hair dying treatments. Concentrations of xylene was affected only by the number of hair styling processes. And finally, the concentrations of formaldehyde were affected by either the number of hair stylings and nail treatments. The number of any processes had no effect the concentrations of acetaldehyde.

Table 3 presents the Pearson correlation coefficients between 6 investigated air pollutants. According to this table, only the correlation between formaldehyde and acetaldehyde ($r = 0.65$) was significant ($p<0.05$), indicating that 65% of formaldehyde and acetaldehyde variations are associated.

According to deterministic risk assessment analyses, the cancer risks of benzene, formaldehyde and acetaldehyde were estimated to be 5.44×10^{-6}, 1.33×10^{-5}, and 6.26×10^{-6}. Hazard ratios for toluene, ethylbenzene, and xylene were 1.60×10^{-4}, 1.20×10^{-3}, and 1.54×10^{-2},

respectively. Figs. 2 and 3 show the results of the stochastic risk assessment for BTEX compounds, formaldehyde and acetaldehyde. The minimum cancer risks of benzene, formaldehyde and acetaldehyde were predicted to be 3.11×10^{-6}, 3.13×10^{-6}, and 2.12×10^{-6}, respectively. The maximum values of cancer risks for benzene, formaldehyde and acetaldehyde were 9.04×10^{-6}, 2.70×10^{-5}, and 1.12×10^{-5}, respectively. The minimum hazard ratios for toluene, ethylbenzene, and xylene were 7.12×10^{-6}, 6.45×10^{-4}, and 8.76×10^{-3}, respectively. The maximum values of hazard ratios predicted for toluene, ethylbenzene, and xylene were $2.57 \times 10{-4}$, 2.05×10^{-3} and 2.49×10^{-2}, respectively.

Discussion

The indoor concentrations of each pollutant were higher than the corresponding values in the local ambient air.

Table 2 Parameters affecting the indoor concentrations of air pollutants

	Parameter	Coefficient	Std. coefficient	Std. Error	P-value	R^2
Benzene	Constant	3.786	–	1.163	–	0.387
	Dying	0.620	0.622	0.184	0.003	
Toluene	Constant	4.768	–	2.146	–	0.204
	Dying	0.729	0.452	0.339	0.046	
Ethylbenzene	–	–	–	–	–	–
Xylene	Constant	13.027	–	2.356	–	0.222
	Hair styling	0.772	0.471	0.341	0.036	
Formaldehyde	Constant	−2.232	–	4.265	–	0.415
	Nail	1.639	0.549	0.556	0.009	
	Hair styling	0.892	0.386	0.431	0.054	
Acetaldehyde	–	–	–	–	–	–

Table 3 Pearson's correlation coefficients between air pollutants

Pollutants	Benzene	Ethylbenzene	Toluene	Xylene	Formaldehyde	Acetaldehyde
Benzene	1.00	−0.43	0.52	−0.04	−0.07	0.16
Ethylbenzene			−0.24	0.45	−0.04	−0.31
Toluene				0.27	0.02	0.13
Xylene					0.27	0.12
Formaldehyde						*0.65*[a]
Acetaldehyde						1.00

[a]$p < 0.05$

This result was expected given that cosmetic products are known emission sources. The I/O ratios were between 1.7 and 2.4 for all measured pollutants. de Gennaro et al. (2014) found very high (> 10) indoor to outdoor (I/O) ratios of VOC concentrations in hair salons [33]. The lower ratios in the present study can be associated with the presence of ventilation systems. de Gennaro et al. (2014) did not discuss the ventilation in their measured salons. Goldin et al. (2014) measured total VOC concentrations in nail salons and reported the median concentration was 4800 ppb [21]. Tsigonia et al. (2010) examined VOCs in beauty salons, and reported that the major detected VOCs were aromatics (toluene, xylene), esters and ketones (ethyl acetate, acetone, etc.), terpenes (pinene, limonene, camphor, menthenol), and camphor. Formaldehyde concentrations were below detection limit of their method [4]. This difference with the present study may be due to differences in the cosmetic products in use and measurements were made in small salons with fewer customers. Chang et al. (2017) investigated indoor air of hairdressing salons in Taipei, and found 387 different ingredients. Their minimum and maximum formaldehyde concentrations were 12.40 and 1.04×10^3 µg/m^3, respectively [22]. In our study, all of the observed formaldehyde concentrations were lower than WHO guideline value of 100 µg/m^3 for 30-min exposures. In case of benzene, no safe level of exposure has been recommended by WHO [12].

Beauty salons with better ventilations had lower concentrations of VOCs. Chang et al. (2017) reported high concentrations of CO_2 in salons with poor ventilation [22]. Goldin et al. (2014) observed higher TVOC and $PM_{2.5}$ concentrations in salons with less ventilation. It appears that salons with open doors, and table or roof fans had lower concentrations of pollutants compared to enclosed buildings with central ventilation systems [21].

Formaldehyde and acetaldehyde were correlated to each other, likely due to common sources. However, acetaldehyde was not related to any ongoing treatments. However, nail treatments and hair styling affected formaldehyde concentrations. An additional linear regression analysis was performed to investigate just the effect of hair styling, the variable that had the lowest P-value in the multiple regression analysis, on acetaldehyde concentration. The fit was marginally significant ($p < 0.1$). The intercept and slope for hair styling were 20.47 and 1.89, respectively. This shows that the number of hair styling treatments affects both formaldehyde and acetaldehyde concentrations, but in different statistical significance levels. In addition, Fig. 1 showed that acetaldehyde concentrations were higher than formaldehyde. This can be due to the content of cosmetic products. Additional studies should be conducted to explore the relationship between the ingredients of cosmetic products and toxic compounds in the air.

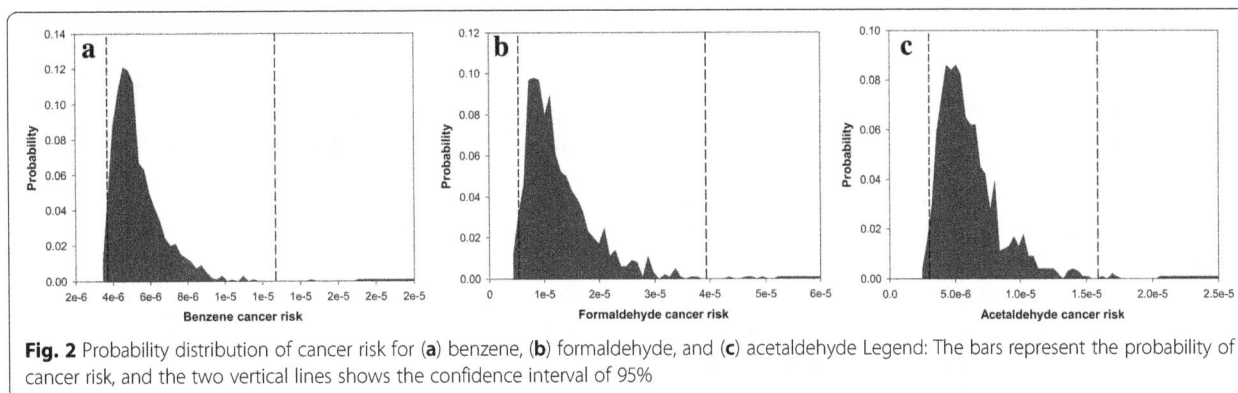

Fig. 2 Probability distribution of cancer risk for (**a**) benzene, (**b**) formaldehyde, and (**c**) acetaldehyde Legend: The bars represent the probability of cancer risk, and the two vertical lines shows the confidence interval of 95%

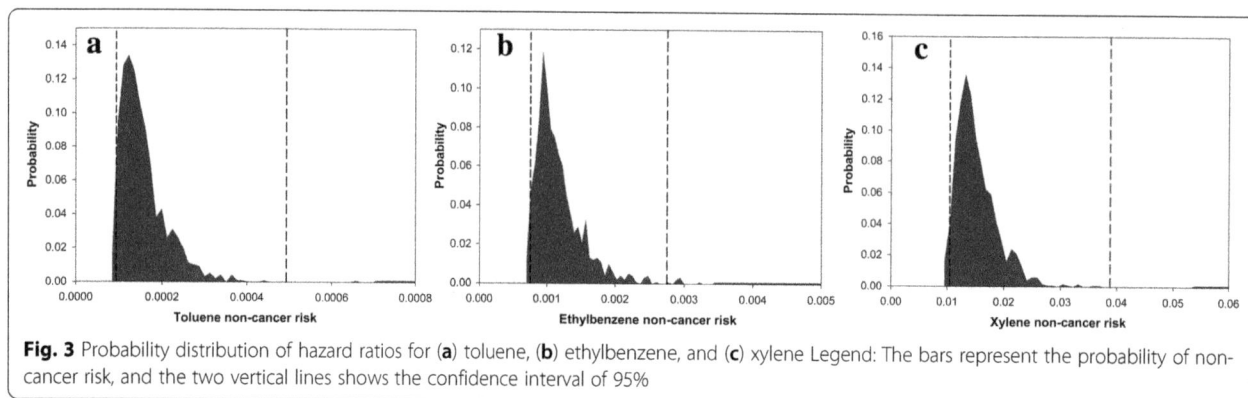

Fig. 3 Probability distribution of hazard ratios for (**a**) toluene, (**b**) ethylbenzene, and (**c**) xylene Legend: The bars represent the probability of non-cancer risk, and the two vertical lines shows the confidence interval of 95%

Temperature and relative humidity were positively correlated with the total VOC concentrations in accordance with prior literature [34, 35]. Higher temperatures increase the evaporation of VOCs from cosmetic products [36]. Therefore, in order to decrease the concentrations of VOCs in beauty salons, the optimum conditions in case of temperature and humidity can be provided. However, Quach et al. (2011) report that temperature was weakly correlated with toluene and isopropyl acetate concentrations. Relative humidity had no relationship with measured concentrations for any of the compounds [37].

Significant relationships were found between compound concentrations and the number of ongoing treatments. The results found relationships between benzene-hair dying, toluene-hair dying, xylene-hair styling, formaldehyde-nail treatment, and formaldehyde-hair styling. Goldin et al. (2014) reported higher TVOC concentrations were observed during nail treatments. However, TVOCs concentrations were independent of the number of ongoing nail treatments [21]. Quach et al. (2011) reported that workers who performed pedicures were more likely to be exposed to higher ethyl acetate values compared with those who applied silk nails and acrylic nails. They found that the number of permanent wave treatments and the number of workers were associated with formaldehyde concentrations [37].

According to previous studies, compounds with an attributable cancer risk more than 1×10^{-4} were defined as a "definite risk", those between 1×10^{-5} and 1×10^{-4} were "probable risk", and between 1×10^{-5} and 1×10^{-6} was a "possible risk". A cancer risk less than 1×10^{-6} is recommended by USEPA as an "acceptable risk" [38]. In this study, minimum, average, and maximum carcinogen risks for benzene, formaldehyde, and acetaldehyde were exceeded 1×10^{-6}. Hence, these compounds represent a possible cancer risk in the beauty salons but does not pose a significant risk. To assess the non-carcinogenic effects of the TEX compounds, an HR below 1 should be considered to be as a negligible risk [39]. The findings

in this study showed average, minimum, and maximum non-carcinogenic risks of toluene, ethylbenzene, and xylene in beauty salons were less than one. Therefore, they can be considered to have negligible non-carcinogenic risks. In addition to the risk attributed to each compound, the total cumulative non-cancer risk can be an important value. By aggregating all the individual values, total cumulative non-cancer risk was 1.70×10^{-2}, that is still less than one.

Conclusions

High inside to outside ratio of air pollutant concentrations demonstrated that the indoor activities were VOC sources. Significant relationships between the concentrations of some compounds (i.e. benzene, toluene, ethylbenzene, and formaldehyde) and the number of different treatments identified possible sources for these compounds. Relationships between air pollutant concentrations and the salon characteristics were analyzed, and effective ventilation was found to reduce exposure. Chronic exposure to a mixture of air pollutants can impose greater adverse health effects rather than single exposures. Thus, to protect the workers, controlling ventilation, it is possible to reduce indoor pollutant concentrations. It would also be possible to use products with little or none of these toxic species as ingredients. To improve health conditions in beauty salons, air quality guidelines or a mandatory occupational regulatory framework is needed. In addition, identifying and prohibiting cosmetic products with potentially toxic emissions could reduce VOC exposures to both workers and customers.

Acknowledgements
This study was has supported by grant No. 6618 from Shahid Beheshti University of Medical Sciences. Also Environmental and Occupational Health Centre of the Ministry of Health and Medical Education has supported this study.

Funding
This study was has supported by grant No. 6618 from Shahid Beheshti University of Medical Sciences.

Authors' contributions
All authors (except for PKH) contributed with study design, data collection, data handling and manuscript preparation. PKH participated in study design, data handling and manuscript preparation. All authors read and approved the final manuscript.

Competing interests
The authors declare that they have no competing interests.

Author details
[1]Research Center for Environmental Determinants of Health (RCEDH), Kermanshah University of Medical Sciences, Kermanshah, Iran. [2]Department of Public Health Sciences, University of Rochester School of Medicine and Dentistry, Rochester, NY 14642, USA. [3]Center for Air Resources Engineering and Science, Clarkson University, Potsdam, NY 13699, USA. [4]Environmental and Occupational Hazards Control Research Center, Shahid Beheshti University of Medical Sciences, Tehran, Iran. [5]Department of Environmental Health Engineering, School of Public Health and Safety, Shahid Beheshti University of Medical Sciences, Tehran, Iran. [6]Environmental and Occupational Health Center, Ministry of Health and Medical Education, Tehran, Iran. [7]Center for Air Pollution Research (CAPR), Institute for Environmental Research (IER), Tehran University of Medical Sciences, Tehran, Iran.

References
1. Leino T. Working conditions and health in hairdressing salons. Appl Occup Environ Hyg. 1999;14:26–33.
2. Labrèche F, Forest J, Trottier M, Lalonde M, Simard R. Characterization of chemical exposures in hairdressing salons. Appl Occup Environ Hyg. 2003; 18:1014–21.
3. Ronda E, Hollund BE, Moen BE. Airborne exposure to chemical substances in hairdresser salons. Environ Monit Assess. 2009;153:83–93.
4. Tsigonia A, Lagoudi A, Chandrinou S, Linos A, Evlogias N, Alexopoulos EC. Indoor air in beauty salons and occupational health exposure of cosmetologists to chemical substances. Int J Environ Res Public Health. 2010;7:314–24.
5. Leino T, Tammilehto L, Hytonen M. Occupational skin and respiratory diseases among hairdressers. Occupat Health Industr Med. 1999;2:88.
6. Halliday-Bell JA, Gissler M, Jaakkola JJ. Work as a hairdresser and cosmetologist and adverse pregnancy outcomes. Occup Med. 2009;59:180–4.
7. Galiotte MP, Kohler P, Mussi G, Figaro Gattás GJ. Assessment of occupational genotoxic risk among Brazilian hairdressers. Ann Occup Hyg. 2008;52:645–51.
8. Czene K, Tiikkaja S, Hemminki K. Cancer risks in hairdressers: assessment of carcinogenicity of hair dyes and gels. Int J Cancer. 2003;105:108–12.
9. Leino T, Tammilehto L, Luukkonen R, Nordman H. Self reported respiratory symptoms and diseases among hairdressers. Occupat Health Industr Med. 1998;3:134–5.
10. Palmer A, Renzetti AD, Gillam D. Respiratory disease prevalence in cosmetologists and its relationship to aerosol sprays. Environ Res. 1979;19: 136–53.
11. Uter W, Gefeller O, Schwanitz H. The influence of skin sensitivity (atopy) and skin protection on the development of hand eczema in hairdressers-first results of a prospective cohort study. Allergologie. 1995;18:312–5.
12. World Health Organization. WHO Guidelines for indoor air quality: selected pollutants. København: WHO Regional Office for Europe; 2010.
13. Mandin C, Trantallidi M, Cattaneo A, Canha N, Mihucz VG, Szigeti T, Mabilia R, Perreca E, Spinazzè A, Fossati S. Assessment of indoor air quality in office buildings across Europe-the OFFICAIR study. Sci Total Environ. 2017;579:169–78.
14. IRIS. Chemical assessment summary: benzene; CASRN 71–43-2. U.S. National Center for Environmental Assessment: Environmental Protection Agency; 2003.
15. IRIS. Chemical Assessment Summary: toluene; CASRN 108–88-3. U.S. National Center for Environmental Assessment: Environmental Protection Agency; 2005.
16. IRIS. Chemical Assessment Summary: Ethylbenzene; CASRN 100–41-4. U.S. National Center for Environmental Assessment: Environmental Protection Agency; 1988.
17. IRIS. Chemical Assessment Summary: xylenes; CASRN 1330-20-7. U.S. National Center for Environmental Assessment: Environmental Protection Agency; 2003.
18. U.S.EPA. Integrated risk information system (IRIS) on formaldehyde. Washington, D.C.: National Center for Environmental Assessment OoRaD; 1989.
19. IARC. Formaldehyde, 2-butoxyethanol and 1-tert-butoxypropan-2-ol. IARC Monogr Eval Carcinog Risks Hum. 2006;88:1–478.
20. U.S.EPA. Integrated risk information system (IRIS) on acetaldehyde. Washington, D.C.: National Center for Environmental Assessment OoRaD; 1999.
21. Goldin LJ, Ansher L, Berlin A, Cheng J, Kanopkin D, Khazan A, Kisivuli M, Lortie M, Peterson EB, Pohl L. Indoor air quality survey of nail salons in Boston. J Immigr Minor Health. 2014;16:508–14.
22. Chang CJ, Cheng SF, Chang PT, Tsai SW. Indoor air quality in hairdressing salons in Taipei. Indoor Air. 2018;28(10):173–80.
23. Hadei M, Hopke PK, Hashemi Nazari SS, Yarahmadi M, Shahsavani A, Alipour MR. Estimation of mortality and hospital admissions attributed to criteria air pollutants in Tehran Metropolis, Iran (2013-2016). Aerosol Air Qual Res. 2017; 17:2474–81.
24. Shahsavani A, Yarahmadi M, Hadei M, Sowlat MH, Naddafi K. Elemental and carbonaceous characterization of TSP and PM10 during middle eastern dust (MED) storms in Ahvaz, Southwestern Iran. Environ Monit Assess. 2017;189:462.
25. Bakhtiari R, Hadei M, Hopke PK, Shahsavani A, Rastkari N, Kermani M, Yarahmadi M, Ghaderpoori A. Investigation of in-cabin volatile organic compounds (VOCs) in taxis; influence of vehicle's age, model, fuel, and refueling. Environ Pollut. 2018;237:348–55.
26. Khamutian R, Najafi F, Soltanian M, Shokoohizadeh MJ, Poorhaghighat S, Dargahi A, Sharafi K, Afshari A. The association between air pollution and weather conditions with increase in the number of admissions of asthmatic patients in emergency wards: a case study in Kermanshah. Med J Islam Repub Iran. 2015;29:229.
27. Dehghani R, Talaee R, Sehat M, Ghamsari NN, Mesgari L. Investigating the influence of mass media on cosmetics usage among women in Kashan during 2015. Iran J Health Safety Environ. 2017;4:695–8.
28. Dehghani R, Talaee R, Sehat M, Ghamsari NN, Mesgari L. Surveying the rate of using cosmetics among the Kashan's women. J Biol Today's World. 2017; 6:27–32.
29. Karimi G, Ziarati P. Heavy metal contamination of popular nail polishes in Iran. Iranian Journal of Toxicology. 2015;9:1290–5.
30. Mousavi Z, Ziarati P, Shariatdoost A. Determination and safety assessment of lead and cadmium in eye shadows purchased in local market in Tehran. J Environ Anal Toxicol. 2013;3:2161–0525.1000193.
31. Eller PM, Cassinelli ME. NIOSH manual of analytical methods: Diane Publishing; 1994.
32. EPA U. Risk assessment guidance for superfund. Volume I: human health evaluation manual (part a). In: EPA/540/1–89/002; 1989.
33. de Gennaro G, de Gennaro L, Mazzone A, Porcelli F, Tutino M. Indoor air quality in hair salons: screening of volatile organic compounds and indicators based on health risk assessment. Atmos Environ. 2014;83:119–26.
34. Wiglusz R, Sitko E, Nikel G, Jarnuszkiewicz I, Igielska B. The effect of temperature on the emission of formaldehyde and volatile organic compounds (VOCs) from laminate flooring—case study. Build Environ. 2002; 37:41–4.
35. Markowicz P, Larsson L. Influence of relative humidity on VOC concentrations in indoor air. Environ Sci Pollut Res. 2015;22:5772–9.
36. Wang R, Moody RP, Koniecki D, Zhu J. Low molecular weight cyclic volatile methylsiloxanes in cosmetic products sold in Canada: implication for dermal exposure. Environ Int. 2009;35:900–4.

37. Quach T, Gunier R, Tran A, Von Behren J, Doan-Billings P-A, Nguyen K-D,
     Okahara L, Lui BY-B, Nguyen M, Huynh J: Characterizing workplace
     exposures in Vietnamese women working in California nail salons. Am J
     Public Health 2011, 101:S271-S276.
38. Robson MG, Toscano WA. Risk Assessment for Environmental Health: John
     Wiley & Sons; 2007.
39. Ramírez N, Cuadras A, Rovira E, Borrull F, Marcé RM. Chronic risk assessment
     of exposure to volatile organic compounds in the atmosphere near the
     largest Mediterranean industrial site. Environ Int. 2012;39:200–9.

24

Health, risk behaviour and consumption of addictive substances among physicians

Dominik Pförringer[1][*][†], Regina Mayer[1][†], Christa Meisinger[2], Dennis Freuer[2] and Florian Eyer[3]

Abstract

Background: Previous studies were able to show that hazardous alcohol and substance abuse among physicians is not rare. Currently no recent data to detect risk groups are available either on the prevalence of hazardous drinking disorders and risky health behaviour among physicians or on influencing factors (age, gender, role, institution, specialization, working hours).

Methods: A 42-item online questionnaire was distributed to 38 university hospitals, 296 teaching hospitals and 1290 physicians in private practice. The questionnaire addressed health behaviour and alcohol/substance consumption as well as demographic and work-related properties.

Results: Out of 1338 a total of 920 questionnaires could be evaluated. 90% of physicians estimate their health status as satisfying. 23% of doctors consume hazard quantities of ethanol, 5% are nicotine addicted, and 8% suffer from obesity. Childlessness ($p = 0,004$; OR = 1,67; KI = 1,17-2,37) for both genders and the role of a resident for females ($p = 0,046$, OR = 3,10, KI = 1,02-9,40) poses a risk factor for hazardous alcohol consumption. Weekly working hours of more than 50 h ($p = 0,009$; OR = 1,56; KI = 1,12-2,18) and a surgical profession ($p < 0,001$; OR = 2,03; KI = 1,47-2,81) may also be a risk factor towards hazardous and risky health behaviour.

Conclusion: A more structured and frequently repeated education on help offerings and specific institutions for addicted and risk groups seems essential.

Keywords: Health, Physicians' health, Addiction, Risk behaviour, Alcohol, Drugs, Consumption, Online survey

Background

Aspects of health attitude and consumption of addictive substances among doctors are frequently found in media and science [1–6]. Not only overburdening workload and burnout but alcohol and medication abuse also play a significant role. One major problem is the taboo status of discussing such behaviour in a group of co-workers exposed to high pressure and stress. Geuenich showed in 2009, that 46% of doctors in Germany suffer from psychological pressure both in the professional as well as the social context [7]. Information on available help and support as well as solutions are not commonly well known, even though they exist [4, 8–10]. In the US,

lifetime prevalence of alcohol abuse and dependence of doctors in 1992 was estimated at 6%, while in Norway hazardous alcohol consumption among doctors increased from 12 to 15% between 1993 and 2000 [11, 12].

However, little scientific information on German doctors exists – prevalence of hazardous alcohol consumption according to Rosta et al. 2008 was 20% [1, 13, 14]. In a survey study, Unrath et al. determined in 2012 that almost every fourth general practitioner in Rhineland-Palatinate consumes alcohol on a daily basis [14]. Burnout and depression among physicians as well as addiction and risky health behaviours are under-represented clinical pictures [15, 16]. Mäulen assumes that alcohol is the most common drug used by doctors [10, 17]. In a survey study in 2008 Rosta found that particularly surgical disciplines and male doctors pose risk groups for hazardous alcohol

* Correspondence: dominik@pfoerringer.de

[†]Dominik Pförringer and Regina Mayer contributed equally to this work.

[1]Department of Trauma Surgery, Technical University of Munich, Ismaningerstrasse 22-, 81675 Munich, Germany

Full list of author information is available at the end of the article

consumption, but age has no significant influence [13]. However, other influencing factors were not investigated, and the influence of age, sex and discipline was not analysed in a multivariable way. In a smaller study in 2009, Voigt et al. studied the smoking behaviour of physicians in Saxony and Brandenburg - 86% were non-smokers [18]. Furthermore, experts estimate that about 0.7% of physicians in Germany use narcotic drugs (BtM), but there is no reliable data regarding this [10]. There is currently no data on general risk-taking and the physical activity and nutrition of physicians in Germany.

Hazardous drinking is defined as the consumption of an amount of alcohol that increases the risk of harmful consequences for the user or others. Harmful drinking on the other hand comes along with actual physical or mental harm [19]. Since the transition between these terms is fluent, we use the term 'hazardous' for both terms [20]. The amount of alcohol which marks hazardous consumption is differently defined. For example, Reid et al. 1999 defined: "21 drinks or more per week for men (or >= 7 drinks per occasion at least 3 times a week) or 14 drinks or more per week for women (or >=5 drinks per occasion at least 3 times a week)" [21]. A more recent study of Wood et al. concluded that the consumption of more than 100 g alcohol per week is risky [22].

The aim of the present work is to update the data on addiction and health behaviour of physicians, as well as to reflect the general risk tolerance. Furthermore, risk groups can be identified to support the development of prevention strategies. The following questions were examined:

- How do doctors evaluate their own health?
- How balanced is a doctor's diet and how regularly do they exercise?
- What is the general willingness of doctors to take risks and how often do they participate in preventive examinations? Do predisposed groups exist?
- What is the prevalence of dangerous alcohol use among physicians and how does it affect their counselling behaviour? Which groups are particularly at risk?
- What is the prevalence of substance use, risk taking and obesity in specific comparison between surgical and non-surgical specialties?

Methods
Design and conduction of survey
This study was conducted as an anonymous survey of physicians in Germany using web-based survey opportunities on the website of pollster SurveyMonkey® (San Mateo, CA) [16]. The survey was reviewed and approved by the Ethics Committee of the Faculty of Medicine of the Technical University of Munich (number: 555 / 15S).

In mid-October 2016, an e-mail cover letter was sent to medical and commercial directors and / or hospital management of the 38 university hospitals in Germany as well as to 296 teaching hospitals [23]. A maximum of nine teaching hospitals were contacted per university.

During the same period, 1290 physicians in 11 German federal states were contacted by e-mail after selection via a multi-stage random procedure, selected on the basis of the online registries of the medical associations. In each case, according to the area of the federal state, a representative sample stratified by discipline was drawn. A multiple of 15 general practitioners and one representative from 23 specialties was selected in total: Bavaria was chosen as a reference state, where a calculated total of 120 general practitioners and 184 members of other disciplines were examined.

The federal states were Bavaria (120/184), Baden-Wuerttemberg (80/115), Saarland (13/23), Rhineland-Palatinate (40/69), Hesse (40/69), Thuringia (40/69), Lower Saxony (90/138), Saxony-Anhalt (40/69), Bremen (6/12), Schleswig-Holstein (30/46) and Hamburg (7/11).

Areas of specialization were anaesthesiology, surgery, dermatology, gynaecology and obstetrics, internal medicine, child and adolescent psychiatry, laboratory medicine, nuclear medicine, pathology, plastic surgery, psychosomatics, urology, radiology, ear nose throat, human genetics, paediatrics, neurology, microbiology, orthopaedics and traumatology, physical and rehabilitative medicine, psychiatry and radiation therapy.

One out of ten in the online directories of the medical associations, sorted by subject, was selected. Since some federal states did not have enough representatives in the smaller subject areas, 21 physicians less were addressed - so a total of 1290 doctors instead of 1311.

To achieve greater participation and to maintain the anonymity of clinics and doctors, confirmation of participation in the survey by the respective clinic or respective physician was waived. The cover letter included a link to the survey (one-time redirection per IP address), a short description of the content and the request for internal and external distribution. The survey was open for participation for a total of 10 weeks (11th October to 19th December 2016). In mid-November 2016, a reminder letter was sent by e-mail to all contacted clinics and doctors. Surveys addressed to the relevant specialist societies in Austria, Switzerland and occasionally in English-speaking countries were not included in the evaluation due to insufficient numbers of participants.

Questionnaire
By including validated tests and using literature, a 42-item questionnaire (41 plus consent) was developed using SurveyMonkey®'s online tool [24–32]. A team of

eight physicians and four clinical researchers from various disciplines not involved in the study at Klinikum rechts der Isar tested the survey for comprehensibility as well as the quality and lack of questions. After evaluating the suggestions for improvement and the modification of six items, the final version was created. Answering the questions averaged about 7 min. The questionnaire can be found in the online supplement.

Included were questions on general health behaviour and attitude, sports, diet and socio-demographic as well as occupational aspects. To examine the nicotine and alcohol consumption behaviour validated tests were used. The former was examined by using the Heaviness of Smoking Index (HSI), a short form of the Fagerström Test for Nicotine Dependence (FTND) [33, 34]. The latter was examined by the AUDIT-C, a short form of the Alcohol Use Disorders Identification Test (AUDIT) with comparable psychometric quality [26, 32, 35]. A cut-off point of 5 or more was used to detect hazardous alcohol consumption – this sum was recommended as cut-off for the German population [36]. Additionally the CAGE questionnaire was integrated, whose answering was voluntary to avoid dropouts [30].

Statistics

The evaluation was carried out by means of the statistical software SPSS (SPSS Statistics Premium 24, IBM). Depending on type of data, mean values with standard deviations or relative and absolute frequencies were calculated for the descriptive analysis. Differences between physicians, surgical and non-surgical disciplines, as well as hazardous and non-hazardous alcohol consumption were analysed with Fisher's exact test, chi-square test or the t-test for two unconnected samples, depending on the scale level. Furthermore, binary logistic regression analyses were performed in multivariate models, adjusted for potential influencing factors.

Results
Return and sample size

Altogether, in the German-language version of 1338 on-line questionnaires 1096 were completely filled out. Completion rate thus equals 81.9%. The response rate itself is not assessable in this study, because we refrained from retracing the participants to ensure anonymity and to achieve a greater number of participants. Twenty-two participants did not agree to the scientific use of their data and had to be excluded. Due to the low number of active doctors in Austria ($n = 25$) and Switzerland ($n = 50$), only 988 participants active in Germany were selected (excluded: other country: 4, missing information: 7). Forty-six people were excluded because they were not doctors or non-medics and another 22 because they gave missing or obviously wrong

answers in the categories analysed here. Thus, the following results are based on the complete information of 920 physicians working in Germany.

The majority of participating physicians were younger than 35 years, whereas more men than women were over 46 years old (43 and 31%, respectively) (Table 1). Significantly more men than women lived with children in the household (52 and 38%, respectively), and they were also significantly more likely to be married (73 and 53%, respectively). Most participants came from internal medicine (21%), from surgery (including orthopaedics and trauma surgery) (18%) and anaesthesiology (16%). Nearly one in two men worked in a leadership position (45%), while just below half of the women were residents (46%). 85% of all responding physicians worked in a clinic. 53% of the female physicians and 71% of the male physicians regularly worked at least 50 h a week.

Examined variables

There was no difference between the subjective perception of health by members of a surgical specialty and a non-surgical specialty. Health was found to be at least satisfactory by almost all (90%) (Table 2). Almost every second surgeon (44%) sometimes or often took risks, significantly more frequently than doctors in non-surgical disciplines (26%). Surgeons also took greater risks because of the fact that only one out of five regularly participated in check-ups. Also the AUDIT-C test suggested that at least 29% of surgeons had at least a hazardous alcohol intake - nearly one in four doctors in total. 8% of participating physicians were severely obese (BMI ≥30) and 5% showed moderate to high nicotine dependence in the Heaviness of Smoking Index.

Response numbers in the category "substance abuse" were too little to allow for valid conclusions. Only five physicians reported regularly taking benzodiazepines, seven regularly consumed Z-drugs (e.g. Zolpidem, Zopiclon and Zaleplon), two opiates and / or opioids, three ecstasy, cocaine and / or amphetamines, and 18 physicians regularly consumed cannabinoids.

Influencing factors

Comparing the group of people with potentially hazardous alcohol consumption with the group of those who did not consume alcohol or whose consumption was rather harmless in regard to certain risk factors, it is noteworthy that significantly more men than women (32 to 13%) showed a hazardous drinking behaviour (Table 3). Childless persons were significantly more likely (26%) to drink more than parents (19%). Alcohol consumption by physicians working less than 50 h a week was less hazardous (83 to 74%). On the other hand, the age as well as the

Table 1 Socio-demographic and occupational characteristics (absolute numbers/frequency in %)

Characteristic	Female physicians ($n = 417$)	Male physicians ($n = 503$)	All ($n = 920$)	P-value
Age group				
18–35	190/46	150/30	340/37	< 0,001
36–45	101/24	135/27	236/26	
46–55	90/22	131/26	221/24	
older than 55	36/9	87/17	123/13	
Marital status				
Unmarried	177/42	120/24	297/32	< 0,001
Married	221/53	365/73	586/64	
Divorced/widowed	19/5	18/4	37/4	
Children (living in the household)				
Yes	159/38	263/52	422/46	< 0,001
No	258/62	240/48	498/54	
Medical speciality				
General practice	32/8	45/9	77/8	< 0,001
Anaesthesiology	66/16	85/17	151/16	
Surgery[a]	28/7	52/10	80/9	
Orthopaedic and trauma surgery	16/4	66/13	82/9	
Internal medicine	87/21	107/21	194/21	
Paediatrics	38/9	21/4	59/6	
Psychiatry/child and adolescent Psychiatry	38/9	35/7	73/8	
Other	112/27	92/18	204/22	
Position/educational level				
Resident	193/46	145/29	338/37	< 0,001
Specialist	117/28	130/26	247/27	
Physician in a leading position	107/26	228/45	335/36	
Establishment				
University hospital	184/44	192/38	376/41	0.110
For-profit/public/non-profit hospital	177/42	224/45	401/44	
Phyiscian in private practice	56/13	87/17	143/16	
Working hours per week				
More than 70 h	24/6	58/12	82/9	< 0,001
60 h - less than 70 h	61/15	129/26	190/21	
50 h - less than 60 h	132/32	164/33	296/32	
40 h - less than 50 h	124/30	119/24	243/26	
30 h - less than 40 h	49/12	25/5	74/8	
Less than 30 h	27/7	8/2	35/4	
Stresses and strains				
Stress/pressure at work and in the private environment	157/38	173/34	330/36	0.590
Stress/pressure at work or in the private environment	210/50	266/53	476/52	
None	50/12	64/13	114/12	

[a] without orthopaedic and trauma surgery

Table 2 Health, risks, consumption of addictive substances in surgical and non-surgical specialties (absolute numbers/frequency in % or means [standard deviations])

Examined variables	Surgical speciality[a] (n = 241)	Non-surgical speciality[a] (n = 679)	All (n = 920)	P-Value
Health condition (subjective)				
Satisfactory/good/very good	217/90	610/90	827/90	1.000
Very poor/poor/less healthy	24/10	69/10	93/10	
Actively taking health risks				
Sometimes/often	107/44	175/26	282/31	< 0,001
Rarely/never	134/56	504/74	638/69	
Preventive check-ups				
Often	41/17	181/27	222/24	0.003
Rarely	200/83	498/73	698/76	
BMI				
	24,5 (3,8)	24,1 (3,5)	24,2 (3,6)	0.160
BMI - categories				
Short/normal weight (BMI < 25)	159/66	444/65	603/66	0.059
Overweight (BMI 25 bis < 30)	55/23	188/28	243/26	
Obesity (BMI ≥ 30)	27/11	47/7	74/8	
Nicotine[b]				
Moderate to high dependence	15/6	29/4	44/5	0.145
Low dependence	27/11	55/8	82/9	
Non-smoker/other[c]	199/83	595/88	794/86	
Alcohol[d]				
Hazardous alcohol consumption	70/29	142/21	212/23	0.013
Harmless/no alcohol consumption	171/71	537/79	708/77	
"How often do you drink alcohol in general?" (Scores)				
4 times or more often per week (4)	38/16	99/15	137/15	
2–3 times per week (3)	81/34	196/29	277/30	
2–4 times per month (2)	80/33	210/31	290/32	
Monthly or less (1)	26/11	111/16	216/24	
Never (0)	16/7	63/9		
"How many units[e] of alcohol do you drink on a typical day when you are drinking?" (Scores)				
10 or more (4)	1/0	1/0	2/0	
7–9 (3)	6/3	9/1	15/2	
5–6 (2)	11/5	20/3	31/3	
3–4 (1)	59/25	113/17	172/19	
1–2 (0)	148/61	473/70	621/68	
I don't drink alcohol at all. (0)	16/7	63/9	79/9	
"How often have you had 6 or more units of alcohol on one day in the last year?" (Scores)				
Daily or almost daily (4)	3/1	1/0	4/0	
Once a week (3)	12/5	21/3	33/4	
Once a month (2)	35/15	64/9	99/11	
Less than monthly (1)	93/39	200/30	293/32	
Never (0)	98/41	393/58	491/53	

[a]Surgical speciality: surgery, gynaecology, urology, ENT, ophthalmology; non-surgical speciality: general practice, anaesthesiology, occupational medicine, dermatology, Internal medicine, laboratory medicine, microbiology, neurology, nuclear medicine, pathology, paediatrics, physical and rehabilitative medicine, psychiatry, psychosomatics, child and adolescent psychiatry, radiology, radiation therapy, geriatrics, human genetics, palliative care, pharmacology, environment medicine
[b]HSI = Heaviness of Smoking Index (≥2 scores: moderate to high dependence)
[c]Other: pipe, cigar, electro cigarette
[d]AUDIT-C test: (≥5 scores: hazardous alcohol consumption)
[e]One unit equals: 350 ml beer / 150 ml wine/champagne / 40 ml spirits

Table 3 Hazardous alcohol consumption: potential influencing factors (absolute numbers/frequency in %)

Potential influencing factors	Harmless/no alcohol consumption (n = 708)	Hazardous alcohol consumption (n = 212)	All n = 920	P-Value
Age				
≤ 35a	251/74	89/26	340	0.089
> 35a	457/79	123/21	580	
Gender				
Female	365/88	52/13	417	< 0,001
Male	343/68	160/32	503	
Maritial status				
Unmarried	215/72	82/28	297	0.075
Married	464/79	122/21	586	
Divorced/widowed	29/78	8/22	37	
Children (living in the household)				
Yes	340/81	82/19	422	0.018
No	368/74	130/26	498	
Position/educational level				
Resident	250/74	88/26	338	0.170
Specialist	199/81	48/19	247	
Physician in a leading position	259/77	76/23	335	
Establishment				
University hospital	284/76	92/26	376	0.657
For-profit/public/non-profit hospital	314/78	87/22	401	
Physician in private practice	110/77	33/23	143	
Working hours per week				
50 h or more	418/74	150/26	568	0.002
Less than 50 h	290/83	62/18	352	

position and the type of institution did not reveal any significant differences.

Consultation behaviour
Doctors who were prone to hazardous alcohol consumption also differed in their counselling pattern (Fig. 1): Regardless of field of study, they rarely or even never advised their patients to abstain from narcotic drugs (surgical: 56%, non-surgical: 32%), compared to doctors without hazardous alcohol consumption.

CAGE questionnaire
The CAGE questionnaire was voluntary (Fig. 2). Nevertheless, just over 50% of all participants answered the questions. Since two or more positive answers indicate a positive test, 115 of the responding physicians (12.5% of the total, n = 920) would be recommended a further consultation on their alcohol consumption.

Figure 3 indicates a positive correlation of the results of the two tests (AUDIT-C; CAGE questionnaire) to evaluate hazardous alcohol consumption. 75% of the

physicians, who gave two positive answers, scored 4 or more points in the AUDIT-C test - likewise in the group of physicians who gave three positive answers in the CAGE questionnaire.

Self-assessment
Four people with a positive AUDIT-C test described their alcohol use as a dependency and another 44 as abusive (Fig. 4).

Regression analysis
To form multivariate logistic regression models, all survey participants were divided into surgical and non-surgical disciplines with regard to their specialization (classification see Table 2). The significant differences in the discipline from Table 2 ("dangerous alcohol consumption", "risky behaviour", "prevention investigations") were further examined with the help of logistic regression. It was adjusted to "age", "gender", "children in the household", "working time", "subject area", "position", "institution", "burdens". These were converted into dichotomous variables. Tables 4, 5 and 6 show only the relevant estimators.

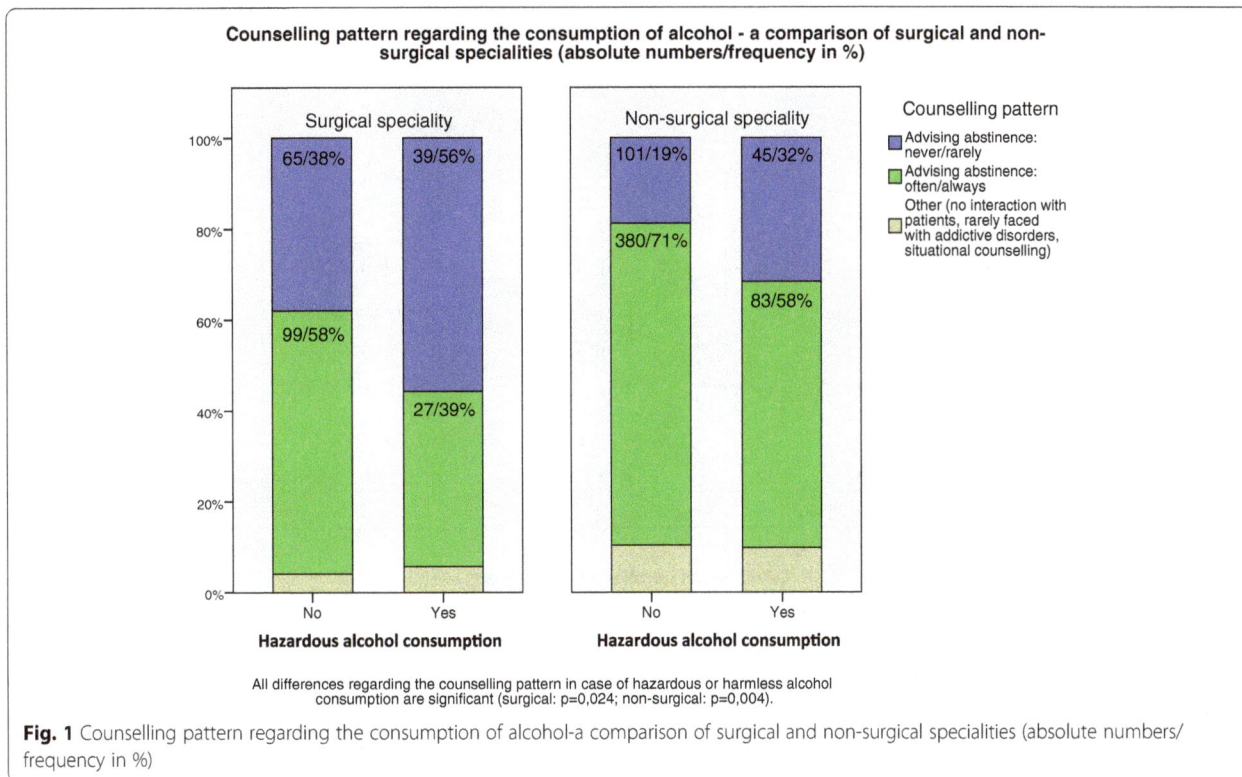

Fig. 1 Counselling pattern regarding the consumption of alcohol-a comparison of surgical and non-surgical specialities (absolute numbers/frequency in %)

In the overall collective, female gender was a significant protective factor against hazardous alcohol consumption (OR = 0.27) (Table 4). However, childless female doctors represented a risk group that was twice as likely to drink alcohol as their female colleagues (OR = 2.16). Female residents even showed three times higher odds compared to their female colleagues in senior positions (OR = 3.10), but there was a large confidence interval of 1.02–9.40, indicating a too small collective. In the case of male

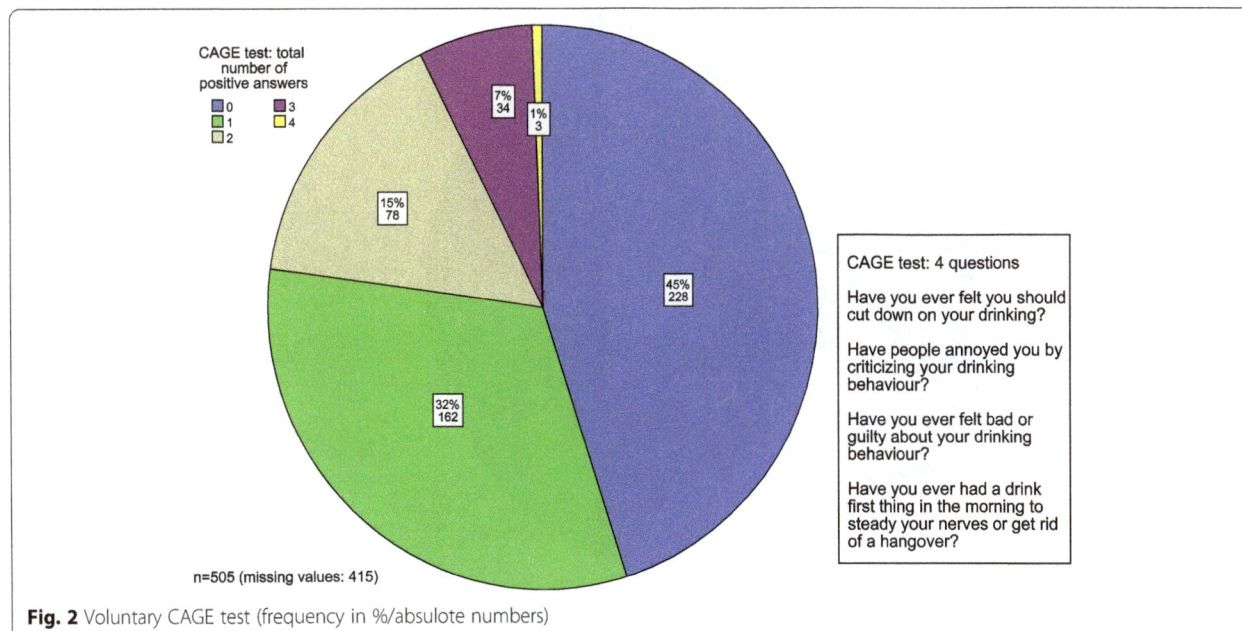

Fig. 2 Voluntary CAGE test (frequency in %/absulote numbers)

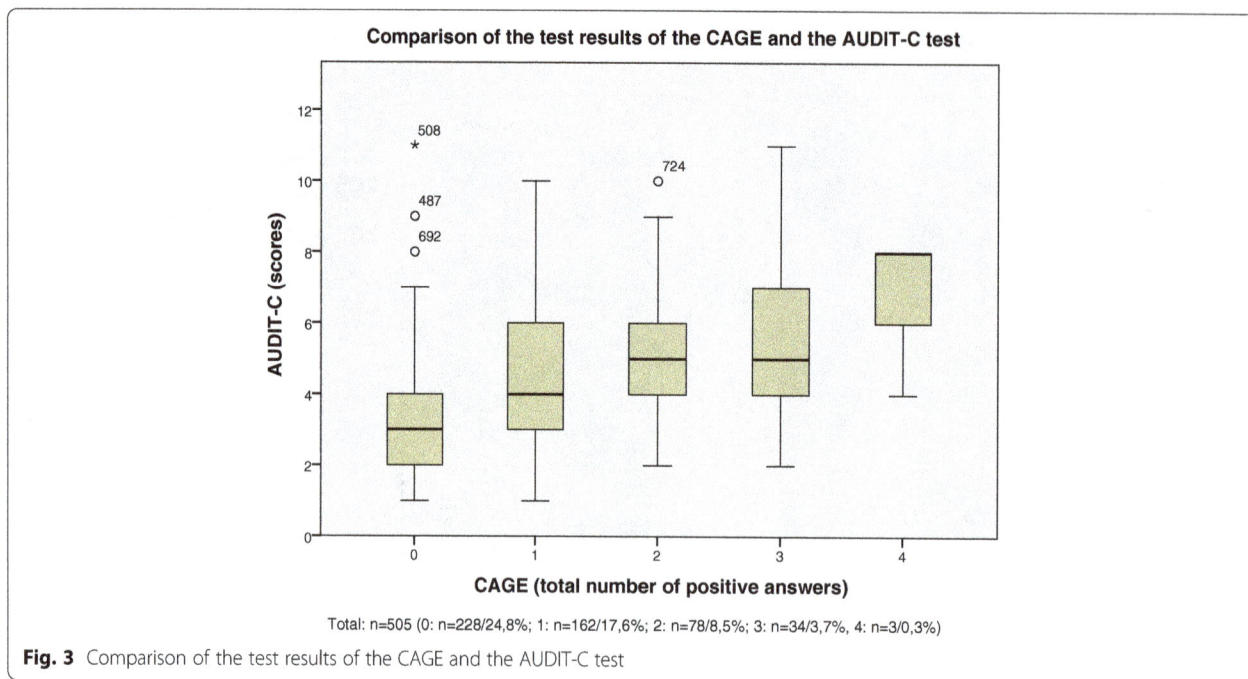

Fig. 3 Comparison of the test results of the CAGE and the AUDIT-C test

physicians, childless physicians had a significantly increased risk of hazardous alcohol consumption (OR = 1.62).

Table 5 shows that surgeons were twice as likely to behave riskily as their non-surgical counterparts (OR = 2.09 for "female doctors" and 2.00 for "doctors"). Childlessness was associated with risky behaviours among male physicians (OR = 1.61). Similarly, women were significantly less

likely to behave riskily than men (OR = 0.46) and physicians who work more than 50 h a week were significantly more likely than their less-active counterparts (OR = 1.56).

Table 6 shows that female doctors attended a significantly higher number of check-ups than male doctors (OR = 0.34). Surgical specialists were less likely to take precautionary measures than their non-surgical counterparts (OR = 1.57). Being a surgeon, especially in

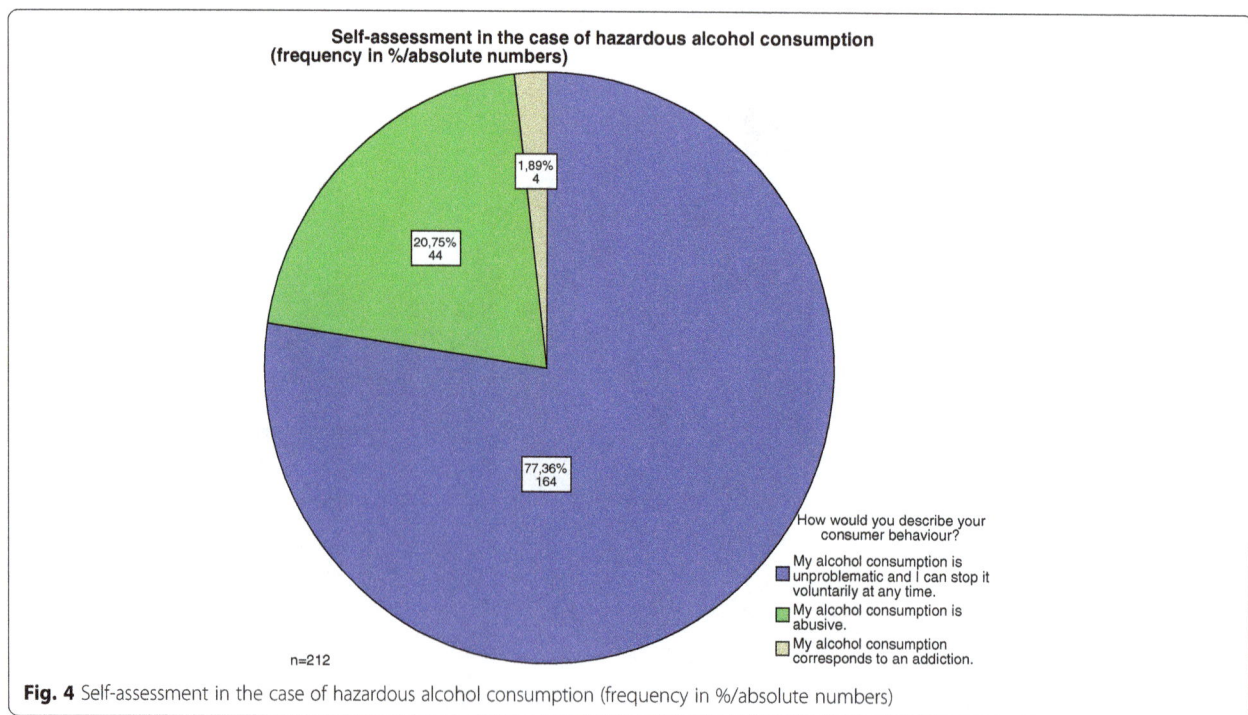

Fig. 4 Self-assessment in the case of hazardous alcohol consumption (frequency in %/absolute numbers)

Table 4 Multivariate logistic regression models[a]: hazardous alcohol consumption

Variables	Odds ratio	95% confidence interval	P-value
Hazardous alcohol consumption (AUDIT C test ≥5 points) - all physicians (n = 920)			
Female gender	0.27	0,19–0,39	< 0,001
No children in the household	1.67	1,17–2,37	0.004
Female physicians (n = 417)			
No children in the household	2.16	1,01–4,62	0.047
Surgical speciality	2.00	0,97–4,12	0.062
Residents[b]	3.10	1,02–9,40	0.046
Specialists[b]	2.61	0,92–7,43	0.071
Male physicians (n = 503)			
No children in the household	1.62	1,08 - 2,43	0.019
Surgical speciality	1.27	0,83 - 1,93	0.270
Residents[b]	1.19	0,62 - 2,27	0.605
Specialists[b]	0.66	0,38 - 1,15	0.141

[a]Depending on examined exposure adjusted to: Gender, age, children in the household, medical specialty, position/level of education, establishment, stresses and strains, working hours per week
[b]Compared to physicians in a leading position

males, was clearly associated with the outcome "rare use of check-ups" (OR = 2.15).

Discussion

Sample and approach

In order to lose as few participants as possible and to maintain anonymity in the context of the topic, it was decided not to collect confirmations of the internal forwarding by the hospital management and to calculate a response rate from this. In particular, international contact attempts (Great Britain and the USA) proved to be difficult, as there were considerable concerns regarding the confidentiality of data or traceability.

More younger physicians took part in the survey, as they may be more Internet affine than their older colleagues [37]. Furthermore, it is also to be assumed that very sick or stressed doctors do not participate in such a survey. All the more surprising is the high number of senior physicians, as they are exposed to a slightly higher number of weekly working hours than medical residents [38].

Literature suggests that distortions due to the effect of social desirability or false responses play a less relevant role in online surveys, the reason for this being that the Internet provides respondents with an anonymous environment [39, 40]. However, it can be assumed that especially physicians with intentionally risky substance use or

Table 5 multivariate logistic regression models[a]: risky behaviour

Variables	Odds ratio	95% confidence interval	P-value
Risky behaviour - all physicians (n = 920)			
Female gender	0.46	0,34–0,63	< 0,001
Working hours per week (> 50 h)	1.56	1,12–2,18	0.009
No children in the household	1.45	1,05–2,00	0.023
Surgical speciality	2.03	1,47–2,81	< 0,001
Female physicians (n = 417)			
Working hours per week (> 50 h)	1.69	0,99–2,88	0.055
No children in the household	1.17	0,65–2,08	0.604
Surgical speciality	2.09	1,18–3,69	0.011
Male physicians (n = 503)			
Working hours per week (> 50 h)	1.53	0,99–2,38	0.057
No children in the household	1.61	1,08–2,38	0.018
Surgical speciality	2.00	1,34–3,00	0.001

[a]Depending on examined exposure adjusted to: Gender, age, children in the household, medical specialty, position/level of education, establishment, stresses and strains, working hours per week

Table 6 Multivariate logistic regression models: preventive check-ups (rare utilization)

Variables	Odds ratio	95% confidence interval	P-value
Preventive check-ups - all physicians (n = 920)			
Female gender	0.34	0,24–0,48	< 0,001
Surgical speciality	1.57	1,05 - 2,35	0.029
Age < 35a	0.68	0,42 - 1,10	0.117
Female physicians (n = 417)			
Surgical speciality	1.22	0,71 - 2,09	0.482
Age < 35a	0.80	0,43 - 1,51	0.490
Male physicians (n = 503)			
Surgical speciality	2.15	1,13 - 4,09	0.020
Age < 35a	0.49	0,22 - 1,10	0.083

*Depending on examined exposure adjusted to: Gender, age, children in the household, medical specialty, position/level of education, establishment, stresses and strains, working hours per week

already diagnosed dependence - in particular with regard to the medical habitus - for reasons of shame, concern about confidentiality of the data and thus labour law consequences do not participate in such online surveys. It may therefore be assumed that there are a certain number of unreported cases, so that the actual prevalence of risky drug use or risk behaviour may be higher than shown in the present work.

For the AUDIT-C, a cut-off score of 5 points was used for men and women, as it could achieve a higher specificity compared with 3 points (0.42 vs. 0.83) [36]. Admittedly Rumpf et al. found a higher sensitivity for at-risk drinking throughout the AUDIT compared to the AUDIT-C, however, specificity of the latter was higher. This was crucial to avoid overestimating the problem. Moreover, it was not expedient to carry out a screening as in the clinical setting, but to minimize the number of false-positive results so as to better map and reflect the reality. Correction of the specificity results was not performed, therefore the results should be interpreted with caution - a survey among Salzburg physicians showed a corrected value of 7% as a prevalence for high-risk alcohol consumption, uncorrected reached a positive value in the AUDIT-C of 27.4% [41].

Since the CAGE questionnaire had to be completed on a voluntary basis in order not to lose participants through personal questions, only just under half of all participants could be evaluated.

As a whole the questionnaire is not validated and thus the results have to be interpreted very carefully. Partially, validated questions were used, though standardised questionnaires to examine physicians' health better lack. This study merely might provide hints on existing difficulties and constitute a first impression of the current situation in Germany.

Investigated variables

With regard to nicotine consumption, Voigt et al. found the same value for the number of non-smokers in 2009 [18]. However, with regard to smoking behaviour, they only determined the number of cigarettes smoked per day. The Heaviness of Smoking Index - a section of the Fagerström test for nicotine addiction - also makes it possible to distinguish the severity of nicotine dependence [42].

With regard to ethanol, male physicians generally seem to drink more than female doctors, but women in the present survey are significantly more influenced by professional factors such as position and discipline in their drinking behaviour. In contrast to Rosta et al. we could not identify affiliation to surgical disciplines as an independent risk factor for hazardous alcohol consumption for men, whereas for women - if there would be a higher number of surgeons - a high risk of surgical subjects could be identified with high probability - the wide confidence interval indicates a low number of female surgeons in this study (p-value 0.062, OR = 2.00, CI: 0.97–4.12) [13, 43]. This corresponds to findings for female surgeons in Norway [43].

Assistants also seem to have a high odd (p-value 0.046, OR = 3.10, CI: 1.02–9.40). This raises the question of whether women are less able to compensate for the burden of working in operational subjects than men.

Finally, we were able to confirm the lack of influence of age on hazardous alcohol consumption as described by Rosta et al. [13].

One risk group still consists of childless physicians: they are more prone to risky behaviour and hazardous alcohol consumption - this could be due to the fact that childless doctors have no obligation to be role models for anyone, have no responsibility in educational and entertainment aspects, and possibly more time for hazardous ventures.

While senior and chief physicians with children in literature have an increased risk of burnout, childlessness and long weekly working hours may predispose to more frequent risky behaviour [44]. Surgical professionals and physicians who work more than 50 h per week seem more risk-averse - a coping mechanism may be responsible.

A surgical discipline leads to less frequent use of preventive examinations in men. Men are generally less likely to seek medical check-ups and tend to be more careless about their own health [45, 46]. Surgeons may argue more than others to have to meet a particular personality profile required by the patient and supervisor: great self-esteem, high resilience, strong stamina. Illness could be interpreted as a sign of weakness and preventive examinations are therefore avoided.

In conclusion, however, risky behaviour, as well as the use of preventive screening and high-risk alcohol consumption, seems to be independent of whether or not respondents suffered from stress at the time of the survey.

For comparison no current data is available regarding the prevalence of hazardous alcohol consumption in certain occupation groups apart from physicians in Germany. Documented data on problems caused by alcohol in the professional environment can provide information on exposed occupation groups: Especially affected seem to be people who are working in the gastronomy. Also the category "delivery of other economic services" which includes temporary work is affected above average [47]. Regarding the total population the following data should be mentioned: the prevalence of alcohol-related disorders by DSM-IV in adults between 18 and 64 years in Germany in 2013 evaluated by Pabst et al. for abuse and dependency in total 6,5%, in men 9,5% and in women 3,5% [48]. A study by the Robert-Koch-Institute from 2008 till 2011 by the means of the AUDIT-C test resulted in a risky consumption of alcohol for 41,6% for the men and 25,6% for the women [49].

Conclusion

Risk groups and factors influencing health-endangering behaviour may further be investigated in future studies and standardised questionnaires for the examination of physicians'health have to be developed. The number of women in the medical profession will continue to increase and so will the need for female doctors in surgical professions [50, 51]. These require a high level of resilience and coping strategies as stress and strain levels increase. There is an urgent need to conduct further studies on the risk for female surgeons for hazardous alcohol consumption.

In Germany aid offers are readily available. Specialist clinics, such as the Oberbergkliniken, provide an anonymous environment and offer structured treatment options [52]. In cooperation with the regional medical associations, there is an intervention program based on the principle "help instead of punishment", which addresses the special circumstances of the medical profession: It guarantees anonymity, regulates practice representation and reimbursement of costs, and offers close outpatient follow-up care [4, 53].

However, the primary prevention should be extended significantly, as many doctors are not familiar with the offers of help and treatment opportunities and, among other things, do not get help for fear of labour-law consequences. To address this, one could also train chief physicians better in the handling and recognition of addiction problems. One could also teach doctors how to interact with and help potentially affected colleagues. There should already be contact persons in the immediate vicinity of the clinic. For example, with the help of an occupational medical burnout screening to identify particularly stressed physicians who have few coping strategies, risk groups could be identified at an early stage.

Key messages

- Nearly one in four physicians consumed alcohol at hazardous levels.
- Female assistants had a three times higher risk of hazardous alcohol use compared to women in senior positions.
- Surgical professionals tended towards risky health habits twice as often compared to their colleagues in non-surgical disciplines.
- There is a need to improve primary prevention.
- The aim should be the identification of the most vulnerable groups followed by early intervention.

Acknowledgements
We would like to thank the team from Unika-T as well as all participants in the survey.

Funding
This work was supported by the German Research Foundation (DFG) and the Technical University of Munich (TUM) in the framework of the Open Access Publishing Program.

Authors' contributions
The authors contributed to the research as follows: Conceptualization: F.E., R.M. and D.P. Methodology: F.E., R.M. and D.P. Software: R.M., C.M. and D.F. Validation: F.E., R.M., C.M., D.F. and D.P. Formal Analysis: F.E., R.M., C.M., D.F. and D.P. Investigation: F.E., R.M. and D.P. Resources: F.E., R.M., C.M., D.F. and D.P. Data Curation: F.E., R.M., C.M., D.F. and D.P. Writing-Original Draft Preparation: R.M., D.P. and F.E. Writing-Review & Editing: F.E., R.M., C.M., D.F. and D.P. Visualization: R.M. and F.E. Supervision: F.E. and D.P. Project Administration: F.E., R.M., C.M., D.F. and D.P. All authors read and approved the final manuscript.

Competing interests
The authors declare that they have no competing interests.

Author details
[1]Department of Trauma Surgery, Technical University of Munich, Ismaningerstrasse 22-, 81675 Munich, Germany. [2]Chair for Epidemiology at UNIKA-T, Ludwig-Maximilians University of Munich, Augsburg, Germany. [3]Klinikum rechts der Isar, Department of Clinical Toxicology, Technical University of Munich, Munich, Germany.

References

1. Rosta J. Prevalence of problem-related drinking among doctors: A review on representative samples. Ger Med Sci. 2005;3:Doc07.

2. Mayall RM. Substance abuse in anaesthetists. BJA Educ. 2016;16:236–41. https://doi.org/10.1093/bjaed/mkv054.

3. NHS doctors turning to substance abuse amid rising levels of stress and burnout. 27.06.2017. https://www.independent.co.uk/news/health/nhs-doctors-substance-abuse-stress-burnout-rising-gps-addiction-health-service-bma-clare-gerada-a7805571.html. Accessed 11 Apr 2018.

4. Bühring P. Suchtkranke Ärzte: Sehr hohe Behandlungsmotivation. Deutsches Ärzteblatt. 2017;114:A-935 / B-785 / C-767.

5. Ärzte: Kranker Job. 30.01.2016. http://www.zeit.de/campus/2016/01/aerzte-krankenhaus-gesundheit-arbeitsbedingungen-ungesund. Accessed 14 Jan 2018.

6. Frankfurter Allgemeine Zeitung GmbH. Burnout am OP-Tisch: „Als Chirurg muss man eben saufen". http://www.faz.net/aktuell/gesellschaft/gesundheit/burnout-am-op-tisch-als-chirurg-muss-man-eben-saufen-1751063.html?printPagedArticle=true#pageIndex_0. Accessed 14 Jan 2018.

7. Geuenich K. Sind Sie Burnout-gefährdet?: Ergebnisse unserer Ärztestudie. Der Hausarzt. 2009:2–4.

8. Diefenbach C, Drexler S, Schön C. Suchterkrankungen bei Ärzten: Sanktionieren und Helfen sind kein Widerspruch. Deutsches Ärzteblatt. 2013; 110:A-1028.

9. Mundle G, Gottschaldt E. Hilfsangebote für suchtkranke Ärzte - Spezifische Behandlungsmaßnahmen ermöglichen eine erfolgreiche Behandlung. Psychoneuro. 2007;33:13–8. https://doi.org/10.1055/s-2007-973731.

10. Mäulen B. Sucht unter Ärzten. In: Badura B, Ducki A, Schröder H, Klose J, Meyer M, editors. Fehlzeiten-Report 2013: Verdammt zum Erfolg - Die süchtige Arbeitsgesellschaft? Berlin: Springer; 2013. p. 143–50. https://doi.org/10.1007/978-3-642-37117-2_16.

11. Hughes PH. Prevalence of substance use among US physicians. JAMA. 1992; 267:2333. https://doi.org/10.1001/jama.1992.03480170059029.

12. Gulbrandsen P, Aasland OG. Endringer i norske legers alkoholvaner 1985-2000. Tidsskr Nor Laegeforen. 2002;122:2791–4.

13. Rosta J. Hazardous alcohol use among hospital doctors in Germany. Alcohol Alcohol. 2008;43:198–203. https://doi.org/10.1093/alcalc/agm180.

14. Unrath M, Zeeb H, Letzel S, Claus M, Escobar Pinzón LC. Identification of possible risk factors for alcohol use disorders among general practitioners in Rhineland-Palatinate, Germany. Swiss Med Wkly. 2012;142:w13664. https://doi.org/10.4414/smw.2012.13664.

15. Braun M, Freudenmann R, Schönfeldt-Lecuona C, Beschoner P. Burnout, Depression und Substanzgebrauch bei Ärzten - Ein Überblick zur derzeitigen Datenlage in Deutschland. psychoneuro. 2007;33:19–22. https://doi.org/10.1055/s-2007-973732.

16. Unrath M. Psychische Gesundheit von Ärzten in Deutschland: Prävalenz psychischer Erkrankungen und Risikofaktoren. Hessisches Ärzteblatt. 2013:86–90.

17. Badura B, Ducki A, Schröder H, Klose J, Meyer M, editors. Fehlzeiten-Report 2013: Verdammt zum Erfolg - Die süchtige Arbeitsgesellschaft? Berlin: Springer; 2013.

18. Voigt K, Twork S, Mittag D, Göbel A, Voigt R, Klewer J, et al. Consumption of alcohol, cigarettes and illegal substances among physicians and medical students in Brandenburg and Saxony (Germany). BMC Health Serv Res. 2009; 9:219. https://doi.org/10.1186/1472-6963-9-219.

19. World Health Organization. WHO | Lexicon of alcohol and drug terms published by the World Health Organization. http://www.who.int/substance_abuse/terminology/who_lexicon/en/. Accessed 27 Jun 2018.

20. Reid MC, Fiellin DA, O'Connor PG. Hazardous and harmful alcohol consumption in primary care. Arch Intern Med. 1999;159:1681. https://doi.org/10.1001/archinte.159.15.1681.

21. Piccinelli M, Tessari E, Bortolomasi M, Piasere O, Semenzin M, Garzotto N, Tansella M. Efficacy of the alcohol use disorders identification test as a screening tool for hazardous alcohol intake and related disorders in primary care: a validity study. BMJ. 1997;314:420–4.

22. Wood AM, Kaptoge S, Butterworth AS, Willeit P, Warnakula S, Bolton T, et al. Risk thresholds for alcohol consumption: combined analysis of individual-participant data for 599 912 current drinkers in 83 prospective studies. Lancet. 2018;391:1513–23. https://doi.org/10.1016/S0140-6736(18)30134-X.

23. Übersicht der Universitätsklinika | Die Deutschen Universitätsklinika. https://www.uniklinika.de/die-deutschen-universitaetsklinika/uebersicht-der-universitaetsklinika/. Accessed 25 Feb 2018.

24. SurveyMonkey: The World's Most Popular Free Online Survey Tool. https://www.surveymonkey.com/. Accessed 11 Apr 2018.

25. WHO: Global Database on Body Mass Index. http://apps.who.int/bmi/index.jsp?introPage=intro_3.html. Accessed 11 Apr 2018.

26. Bush K. The AUDIT alcohol consumption questions (AUDIT-C)<subtitle>an effective brief screening test for problem drinking</subtitle>. Arch Intern Med. 1998;158:1789. https://doi.org/10.1001/archinte.158.16.1789.

27. Jacob R, Heinz A, Décieux JP. Umfrage: Einführung in die Methoden der Umfrageforschung. 3rd ed. München: Oldenbourg; 2013.

28. John U, Meyer C, Schumann A, Hapke U, Rumpf H-J, Adam C, et al. A short form of the Fagerström test for nicotine dependence and the heaviness of smoking index in two adult population samples. Addict Behav. 2004;29:1207–12. https://doi.org/10.1016/j.addbeh.2004.03.019.

29. Raab-Steiner E, Benesch M. Der Fragebogen: Von der Forschungsidee zur SPSS-Auswertung. 4th ed. Wien: Facultas; 2015.

30. Mayfield D, McLeod G, Hall P. The CAGE questionnaire: validation of a new alcoholism screening instrument. Am J Psychiatry. 1974;131:1121–3. https://doi.org/10.1176/ajp.131.10.1121.

31. Eveleth PB, Andres R, Chumlea WC, Eiben O, Ge K, Harris T, et al. Uses and interpretation of anthropometry in the elderly for the assessment of physical status. Report to the nutrition unit of the World Health Organization: the expert subcommittee on the use and interpretation of anthropometry in the elderly. J Nutr Health Aging. 1998;2:5–17.

32. Babor TF, Higgins-Biddle JC, Saunders JB, Monteiro MG, World Health Organisation (WHO). AUDIT: the alcohol use disorders identification test: guidelines for use in primary health care. 2nd ed. Geneva: World Health Organisation; 2001.

33. Heatherton TF, Kozlowski LT, Frecker RC, Fagerström KO. The Fagerström test for nicotine dependence: a revision of the Fagerström tolerance questionnaire. Br J Addict. 1991;86:1119–27.

34. Heatherton TF, Kozlowski LT, Frecker RC, Rickert W, Robinson J. Measuring the heaviness of smoking: using self-reported time to the first cigarette of the day and number of cigarettes smoked per day. Br J Addict. 1989;84:791–9.

35. de Meneses-Gaya C, Zuardi AW, Loureiro SR, Crippa JAS. Alcohol use disorders identification test (AUDIT): an updated systematic review of psychometric properties. Psychol Neurosci. 2009;2:83–97. https://doi.org/10.3922/j.psns.2009.1.12.

36. Rumpf H-J, Hapke U, Meyer C, John U. Screening for alcohol use disorders and at-risk drinking in the general population: psychometric performance of three questionnaires. Alcohol Alcohol. 2002;37:261–8.

37. von Baur N, Florian MJ. Stichprobenprobleme bei Online-Umfragen. In: Jackob N, Schoen H, Zerback T, editors. Sozialforschung im Internet: Methodologie und Praxis der Online-Befragung. 1st ed. Wiesbaden: VS Verlag für Sozialwissenschaften / GWV Fachverlag GmbH Wiesbaden; 2009. p. 109–28. https://doi.org/10.1007/978-3-531-91791-7_7.

38. Rosta J. Hospital Doctors´ Working Hours in Germany: Preliminary Data from a National Survey in Autumn 2006. Deutsches Ärzteblatt. 2007;104:A-2417.

39. Dodou D, de Winter JCF. Social desirability is the same in offline, online, and paper surveys: a meta-analysis. Comput Hum Behav. 2014;36:487–95. https://doi.org/10.1016/j.chb.2014.04.005.

40. Crutzen R, Göritz AS. Social desirability and self-reported health risk behaviors in web-based research: three longitudinal studies. BMC Public Health. 2010;10:720. https://doi.org/10.1186/1471-2458-10-720.

41. Wurst FM, Rumpf H-J, Skipper GE, Allen JP, Kunz I, Beschoner P, Thon N. Estimating the prevalence of drinking problems among physicians. Gen Hosp Psychiatry. 2013;35:561–4. https://doi.org/10.1016/j.genhosppsych.2013.04.018 .

42. Schnoll RA, Goren A, Annunziata K, Suaya JA. The prevalence, predictors and associated health outcomes of high nicotine dependence using three measures among US smokers. Addiction. 2013;108:1989–2000. https://doi.org/10.1111/add.12285.

43. Rosta J, Aasland OG. Female surgeons' alcohol use: a study of a national sample of norwegian doctors. Alcohol Alcohol. 2005;40:436–40. https://doi.org/10.1093/alcalc/agh186.

44. Wegner R, Kostova P. Belastung und Beanspruchung von Krankenhausärzten zwischen 1975 und 2007. Arbeitsbedingungen und Befinden von Ärztinnen und Ärzten Befunde und Interventionen. 2010:243–51.

45. Starker A, Saß A-C. Inanspruchnahme von Krebsfrüherkennungsuntersuchungen: Ergebnisse der Studie zur Gesundheit Erwachsener in Deutschland (DEGS1). Bundesgesundheitsblatt Gesundheitsforschung Gesundheitsschutz. 2013;56: 858–67. https://doi.org/10.1007/s00103-012-1655-4.

46. Robert Koch-Institut. Gesundheitliche Lage der Männer in Deutschland | Beiträge zur Gesundheitsberichterstattung des Bundes.

47. Deutsche Hauptstelle für Suchtfragen e.V., DHS, www.dhs.de. Berufsgruppen mit erhöhtem Risiko. http://www.sucht-am-arbeitsplatz.de/themen/ vorbeugung/zahlen-daten-fakten/berufsgruppen-mit-erhoehtem-risiko/. Accessed 27 Jun 2018.

48. Pabst A, Kraus L, EGd M, Piontek D. Substanzkonsum und substanzbezogene Störungen in Deutschland im Jahr 2012. SUCHT. 2013;59: 321–31. https://doi.org/10.1024/0939-5911.a000275.

49. Hapke U, V der Lippe E, Gaertner B. Riskanter Alkoholkonsum und Rauschtrinken unter Berücksichtigung von Verletzungen und der Inanspruchnahme alkoholspezifischer medizinischer Beratung: Ergebnisse der Studie zur Gesundheit Erwachsener in Deutschland (DEGS1). Bundesgesundheitsblatt Gesundheitsforschung Gesundheitsschutz. 2013;56: 809–13. https://doi.org/10.1007/s00103-013-1699-0.

50. Jefferson L, Bloor K, Maynard A. Women in medicine: historical perspectives and recent trends. Br Med Bull. 2015;114:5–15. https://doi. org/10.1093/bmb/ldv007.

51. Healthcare personnel statistics - physicians - Statistics Explained. http://ec. europa.eu/eurostat/statistics-explained/index.php/Healthcare_personnel_ statistics_-_physicians. Accessed 11 Apr 2018.

52. Oberbergklinik. 05.03.2018. https://www.oberbergkliniken.de/. Accessed 17 Mar 2018.

53. Arzt und Sucht. http://www.blaek.de/arzt_und_sucht/. Accessed 17 Mar 2018.

25

Leadership position and physician visits –results of a nationally representative longitudinal study in Germany

Katrin Christiane Reber, Hans-Helmut König and André Hajek[*] (iD)

Abstract

Background: So far, studies within the occupational field have largely concentrated on working conditions and job stressors and staff members' or subordinate health. Only a few have focused on managers in this context, but studies are missing that explicitly look at the relation between leadership position and health care use (HCU). Thus, the purpose of this study was to examine the potential effects of a change in leadership position on HCU in women and men longitudinally.

Methods: Data were drawn from a nationally representative longitudinal study in Germany (German Socio-Economic Panel, GSOEP). Data from 2009 and 2013 were used. Leadership position was divided into (i) top management, (ii) middle management, (iii) lower management, and (iv) a highly qualified specialist position. The number of physician visits in the preceding 3 months were used to quantify HCU (n = 2140 observations in regression analysis; 69% male).

Results: Adjusting for various potential confounders (e.g., age, self-rated health, chronic conditions, and personality factors), Poisson FE regression analysis revealed that changes from a highly qualified specialist position to the top management were associated with a *decrease* in the number of physician visits in men ($\beta = .47$, $p < .05$), but not in women. Gender differences (gender x leadership position) were significant.

Conclusions: Findings of this study emphasize the impact of leadership positions on the number of physician visits in men. Further study is required to elucidate the underlying mechanisms.

Keywords: Leadership position, Health care utilization, Longitudinal studies, Germany

Background

There is unequivocal evidence that socioeconomic position, commonly measured by occupational class, education or income, is a leading determinant of health. Lower socioeconomic positions have generally been linked to unhealthier behaviors compared to higher positions [1]. Several studies have shown that health and health–related outcomes vary considerably by occupation [2, 3]. Occupational rank/position and employment conditions were identified as important factors in creating these health differentials [4]. Occupational position has been reported to be associated with both physical and psychological health and the association between job status and health appeared to be quite robust across different countries and settings and after adjusting for other socioeconomic position measures like education or income (though these measures will be interrelated [5, 6]) [7]. There is further evidence that the magnitude of the association between occupational position and health differs between men and women. In women, the relationship between occupational position and self-perceived health was less pronounced than in men [8]. These gender differences in the prevalence of unfavorable physical and mental health outcomes have been at least partly attributed to gender discrimination in the labor market [9–11].

In addition to inequalities in health outcomes between different socioeconomic groups as well as between men and women, numerous studies have shown that socioeconomic position affects use of health care services. Findings from Germany and other European countries

* Correspondence: a.hajek@uke.de
Department of Health Economics and Health Services Research, University Medical Center Hamburg-Eppendorf, Hamburg Center for Health Economics, Hamburg, Germany

indicated a general tendency toward higher health services use among lower socioeconomic groups [12–14]. Furthermore, studies generally assumed a directionality from work to health or use of health care services, and not vice versa [15, 16].

Previous research has also suggested that changes in occupational position may affect an individual's health status. For example, Halleröd and Gustafsson [17] found a link between changes in occupational prestige and changes in morbidity such that a more prestigious career development resulted in more favorable health outcomes. Both short- and long-term negative health consequences of experienced or anticipated job change have also been confirmed by other studies [18, 19]. For example, poorer self-rated health and an increased risk of minor psychiatric disorders have been reported by white collar civil service employees when compared to those not affected by job change [18, 19]. However, these effects were found to be different for men and women and to depend on occupational grade. In particular, men and women in the highest employment grade as well as men in the middle grade reported significantly more psychiatric disorders and poorer health [18]. Though contrary to previous suggestions that negative health effects are more common among persons of lower income positions [20], also another study found health effects and the risk of sick leave to be greater amongst higher income positions [21]. Poorer health status among higher grade employees / managers could thus lead to increased health care use (HCU). However, since higher positions generally come along with greater responsibilities and workload, less time or other factors e.g., fear of loss of power (an increase in the power of subordinates might reduce their own [22]) may prevent them from using health care services. As regards gender differences in the context of change in leadership position and HCU knowledge is limited. Inconclusive results have been found when investigating gender-specific health effects in times of organizational change [18, 23]. Yet, it has been noted that gender bias may be aggravated during phases of organizational and job change and this bias is possibly more obvious at positions that are higher in hierarchy [24] - not only in terms of hiring bias but also in terms of job promotion or career progression as well as in terms of destabilization of professional careers in times of organizational change [25].

While the relation between socio-economic position and HCU has received quite some attention, there is little research investigating the association between occupational position and HCU when employed in similar circumstances, experiencing a similar work or job "role", i.e., leadership position.

So far, studies within the occupational field have largely concentrated on working conditions and job stressors and staff members' or subordinate health [26]. Only a few have focused on managers in this context [27, 28] but studies are missing that explicitly look at the relation between leadership position and HCU. However, the health of an organization's leader /manager is of crucial importance for the leader, for the organization and for its staff, because managers' poor health can negatively affect both team and an organization's performance [28, 29]. Consequently, based on a large nationally representative sample, the purpose of this study was to examine whether changes in leadership position (e.g., from middle management to the top management) are associated with changes in HCU (i.e., physician visits) among women and men using a longitudinal approach.

We hypothesize that a change to a higher leadership position is accompanied by more responsibilities, higher workload, but also more power and prestige. On the one hand, we hypothesize that more responsibilities and higher workload result in higher stress or poorer health status and thus increase physician visits. On the other hand, we hypothesize that prestigious positions are accompanied by less time for physician visits. In addition, individuals in these leadership positions might have better coping strategies to handle potential health problems or job stress [30].

There are well-known gender differences in socioeconomic position, particularly in occupational position and due to extensive evidence that gender matters in HCU – as reported in a recent systematic review [31]. For example, based on American or Australian samples it has been shown that women were more likely to consult a physician [32, 33]. Consequently, we conducted analyses separately for women and men. It was further tested whether gender moderates the impact of the leadership position on the number of physician visits.

Methods

Sample

Data were drawn from the German Socio-Economic Panel (GSOEP), located at the German Institute for Economic Research (DIW Berlin), beginning in 1984. It is a nationally representative survey of the German population. Above 20,000 individuals (about 11,000 households) were interviewed on an annual basis. A very broad range of topics is covered in the GSOEP such as occupational status, subjective well-being, health or attitudes. It has been shown that survey attrition is low and re-interview response rates are very high in the GSOEP [34, 35]. For further details concerning the GSOEP (e.g., sample composition or subsamples), please see Wagner et al. [36]. In the present study, data from two waves (2009 and 2013) were used for reasons of data availability. Thus, mid-term associations between changes in leadership positions and HCU were analyzed. In other words: We restricted our sample to individuals who changed their leadership position from 2009 and 2013.

Outcome measure: Physician visits

The self-reported number of physician visits in the preceding 3 months was used to measure the number of outpatient physician visits.

Independent variables

Based on the behavioral model developed by Andersen et al. [37], explanatory variables were selected. The Andersen model distinguishes between predisposing characteristics (e.g., sex and age), enabling resources (e.g., income) and need factors (e.g., self-rated health or chronic illnesses).

For *predisposing characteristics*, age, gender family status, and the kinds of leadership position were included.

The self-reported kinds of leadership position were divided into

- Top management (for example, executive board, business director, division manager)
- Middle management (for example, department head, regional director)
- Lower management (for example, group supervisor, section head, management of a small branch office / small business)
- Highly qualified specialist position (for example, project head)

We note that we only analyzed individuals who fell in one of the above categories. Changes in the leadership position from 2009 to 2013 were analyzed.

Family status was dichotomized into those married or living together with a partner and those not living with a partner, i.e. divorced, widowed or single. As regards *need factors*, self-rated health (1 = "bad" and 5 = "very good") and a count score of chronic conditions was used (diabetes, asthma, cardiac disease, cancer, heart attack, migraine, high blood pressure and dementia). The self-rated health single item measure has widely been used in previous studies [38].

There are some personality traits which literature has well documented to be related to leadership position (e.g. extraversion). Moreover, evidence exists showing that personality traits affect physical and mental health, and play a role in pursuing (un)healthy behaviors and in achieving (un)favorable health outcomes [39, 40]. Studies have further shown that personality (e.g., neuroticism) is important in HCU [41–43]. Personality is commonly divided into five big traits [44]. These big traits are agreeableness, conscientiousness, extraversion, neuroticism and openness to experience. Agreeableness refers to the tendency to get along well with others. Conscientiousness

refers to the tendency to be well organized. Extraversion refers to the tendency to be talkative or sociable. Neuroticism refers to the tendency to be insecure or anxious. Openness to experience refers to the tendency to take risks or to be imaginative. In the GSOEP, the short version of the Big Five Inventory (BFI-S) was used. Three items per dimension were used. Each item was rated on a seven-point Likert scale ranging from 1 = "does not apply to me at all" to 7 = "applies to me perfectly". It has been demonstrated that the BFI-S has satisfactory psychometric properties [45]. While those traits have predominantly been considered to remain stable over time, more recent findings point to the dynamic effects of personality change and their implications for the personality-health link [39, 46]. Therefore, these factors were included in regression analysis as time-varying variables.

Statistical analysis

First, descriptive statistics for the analytical sample were computed. Second, panel regression models were used to assess the longitudinal association between change in leadership positions and HCU, adjusting for potential confounders (age, marital status, self-rated health, number of chronic diseases, and personality traits).

In large survey studies, unobserved heterogeneity (time-constant unobserved factors such as genetic disposition) is a key problem. For example, it is almost impossible to control for differences between individuals in genetic factors in these studies [47]. This is a critical problem when these unobserved factors are systematically correlated with the explanatory variables. The reason is that most of the widely used panel regression models such as random effects regressions produce inconsistent estimates when this correlation is present. Or, to put it another way: These panel regression models rest on the assumption of no correlation between the explanatory variables and the time-constant unobserved factors [48]. In contrast to these panel regression models, FE regression produce consistent estimates even if this strong assumption is violated. Thus, FE regressions were used in the present study. This choice was supported by a Hausman-test [49] – the Hausman test statistic was statistically significant, with $p < .001$. This test indicated that the effects are associated with the explanatory variables and thus the RE model cannot be estimated consistently.

FE regressions ("Within-estimator") only exploit transitions within individuals over time. Hence, the results can be interpreted as "Average Treatment Effect on the Treated" (ATET) [47]. In other words: Our findings are not generalizable to the whole population.

For example, it is worth emphasizing that changes from a "highly qualified specialist position" to "lower management" within an individual over time were examined in our study. Factors constant within individuals over time such as gender can only be included as moderating variables (e.g., gender x leadership position).

Due to power issues in our FE regression analysis changes in both directions were covered, i.e., changes from lower level leadership positions to higher level leadership positions as well as changes from higher level leadership positions to lower level leadership positions.

In the current study, cluster robust standard errors were computed [50]. A P value less than 0.05 was deemed statistically significant. Analyses were conducted using Stata 15.0 (Stata Corp., College Station, Texas).

In sensitivity analysis, satisfaction with free time, family life, and job (if employed) (each variables ranges from 0 = 'totally unhappy' to 10 = 'totally happy') were added to the main model. In further sensitivity analysis, concerns about the job security (if employed) (1 = very concerned; 2 = somewhat concerned; 3 = not concerned at all) and the difficulty of finding an appropriate position ("If you were currently looking for a new job: Is it or would it be easy, difficult, or almost impossible to find an appropriate position?"; 1 = easy; 2 = difficult; 3 = "almost impossible") were added to the main model. In other sensitivity analyses, (log) equivalence income and working hours per week were added to our main model. In another robustness

check, negative binomial fixed effects (FE) regressions were used.

Results
Sample characteristics
Pooled sample characteristics for individuals included in FE regression analysis with physician visits in the past 3 months as outcome variable are depicted in Table 1 (stratified by gender, men: 1476 observations; women: 664 observations).

About two-thirds were male. The average age for men was 48.3 years, and for women, the average age was 46.2 years. While in men approximately one half were in the middle or top management, less than 40% held these positions in women. In men, the average number of physician visits in the past 3 months equaled 2.1, the average number was 2.5 in women. Further details are provided in Table 1.

It is worth noting that the average number of doctor visits (GP and specialist visits) is about 8.5 among the adult population in Germany per year [51].

Regression analysis
Results of Poisson FE regressions are depicted in Table 2. In Table 2, Poisson coefficients with cluster-robust standard errors were reported. In total, 390 intraindividual

Table 1 Sample characteristics for individuals included in fixed effects regressions (Wave 2009 and 2013, pooled; 2140 observations)

	Men (1476 observations)		Women (664 observations)	
	N/Mean	%/SD	N/Mean	%/SD
Age (in years)	48.3	9.4	46.2	9.3
Married, living together with spouse	372	25.2%	288	43.4%
Self-rated health (from 1 = "very good" to 5 = "bad")	2.5	0.8	2.5	0.8
Number of chronic diseases	0.4	0.7	0.5	0.7
Number of chronic diseases: 0	944	64.0%	422	63.5%
Number of chronic diseases: 1	420	28.4%	182	27.4%
Number of chronic diseases: 2	94	6.4%	43	6.5%
Number of chronic diseases: 3	16	1.1%	16	2.4%
Number of chronic diseases: > 3	2	0.1%	1	0.2%
- Agreeableness	15.4	2.9	16.0	2.9
- Conscientiousness	17.6	2.5	18.2	2.4
- Extraversion	14.5	3.3	15.4	3.3
- Openness to experience	13.6	3.3	14.2	3.5
- Neuroticism	10.1	3.4	11.3	3.5
Physician visits in the preceding 3 months	2.1	3.2	2.5	3.0
Leadership position				
Top management	319	21.6%	91	13.7%
Middle management	416	28.2%	161	24.3%
Lower management	477	32.3%	283	42.6%
Highly qualified specialist position	264	17.9%	129	19.4%

Table 2 Determinants of physician visits in the past three months. Results of FE poisson regressions

Independent variables	(1)	(2)	(3)	(4)
	Doctor visits – Total sample	Doctor visits - Men	Doctor visits - Women	Doctor visits – with interaction
Age (in years)	−0.01	− 0.00	− 0.04*	− 0.02
	(0.01)	(0.01)	(0.02)	(0.01)
Other marital statuses (Ref.: Married, living together with spouse)	−0.15	− 0.02	− 0.40*	− 0.16
	(0.14)	(0.19)	(0.16)	(0.14)
Self-rated health (from 'very good' to 'bad')	0.52***	0.55***	0.43***	0.51***
	(0.05)	(0.07)	(0.08)	(0.05)
Number of chronic diseases	0.16**	0.14+	0.22+	0.17**
	(0.06)	(0.07)	(0.12)	(0.06)
Neuroticism (higher values indicate higher neuroticsm)	0.01	0.01	0.00	0.01
	(0.01)	(0.02)	(0.02)	(0.01)
Extraversion (higher values indicate higher extraversion)	−0.02	−0.01	−0.03	−0.01
	(0.02)	(0.02)	(0.03)	(0.02)
Openness to experience (higher values indicate higher openness)	−0.00	0.01	−0.01	−0.00
	(0.01)	(0.02)	(0.02)	(0.01)
Agreeableness (higher values indicate higher agreeableness)	−0.01	0.00	−0.04	− 0.01
	(0.02)	(0.02)	(0.03)	(0.02)
Conscientiousness (higher values indicate higher conscientiousness)	0.01	0.02	0.01	0.01
	(0.02)	(0.03)	(0.02)	(0.02)
Leadership position: - Middle management (Ref.: Top Management)	0.14	0.22	−0.03	0.23
	(0.16)	(0.20)	(0.28)	(0.20)
- Lower management	0.15	0.41+	−0.36	0.43*
	(0.16)	(0.22)	(0.23)	(0.21)
- Highly qualified specialist position	0.25	0.47*	−0.24	0.49*
	(0.18)	(0.22)	(0.31)	(0.21)
Gender (Ref.: male) x Middle management				−0.32
				(0.34)
Gender (Ref.: male) x Lower management				−0.83**
				(0.31)
Gender (Ref.: male) Highly qualified specialist position				−0.78*
				(0.38)
Observations	2140	1476	664	2140
Number of Individuals	1070	738	332	1070

First column: total sample; second column: men; third column: women; fourth column: total sample, with interaction term gender x leadership position; Poisson coefficients were reported; cluster-robust standard errors in parentheses
*** $p < 0.001$; ** $p < 0.01$; * $p < 0.05$; + $p < 0.10$

changes in leadership positions were used in FE regression analysis. Changes from a 'highly qualified specialist position' to 'top management' from 2009 to 2013 were associated with a decrease in the number of physician visits in the preceding 3 months in men ($\beta = .47$, $p < .05$), but not in women (with significant gender differences: $p = .008$).

While worsening self-rated health was associated with an increase in the outcome measure in the total sample and in both genders, an increase in the number of chronic diseases was only associated with an increase in the outcome measure in the total sample. Moreover, increasing age and changes from 'married' to another marital status were associated with a decrease in the outcome measure in women, but not in men. None of the personality factors reached statistical significance.

Sensitivity analysis

In sensitivity analysis (results of sensitivity analysis are not shown, but are available upon request), satisfaction with (i) free time, (ii) family life and (iii) job were added to the main model. However, findings with regard to the leadership position remained virtually the same. In further sensitivity analysis, concerns about the job security and the difficulty of finding an appropriate position were added to the main model. In another robustness check, it was additionally adjusted for income. In additional sensitivity analysis, it was adjusted for working hours per week. Again, our results remained almost the same.

Moreover, robustness was checked by using negative binomial FE regression models. In terms of significance, the relation between leadership position and physician visits was nearly identical.

Discussion

Main findings

The aim of the present study was to investigate the association between leadership position and HCU in women and men longitudinally. Adjusting for various potential confounders such as self-rated health, FE regression analysis revealed that changes from a highly qualified specialist position to the top management were associated with a *decrease* in the number of physician visits in men, but not in women. Gender differences (gender x kind of leadership) achieved statistical significance.

Possible explanations of how (change in) leadership position contributes to healthcare use

Inconsistent findings have been reported regarding the relationship between socioeconomic status and healthcare use (outpatient and inpatient) in Germany based on cross-sectional studies [13, 14]. However, these cross-sectional findings are not directly comparable to ours as we consider leadership position and not socioeconomic status in general as explanatory variable using a specific sample of the German labor force as well as a longitudinal approach. In addition, we specifically examined physician visits and not general healthcare use as outcome measure. More generally, studies are missing which explicitly focus on the relation between *leadership position* and healthcare use both cross-sectionally and longitudinally. In conclusion, our findings are difficult to compare with previous studies.

As regards possible explanations, it could be that a change in leadership is accompanied by a change in one's own perceptions of discomfort or chronic conditions [52]. Due to workload and time constraints, symptoms may be ignored. This change in perception might cause the decrease in physician visits. Moreover, it might be that the change in leadership position (from lower to higher) heavily restricts managers' time available, e.g., to use health care services, and therefore physician visits will decrease [53]. For example, in our analytical sample, the lower the leadership position is, the higher is the leisure time in hours (association between leisure time in hours and leadership position (from 1 = top management to 4 = highly

qualified specialist position): Spearman's rho = .08, $p < .001$) and the lower are the working hours (association between working hours per week and leadership position: Spearman's rho = $-.28$, $p < .001$).

High-status professionals may also have more resources available to buffer the potentially negative impact of work stress. It has been previously suggested that individuals in higher occupational positions feel less burdened by high job stress compared to those in lower occupational positions [54, 55]. Possibly, the change to (higher) leadership position in *men* is associated with an increased engagement in health behaviors (e.g., physical activity or healthy diet) to cope with increased stress levels in the leadership position [56]. Thus, their health status will be less affected and consequently, the change in leadership position in men might lead to decreases in physician visits. However, the change to a higher position frequently comes along not only with more responsibilities but also higher stakes and increased level of work stress. Therefore, self-selection is likely to play a role; and individuals who consider themselves suitable and able to tolerate high levels of stress may be more likely to move into higher management positions [57].

Another explanation could be that individuals in top management positions may have access to a broader network through which they may get more social support [58] which could positively influence health. Changes to higher leadership positions may also come along with positive feelings of appreciation and thus higher levels of job satisfaction [59]. This may eventually result in reduced HCU. However, our findings remained almost the same, when we included various types of satisfaction (i.e., job, family, leisure time) in sensitivity analysis.

Possibly, higher-rank managers expect a tenured, more secure position and hence will be more involved in their jobs [60]. At the same time they may face higher job demands and responsibilities but also more competitive pressure within these ranks. This could translate in greater fear of job degradation and thus result in fewer physician visits (for example to avoid absence from work due to illness). In a similar vein, higher-level managers may feel more committed to the organization and thus could be more inclined to sacrifice own interests and needs for the good of the organization. Consequently, they may use physician services less.

Several speculative explanations are possible why changes in leadership positions were not associated with HCU in *women*. First, there might be heterogeneous effects in female managers. While changes from the lower management to the top management might be associated with an *increase* in HCU among some women who score high in prudence (for example, to avoid negative health effects on their children or family), it might *decrease* HCU in other women who score high in competitiveness. Future studies are needed to clarify this issue.

While one may argue that the combinations of career and family obligations could lead to more HCU in women compared to men, research found that multiple roles and a challenging job may buffer against stress and entail positive health effects [61–63]. As a result, these women may not need physician services and decrease their use. However, future studies are required to investigate this in depth. Another more general explanation might be that women's health care use is typically affected by need factors rather than external circumstances [31].

Furthermore, the non-significant association might be explained by a lack of statistical power (small number of changes in leadership positions among women), but the number is increasing steadily [64]. Particularly in women, a hiring bias may still be present despite advancement of equality between genders in leadership positions [24]. Yet, it could also be that women have different preferences and are less likely to opt for these positions compared to their male counterparts due to double burden of family and working life [65]. Thus, future research with greater statistical power is required.

While personality traits have been suggested to predict health outcomes [46], this could not be confirmed in our study for HCU. This might be explained by a lack of statistical power. Moreover, a recent study showed that only high neuroticism was associated with HCU among Dutch young adults [66], whereas the other personality factors were not associated with high GP costs (dichotomized outcome measure with low and high GP costs). However, we expect that significant associations between personality factors and HCU (particularly with mental HCU [67]) might appear in a large sample representing the general population [41].

Strengths and limitations

To the best of our knowledge, this is the first study examining the association between leadership position and HCU in women and men longitudinally. Data were drawn from a nationally representative sample. Four kinds of leadership positions were used. In addition, one of the main challenges in large survey studies - the problem of unobserved heterogeneity - was reduced using FE regressions. In accordance with recommendations [68] and in line with previous studies investigating the determinants of HCU [31], a short recall period (3 months) was used for physician visits. Consequently, we assume that the recall bias was small and many health-related events were covered in the current study. Panel attrition is a common source of bias in longitudinal studies. However, it has been demonstrated that panel attrition is only a minor problem in the GSOEP [34]. Leadership position was based on self-reports on a scale specifically developed for the SOEP (personal communication), which is a potential limitation.

While we cannot dismiss the possibility of an endogeneity bias (physician visits affect leadership position), we strongly believe that this is rarely the case. Moreover, findings from other longitudinal studies showed that the social gradient was mainly explained by the path from work to health ("causal effect") and not by the reverse pathway from health to work ("health selection effect") [15, 16]. Our findings are restricted to two waves (2009 and 2013) for reasons of data availability. Furthermore, changes in job status may take time to affect HCU. Consequently, further studies are required considering a longer period of time to determine long-term or dynamic effects. While we examined changes in leadership positions in general due to power issues, future research might look at differences between industries. Furthermore, the reason for changes in leadership position (e.g., whether the change was compulsory or the individual elected to change voluntarily) should be analyzed in future studies.

Conclusion

Findings of the present study emphasize the impact of leadership positions on the number of physician visits in men. Further studies are required to elucidate the underlying mechanisms (e.g., working conditions) between changes in leadership positions and physician visits in men.

Acknowledgements

The data used in this publication were made available to us by the German Socio-Economic Panel Study (SOEP) at the German Institute for Economic Research (DIW), Berlin.

Funding

None.

Availability of data and materials

GSOEP data access must comply with high security standards for maintaining confidentiality and protecting personal privacy. The data are also subject to regulations limiting their use to scientific purposes, that is, they are only made available to the scientific community (in German language only). After conclusion of a data distribution contract with DIW Berlin, the data of every new wave will be available on request either via personalized encrypted download or via certified mail on a DVD. Please see for further information: https://www.diw.de/en/diw_02.c.238237.en/conditions.html.

Authors' contributions

KCR, HHK, AH: Design and concept of analyses, preparation of data, statistical analysis and interpretation of data, preparing of the manuscript. All authors critically reviewed the manuscript, provided significant editing of the article and approved the final manuscript.

Competing interests
The authors declare that they have no competing interests.

References

1. Cockerham WC. Social causes of health and disease: Polity; 2007.
2. Marmot MG, Smith GD, Stansfeld S, Patel C, North F, Head J, et al. Health inequalities among British civil servants: the Whitehall II study. Lancet (London, England). 1991;337(8754):1387–93.
3. Mackenbach JP, Stirbu I, AJR R, Schaap MM, Menvielle G, Leinsalu M, et al. Socioeconomic inequalities in health in 22 European countries. N Engl J Med. 2008;358(23):2468–81.
4. Siegrist J, Theorell T. Socio-economic position and health: the role of work and employment. In: Siegrist J, Marmot M, editors. Social inequalities in health. Oxford; 2006. p. 73–100.
5. Lahelma E, Martikainen P, Laaksonen M, Aittomaki A. Pathways between socioeconomic determinants of health. J Epidemiol Community Health. 2004;58(4):327–32.
6. Geyer S, Hemstrom O, Peter R, Vagero D. Education, income, and occupational class cannot be used interchangeably in social epidemiology. Empirical evidence against a common practice. J Epidemiol Community Health. 2006;60(9):804–10.
7. Clougherty JE, Souza K, Cullen MR. Work and its role in shaping the social gradient in health. Ann N Y Acad Sci. 2010;1186:102–24.
8. Volkers AC, Westert GP, Schellevis FG. Health disparities by occupation, modified by education: a cross-sectional population study. BMC Public Health. 2007;7(1):196.
9. Sekine M, Chandola T, Martikainen P, Marmot M, Kagamimori S. Socioeconomic inequalities in physical and mental functioning of British, Finnish, and Japanese civil servants: role of job demand, control, and work hours. Soc Sci Med. 2009;69(10):1417–25.
10. Palencia L, Malmusi D, De Moortel D, Artazcoz L, Backhans M, Vanroelen C, et al. The influence of gender equality policies on gender inequalities in health in Europe. Soc Sci Med. 2014;117:25–33.
11. Julià M, Ollé-Espluga L, Vanroelen C, Moortel DD, Mousaid S, Vinberg S, et al. Employment and labor market results of the SOPHIE project. Int J Health Serv. 2017;47(1):18–39.
12. Fjaer EL, Balaj M, Stornes P, Todd A, McNamara CL, Eikemo TA. Exploring the differences in general practitioner and health care specialist utilization according to education, occupation, income and social networks across Europe: findings from the European social survey (2014) special module on the social determinants of health. Eur J Pub Health. 2017;27(suppl_1):73–81.
13. Hoebel J, Rattay P, Prutz F, Rommel A, Lampert T. Socioeconomic status and use of outpatient medical care: the case of Germany. PLoS One. 2016;11(5): e0155982.
14. Klein J, Hofreuter-Gätgens K, von dem Knesebeck O. Socioeconomic status and the utilization of health services in Germany: a systematic review. Health care utilization in Germany: Springer; 2014. p. 117–43.
15. Ibrahim S, Smith P, Muntaner C. A multi-group cross-lagged analyses of work stressors and health using Canadian national sample. Soc Sci Med. 2009;68(1):49–59.
16. Chandola T, Bartley M, Sacker A, Jenkinson C, Marmot M. Health selection in the Whitehall II study, UK. Soc Sci Med. 2003;56(10):2059–72.
17. Halleröd B, Gustafsson J-E. A longitudinal analysis of the relationship between changes in socio-economic status and changes in health. Soc Sci Med. 2011; 72(1):116–23.
18. Falkenberg H, Fransson EI, Westerlund H, Head JA. Short-and long-term effects of major organisational change on minor psychiatric disorder and self-rated health: results from the Whitehall II study. Occup Environ Med. 2013;70(10):688–96.
19. Ferrie JE, Shipley MJ, Marmot MG, Stansfeld S, Smith GD. Health effects of anticipation of job change and non-employment: longitudinal data from the Whitehall II study. BMJ. 1995;311(7015):1264–9.
20. Vahtera J, Kivimaki M, Pentti J. Effect of organisational downsizing on health of employees. Lancet. 1997;350(9085):1124–8.
21. Vahtera J, Kivimäki M, Pentti J, Theorell T. Effect of change in the psychosocial work environment on sickness absence: a seven year follow up of initially healthy employees. J Epidemiol Community Health. 2000;54(7):484–93.
22. Fenton-O'Creevy M. Employee involvement and the middle manager: evidence from a survey of organizations. J Org Behav. 1998;19(1):67–84.
23. Kivimäki M, Vahtera J, Pentti J, Ferrie JE. Factors underlying the effect of organisational downsizing on health of employees: longitudinal cohort study. BMJ. 2000;320(7240):971–5.
24. Karambayya R. Caught in the crossfire: women and corporate restructuring. Can J Adm Sci. 1998;15(4):333.
25. Pochic S, Guillaume C. Les carrières de cadres au cœur des restructurations: la recomposition des effets de genre? L'internationalisation d'un groupe français en Angleterre et en Hongrie. Sociologie du travail. 2009;51(2):275–99.
26. Clougherty JE, Souza K, Cullen MR. Work and its role in shaping the social gradient in health. Ann N Y Acad Sci. 2010;1186(1):102–24.
27. Björklund C, Lohela-Karlsson M, Jensen I, Bergström G. Hierarchies of health: health and work-related stress of managers in municipalities and county councils in Sweden. J Occup Environ Med. 2013;55(7):752–60.
28. Little LM, Simmons BL, Nelson DL. Health among leaders: positive and negative affect, engagement and burnout, forgiveness and revenge. J Manag Stud. 2007;44(2):243–60.
29. Quick JC, Macik-Frey M, Cooper CL. Managerial dimensions of organizational health: the healthy leader at work*. J Manag Stud. 2007;44(2):189–205.
30. Romswinkel EV, König HH, Hajek A. The role of optimism in the relationship between job stress and depressive symptoms. Longitudinal findings from the German ageing survey. J Affect Disord. 2018;241:249–55.
31. Babitsch B, Gohl D, von Lengerke T. Re-visiting Andersen's behavioral model of health services use: a systematic review of studies from 1998–2011. Psychosoc Med. 2012;9:Doc11.
32. Dhingra SS, Zack M, Strine T, Pearson WS, Balluz L. Determining prevalence and correlates of psychiatric treatment with Andersen's behavioral model of health services use. Psychiatr Serv. 2010;61(5):524–8.
33. Parslow R, Jorm A, Christensen H, Jacomb P. Factors associated with young adults' obtaining general practitioner services. Aust Health Rev. 2002;25(6):109–18.
34. Lipps O. Attrition of households and individuals in panel surveys. 2009.
35. Schoeni RF, Stafford F, Mcgonagle KA, Andreski P. Response rates in national panel surveys. Ann Am Acad Pol Soc Sci. 2013;645(1):60–87.
36. Wagner G, Frick J, Schupp J. The German socio-economic panel study (SOEP) – scope, evolution and enhancements. Schmollers Jahrbuch : journal of applied social science studies / Zeitschrift für Wirtschafts- und Sozialwissenschaften. 2007;127(1):139–69.
37. Andersen RM. Revisiting the behavioral model and access to medical care: does it matter? J Health Soc Behav. 1995;36(1):1–10.
38. Jylhä M. What is self-rated health and why does it predict mortality? Towards a unified conceptual model. Soc Sci Med. 2009;69(3):307–16.
39. Smith TW. Personality as risk and resilience in physical health. Curr Dir Psychol Sci. 2006;15(5):227–31.
40. Smith TW, Gallo LC. Personality traits as risk factors for physical illness. In: Baum A, Revenson TA, Singer J, editors. Handbook of health psychology. Hillsdale: Lawrence Erlbaum; 2001. p. 39–172.
41. Hajek A, Bock J-O, König H-H. The role of personality in health care use: results of a population-based longitudinal study in Germany. PLoS One. 2017;12(7):e0181716.
42. McWilliams LA, Cox BJ, Enns MW, Clara IP. Personality correlates of outpatient mental health service utilization. Soc Psychiatry Psychiatr Epidemiol. 2006;41(5):357–63.
43. ten Have M, Oldehinkel A, Vollebergh W, Ormel J. Does neuroticism explain variations in care service use for mental health problems in the general population? Results from the Netherlands mental health survey and incidence study (NEMESIS). Soc Psychiatry Psychiatr Epidemiol. 2005; 40(6):425–31.
44. Goldberg LR. The structure of phenotypic personality traits. Am Psychol. 1993;48(1):26.
45. Hahn E, Gottschling J, Spinath FM. Short measurements of personality- validity and reliability of the GSOEP big five inventory (BFI-S). J Res Pers. 2012;46(3):355–9.
46. Turiano NA, Pitzer L, Armour C, Karlamangla A, Ryff CD, Mroczek DK. Personality trait level and change as predictors of health outcomes: findings from a National Study of Americans (MIDUS). J Gerontol B. 2012;67B(1):4–12.
47. Brüderl J, Ludwig V. Fixed-effects panel regression. In: Wolf C, editor. The Sage handbook of regression analysis and causal inference. Los Angeles: SAGE; 2015. p. 327–57.
48. Cameron AC, Trivedi PK. Microeconometrics: methods and applications. New York: Cambridge University Press; 2005.
49. Hausman JA. Specification tests in econometrics. Econometrica. 1978:1251–71.

50. Stock JH, Watson MW. Heteroskedasticity-robust standard errors for fixed effects panel data regression. Econometrica. 2008;76(1):155–74.

51. Van Doorslaer E, Masseria C, Koolman X. Inequalities in access to medical care by income in developed countries. Can Med Assoc J. 2006;174(2):177–83.

52. Hobson J, Beach J. An investigation of the relationship between psychological health and workload among managers. Occup Med. 2000; 50(7):518–22.

53. Manning MR, Jackson CN, Fusilier MR. Occupational stress and health care use. J Occup Health Psychol. 1996;1(1):100.

54. McCann L, Hughes CM, Adair CG, Cardwell C. Assessing job satisfaction and stress among pharmacists in Northern Ireland. Pharm World Sci. 2009;31(2):188.

55. Kawakami N, Haratani T, Kobayashi F, Ishizaki M, Hayashi T, Fujita O, et al. Occupational class and exposure to job stressors among employed men and women in Japan. J Epidemiol. 2004;14(6):204–11.

56. Mustard CA, Vermeulen M, Lavis JN. Is position in the occupational hierarchy a determinant of decline in perceived health status? Soc Sci Med. 2003;57(12):2291–303.

57. Sherman GD, Lee JJ, Cuddy AJ, Renshon J, Oveis C, Gross JJ, et al. Leadership is associated with lower levels of stress. Proc Natl Acad Sci U S A. 2012;109(44):17903–7.

58. Van Der Gaag M, Snijders TAB. The resource generator: social capital quantification with concrete items. Soc Networks. 2005;27(1):1–29.

59. Fujishiro K, Xu J, Gong F. What does "occupation" represent as an indicator of socioeconomic status?: exploring occupational prestige and health. Soc Sci Med. 2010;71(12):2100–7.

60. Brown SP. A meta-analysis and review of organizational research on job involvement: American Psychological Association; 1996.

61. Lundberg U, Frankenhaeuser M. Stress and workload of men and women in high-ranking positions. J Occup Health Psychol. 1999;4(2):142.

62. Barnett RC. Women and multiple roles: myths and reality. Harv Rev Psychiatry. 2004;12(3):158–64.

63. Barnett R, Marshall NL, Sayer A. Positive-spillover effects from job to home: a closer look. Women Health. 1992;19(2–3):13–41.

64. Holst E, Friedrich M. Führungskräfte-Monitor 2017: Update 1995–2015. DIW Berlin: Politikberatung kompakt; 2017. p. Report No.: 3946417132.

65. Richter A, Kostova P, Harth V, Wegner R. Children, care, career–a cross-sectional study on the risk of burnout among German hospital physicians at different career stages. J Occup Med Toxicol. 2014;9(1):41.

66. Kraft M, Arts K, Traag T, Otten F, Bosma H. Is personality a driving force for socioeconomic differences in young adults' health care use? A prospective cohort study. Int J Public Health. 2017;62(7):795–802.

67. Goodwin RD, Hoven CW, Lyons JS, Stein MB. Mental health service utilization in the United States. Soc Psychiatry Psychiatr Epidemiol. 2002;37(12):561–6.

68. Bhandari A, Wagner T. Self-reported utilization of health care services: improving measurement and accuracy. Med Care Res Rev. 2006;63(2):217–35.

Permissions

The contributors of this book come from diverse backgrounds, making this book a truly international effort. This book will bring forth new frontiers with its revolutionizing research information and detailed analysis of the nascent developments around the world.

We would like to thank all the contributing authors for lending their expertise to make the book truly unique. They have played a crucial role in the development of this book. Without their invaluable contributions this book wouldn't have been possible. They have made vital efforts to compile up to date information on the varied aspects of this subject to make this book a valuable addition to the collection of many professionals and students.

This book was conceptualized with the vision of imparting up-to-date information and advanced data in this field. To ensure the same, a matchless editorial board was set up. Every individual on the board went through rigorous rounds of assessment to prove their worth. After which they invested a large part of their time researching and compiling the most relevant data for our readers.

The editorial board has been involved in producing this book since its inception. They have spent rigorous hours researching and exploring the diverse topics which have resulted in the successful publishing of this book. They have passed on their knowledge of decades through this book. To expedite this challenging task, the publisher supported the team at every step. A small team of assistant editors was also appointed to further simplify the editing procedure and attain best results for the readers.

Apart from the editorial board, the designing team has also invested a significant amount of their time in understanding the subject and creating the most relevant covers. They scrutinized every image to scout for the most suitable representation of the subject and create an appropriate cover for the book.

The publishing team has been an ardent support to the editorial, designing and production team. Their endless efforts to recruit the best for this project, has resulted in the accomplishment of this book. They are a veteran in the field of academics and their pool of knowledge is as vast as their experience in printing. Their expertise and guidance has proved useful at every step. Their uncompromising quality standards have made this book an exceptional effort. Their encouragement from time to time has been an inspiration for everyone.

The publisher and the editorial board hope that this book will prove to be a valuable piece of knowledge for researchers, students, practitioners and scholars across the globe.

List of Contributors

Roland Diel
Institute for Epidemiology, University Medical Hospital Schleswig-Holstein, Airway Research Center North (ARCN), Niemannsweg 11, 24015 Kiel, Germany

Robert Loddenkemper
German Central Committee against Tuberculosis, Berlin, Germany

Albert Nienhaus
Institute for Health Services Research in Dermatology and Nursing, University Medical Center, Hamburg-Eppendorf, Germany
Institution for Statutory Accident Insurance and Prevention in the Health and WelfareServices (BGW), Hamburg, Germany

Eileen M. Wanke, Doris Klingelhöfer, Daniela Ohlendorf and David A. Groneberg
Institute of Occupational Medicine, Social Medicine and Environmental Medicine, Goethe-University, Theodor-Stern-Kai 7, 60590 Frankfurt am Main, Germany

Mike Schmidt
Department of Sports and Exercise Medicine, Institute of Human Movement Science University of Hamburg, Mollerstraße 10, 20148 Hamburg, Germany

Jeremy Leslie-Spinks
School of Performing Arts, University of Wolverhampton, Gorway Rd, Walsall, West Midlands WS1 3BD, England

Zorawar Singh
Department of Zoology, Khalsa College, G.T. Road, Amritsar, Punjab 143001, India

Pooja Chadha
Department of Zoology, Guru Nanak Dev University, Amritsar, Punjab, India

Peter Koch and Jan Felix Kersten
Centre of Excellence for Epidemiology and Health Services Research for Healthcare Professionals (CVcare), University Medical Centre Hamburg-Eppendorf, Martinistraße 52, Hamburg 20246, Germany

Albert Nienhaus
Centre of Excellence for Epidemiology and Health Services Research for Healthcare Professionals (CVcare), University Medical Centre Hamburg-Eppendorf, Martinistraße 52, Hamburg 20246, Germany

Health Protection Division (FBG), Institution for Statutory Accident Insurance and Prevention in the Health and Welfare Services (BGW), Pappelallee 33, Hamburg 22089, Germany

Johanna Stranzinger
Health Protection Division (FBG), Institution for Statutory Accident Insurance and Prevention in the Health and Welfare Services (BGW), Pappelallee 33, Hamburg 22089, Germany

Yuanhai Zhang, Jianfen Zhang, Xinhua Jiang, Liangfang Ni and Chunjiang Ye
Department of Burns and Plastic Surgery, Zhejiang Quhua Hospital, Quzhou 324004, China

Chunmao Han and Xingang Wang
Department of Burns and Wound Care Center, Second Affiliated Hospital of Zhejiang University College of Medicine, Hangzhou 310009, China

Komal Sharma
Zhejiang University School of Medicine, Hangzhou 310000, China

Alice Freiberg, Maria Girbig, Ulrike Euler, Julia Scharfe and Andreas Seidler
1Institute and Policlinic of Occupational and Social Medicine, Medical Faculty Carl Gustav Carus, Technische Universität Dresden, Fetscherstr. 74, Dresden 01307, Germany

Sonja Freitag
Department of Occupational Health Research, German Social Accident Insurance Institution for the Health and Welfare Service, Pappelallee 33-37, Hamburg 22089, Germany

Albert Nienhaus
Department of Occupational Health Research, German Social Accident Insurance Institution for the Health and Welfare Service, Pappelallee 33-37, Hamburg 22089, Germany
Institute for Health Service Research in Dermatology and Nursing, University Clinics Hamburg Eppendorf, Martinistr. 52, Hamburg 20246, Germany

Giuseppe Mastrangelo and Sofia Pavanello
Department of Cardiac, Thoracic, and Vascular Sciences, Unit of Occupational Medicine, University of Padova, Via Giustiniani 2 -, 35128 Padova, Italy

Angela Carta and Cecilia Arici
Department of Medical and Surgical Specialties, Radiological Sciences and Public Health, Section of Public Health and Human Sciences, University of Brescia, Brescia, Italy
University Research Center "Integrated Models for Prevention and Protection in Environmental and Occupational Health", University of Brescia, Brescia, Italy

Stefano Porru
University Research Center "Integrated Models for Prevention and Protection in Environmental and Occupational Health", University of Brescia, Brescia, Italy
Department of Diagnostics and Public Health, Section of Occupational Health, University of Verona, Verona, Italy

Gabriele Berg-Beckhoff
Unit for Health Promotion Research, University of Southern Denmark, Niels Bohrs Vej 9, 6700 Esbjerg, Denmark

Helle Østergaard and Jørgen Riis Jepsen
Centre of Maritime Health and Society, University of Southern Denmark, Niels Bohrs Vej 9, Esbjerg 6700, Denmark

Susel Rosário
Doctoral Programme in Occupational Safety and Health, Faculty of Engineering of the University of Porto, Rua Dr. Roberto Frias, s/n 4200-465 Porto, Portugal

João A. Fonseca
Doctoral Programme in Occupational Safety and Health, Faculty of Engineering of the University of Porto, Rua Dr. Roberto Frias, s/n 4200-465 Porto, Portugal
CINTESIS – Centre for Research in Health Technologies and Information Systems and Information and Decision Sciences Department, Faculty of Medicine of the University of Porto, Rua Dr. Plácido da Costa, s/n 4200-450 Porto, Portugal
Allergy Unit, CUF Porto Institute and Hospital, Estrada da Circunvalação 14341, 4100-180; Rua Fonte das Sete Bicas 170, 4460-188 Porto, Portugal

José Torres da Costa
Doctoral Programme in Occupational Safety and Health, Faculty of Engineering of the University of Porto, Rua Dr. Roberto Frias, s/n 4200-465 Porto, Portugal
Faculty of Medicine of the University of Porto, Alameda Prof. Hernâni Monteiro, 4200-319 Porto, Portugal

LAETA – Associated Laboratory for Energy, Transport and Aeronautics, Faculty of Engineering of the University of Porto, Rua Dr. Roberto Frias, s/n 4200-465 Porto, Portugal

Albert Nienhaus
Doctoral Programme in Occupational Safety and Health, Faculty of Engineering of the University of Porto, Rua Dr. Roberto Frias, s/n 4200-465 Porto, Portugal
Centre of Excellence for Epidemiology and Health Services Research for Healthcare Professionals (CVcare), University Medical Center Hamburg-Eppendorf, Institute for Health Services Research in Dermatology and Nursing (IVDP), Martinistraβe 52, 20246 Hamburg, Germany
Principles of Prevention and Rehabilitation Department (GPR), Institute for Statutory Accident Insurance and Prevention in the Health and Welfare Services (BGW), Hamburg, Germany

Luís F. Azevedo
CINTESIS – Centre for Research in Health Technologies and Information Systems and Information and Decision Sciences Department, Faculty of Medicine of the University of Porto, Rua Dr. Plácido da Costa, s/n 4200-450 Porto, Portugal
Department of Health Information and Decision Sciences (CIDES), Faculty of Medicine of the University of Porto, Rua Dr.Plácido da Costa, s/n 4200-450 Porto, Portugal
National Observatory of Pain– NOPain, Faculty of Medicine of the University of Porto, Alameda Prof. Hernâni Monteiro, 4200-319 Porto, Portugal
Faculty of Medicine of the University of Porto, Alameda Prof. Hernâni Monteiro, 4200-319 Porto, Portugal

Matthias Nübling
Freiburg Research Centre for Occupational Sciences (FFAW GmbH), Bertoldstr. 63, 79098 Freiburg, Germany

Christoph Gyo, Michael Boll, Dörthe Brüggmann, Doris Klingelhöfer, David Quarcoo and David A. Groneberg
The Institute of Occupational Medicine, Social Medicine and Environmental Medicine, School of Medicine, Goethe University Frankfurt, Theodor-Stern-Kai 7, 60590 Frankfurt, Germany

Gary M. Marsh, Sarah D. Zimmerman, Yimeng Liu and Lauren C. Balmert
Center for Occupational Biostatistics and Epidemiology and Department of Biostatistics, Graduate School of Public Health, University of Pittsburgh, 130 DeSoto Street, Pittsburgh, PA 15261, USA

Peter Morfeld
Institute and Policlinic for Occupational Medicine, Environmental Medicine and Preventive Research, University of Cologne, Cologne, Germany
Institute for Occupational Epidemiology and Risk Assessment of Evonik Industries, Essen, Germany

Graziana Intranuovo, Chiara Monica Guastadisegno, Maria Luisa Congedo, Gianfranco Lagioia, Maria Cristina Loparco, Vincenzo Corrado, Domenica Cavone, Luigi Vimercati and Nunzia Schiavulli
Department of Interdisciplinary Medicine (DIM), Section "B. Ramazzini", Regional University Hospital "Policlinico - Giovanni XXIII°", Unit of Occupational Medicine, University of Bari, Piazza G. Cesare, 11, 70124 Bari, Italy

Giovanni Maria Ferri
Department of Interdisciplinary Medicine (DIM), Section "B. Ramazzini", Regional University Hospital "Policlinico - Giovanni XXIII°", Unit of Occupational Medicine, University of Bari, Piazza G. Cesare, 11, 70124 Bari, Italy
Interdisciplinary Department of Medicine (DIM), University Hospital. Policlinico-Giovanni XXIII, University of Bari, Piazza Giulio Cesare, 11, 70124 Bari, Italy

Giorgina Specchia, Annamaria Giordano, Tommasina Perrone and Francesco Guadio
Department of Emergency and Transplantation (DETO), Regional Universitary Hospital "Policlinico - Giovanni XXIII°, Unit of Hematology, University of Bari, Piazza G.Cesare, 11, 70124 Bari, Italy

Patrizio Mazza, Caterina Spinosa, Carla Minoia, Lucia D'Onghia and Michela Strusi
ASL Taranto, Moscati Hospital, Unity of Haematology, Via Paisiello 1, 74100 Taranto, Italy

Giuseppe Ingravallo
Department of Emergency and Transplantation (DETO), Regional University Hospital "Policlinico – Giovanni XXIII° ", Unit of Pathology, University of Bari, Piazza G. Cesare, 11, 70124 Bari, Italy

Pierluigi Cocco
Department of Public Health, Clinical and Molecular Medicine, Occupational Health Section, University of Cagliari, 09100 Cagliari, Italy

Devendra Bhattarai, Dharanidhar Baral, Ram Bilakshan Sah, Shyam Sundar Budhathoki and Paras K. Pokharel
School of Public Health and Community Medicine, B P Koirala Institute of Health Sciences, Ghopa 18, Dharan, Nepal

Suman Bahadur Singh
Lifeline Institute of Health Sciences, Damak, Nepal

Denis Vinnikov
Department of Internal Medicine, Occupational Diseases and Hematology, Kyrgyz State Medical Academy, Akhunbaev street 92, Bishkek 720020, Kyrgyzstan

Daniel Haile Chercos and Demeke Berhanu
Department of Environmental and Occupational Health and Safety, Institute of Public Health, University of Gondar, Gondar, Ethiopia

Xiangning Fan and Sebastian Straube
Division of Preventive Medicine, Department of Medicine, Faculty of Medicine and Dentistry, University of Alberta, 5-30F University Terrace, 8303-112 Street, Edmonton, AB T6G 2T4, Canada

Charl Els
Department of Psychiatry, Faculty of Medicine and Dentistry, University of Alberta, Edmonton, AB, Canada

Kenneth J. Corbet
Department of Community Health Sciences, Cumming School of Medicine, University of Calgary, Calgary, AB, Canada

Magnus Flondell, Birgitta Rosén, Lars B. Dahlin and Anders Björkman
Department of Hand Surgery, Skåne University Hospital, Jan Waldenströms gata 5, 20502 Malmö, SE, Sweden
Department of Translational Medicine – Hand Surgery, Lund University, Malmö, Sweden

Gert Andersson
Departments of Neurophysiology, Skåne University Hospital, Malmö, Sweden
Department of Clinical Sciences, Lund University, Lund, Sweden

Tommy Schyman
Department of Clinical Studies Sweden – Forum South, Skåne University Hospital, Malmö, Sweden

Anja Schablon
Centre of Excellence for Epidemiology and Health Care Research for Health Care Workers (CVcare), University Medical Center Hamburg-Eppendorf (UKE), Martinistr. 41a, 20521 Hamburg, Germany

Melanie Klein
Centre of Excellence for Epidemiology and Health Care Research for Health Care Workers (CVcare), University Medical Center Hamburg-Eppendorf (UKE), Martinistr. 41a, 20521 Hamburg, Germany

DAK-Gesundheit (Health Insurance Fund, Board Manager for Health Care Research, Nagelsweg 27-31, 20097 Hamburg, Germany

Albert Nienhaus
Centre of Excellence for Epidemiology and Health Care Research for Health Care Workers (CVcare), University Medical Center Hamburg-Eppendorf (UKE), Martinistr. 41a, 20521 Hamburg, Germany
Department of Occupational Health Research, German Social Accident Insurance Institution for the Health and Welfare Services, Pappelallee 33-37, 22089 Hamburg, Germany

Stefanie Wobbe-Ribinski
DAK-Gesundheit (Health Insurance Fund, Board Manager for Health Care Research, Nagelsweg 27-31, 20097 Hamburg, Germany

Anika Buchholz
Institute of Medical Biometry and Epidemiology (IMBE), University Medical Center Hamburg-Eppendorf (UKE), Martinistr. 52, 20246 Hamburg, Germany

Reinhard Müller
Justus-Liebig-Universität Giessen, Aulweg 123, 35392 Giessen, Germany

Joachim Schneider
Institut und Poliklinik für Arbeits- und Sozialmedizin am Universitätsklinikum Giessen und Marburg, Aulweg 129, Giessen 35392, Germany

Jian Li, Adrian Loerbroks and Peter Angerer
Institute of Occupational, Social and Environmental Medicine, Centre for Health and Society, Faculty of Medicine, University of Düsseldorf, Universitätsstraße 1, 40225 Düsseldorf, Germany

Martin Bidlingmaier
Endocrine Research Unit, Medizinische Klinik und Poliklinik IV, Ludwig-Maximilians-University, Munich, Germany

Raluca Petru
Institute and Outpatient Clinic for Occupational, Social and Environmental Medicine, WHO Collaborating Centre for Occupational Health, Ludwig-Maximilians-University, Munich, Germany

Francisco Pedrosa Gil
Clinic for Psychiatry, Psychotherapy and Psychosomatics, Helios Vogtland Clinical Center, Plauen, Germany

Nuwadatta Subedi
Department of Forensic Medicine, Gandaki Medical College, Pokhara 33700, Nepal

Ishwari Sharma Paudel
Department of Community Medicine, Gandaki Medical College, Pokhara, Nepal

Ajay Khadka, Umesh Shrestha, Vipul Bhusan Mallik and K. C. Ankur
Gandaki Medical College, Pokhara, Nepal

Saara Taponen
Finla Occupational Health, Satakunnankatu 18 B, 33210 Tampere, Finland
Faculty of Medicine and Life Sciences, University of Tampere, 33014 Tampere, Finland

Lauri Lehtimäki
Allergy Centre, Tampere University Hospital, 33521 Tampere, Finland
Faculty of Medicine and Life Sciences, University of Tampere, 33014 Tampere, Finland

Jukka Uitti
Faculty of Medicine and Life Sciences, University of Tampere, 33014 Tampere, Finland
Finnish Institute of Occupational Health, 00251 Helsinki, Finland

Kirsi Karvala
Finnish Institute of Occupational Health, 00251 Helsinki, Finland

Ritva Luukkonen
Clinicum, Faculty of Medicine, University of Helsinki, 00014 Helsinki, Finland

Mostafa Hadei
Research Center for Environmental Determinants of Health (RCEDH), Kermanshah University of Medical Sciences, Kermanshah, Iran

Philip K Hopke
Department of Public Health Sciences, University of Rochester School of Medicine and Dentistry, Rochester, NY 14642, USA
Center for Air Resources Engineering and Science, Clarkson University, Potsdam, NY 13699, USA

Mahbobeh Moradi4 and Baharan Emam4
Environmental and Occupational Hazards Control Research Center, Shahid Beheshti University of Medical Sciences, Tehran, Iran

Abbas Shahsavani
Environmental and Occupational Hazards Control Research Center, Shahid Beheshti University of Medical Sciences, Tehran, Iran
Department of Environmental Health Engineering, School of Public Health and Safety, Shahid Beheshti University of Medical Sciences, Tehran, Iran

Maryam Yarahmadi
Environmental and Occupational Health Center, Ministry of Health and Medical Education, Tehran, Iran

Noushin Rastkari
Environmental and Occupational Health Center, Ministry of Health and Medical Education, Tehran, Iran
Center for Air Pollution Research (CAPR), Institute for Environmental Research (IER), Tehran University of Medical Sciences, Tehran, Iran

Dominik Pförringer and Regina Mayer
Department of Trauma Surgery, Technical University of Munich, Ismaningerstrasse 22-, 81675 Munich, Germany

Christa Meisinger and Dennis Freuer
Chair for Epidemiology at UNIKA-T, Ludwig-Maximilians University of Munich, Augsburg, Germany

Florian Eyer
Klinikum rechts der Isar, Department of Clinical Toxicology, Technical University of Munich, Munich, Germany

Katrin Christiane Reber, Hans-Helmut König and André Hajek
Department of Health Economics and Health Services Research, University Medical Center Hamburg-Eppendorf, Hamburg Center for Health Economics, Hamburg, Germany

Index

www.ingramcontent.com/pod-product-compliance
Lightning Source LLC
Chambersburg PA
CBHW080524200326
41458CB00012B/4323